SO-AWV-399

Progress in Neuropharmacology and Neurotoxicology
of Pesticides and Drugs

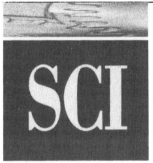

Society of Chemical Industry

Founded in 1881, SCI is an international, interdisciplinary association.

SCI seeks to improve the exchange of information and opinion between industry, academia and the consumer, and to advance society's interest in the application of science.

http://sci.mond.org

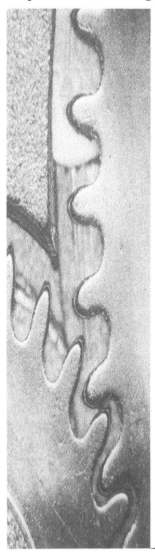

- publishes four peer-reviewed journals
  Journal of the Science of Food and Agriculture
  Journal of Chemical Technology & Biotechnology
  Pesticide Science
  Polymer International
  publishes a range of specialist books
- publishes the *Lecture Papers Series*
- publishes the magazine, *Chemistry & Industry*
- provides a free science and business news service
  News Direct - on the Web at **http://ci.mond.org**
- organises international meetings and conferences
  on a range of science and business issues
- organises *Open Forum* public debates on
  topical subjects
- hosts two Websites:
  http://sci.mond.org; http://ci.mond.org
- supports its members in a diverse range of
  special interest Groups and geographical Sections
- provides core funding for innovative primary science
  teacher training at **SCIcentre**
- confers a range of medals, awards and grants across
  the world to leading industrialists and researchers,
  and to outstanding newcomers
- hosts e-mail discussion forums, eg the *Tomorrow's
  Leaders* project for young professionals across Europe

**For further information on SCI and the benefits
of joining its worldwide membership, contact:
SCI Member Services
Email: members@chemind.demon.co.uk
Fax: +44 (0) 171 823 1698**

*Connecting science and
industry worldwide*

Progress in Neuropharmacology and Neurotoxicology of Pesticides and Drugs

Edited by

D. J. Beadle
Oxford Brookes University, Oxford, UK

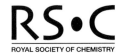

Sep/ae
CHEM

5ª
9/23/49

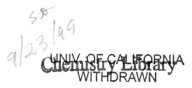

UNIV. OF CALIFORNIA
Chemistry Library
WITHDRAWN

The proceedings of Neurotox '98: Progress in Neuropharmacology and Neurotoxicology of Pesticides and Drugs, organised by the SCI and held at St Catherine's College, Oxford, UK on 28–31 July 1998.

Special Publication No. 232

ISBN 0-85404-729-8

A catalogue record for this book is available from the British Library

© Society of Chemical Industry 1999

All rights reserved.

Apart from any fair dealing for the purpose of research or private study, or criticism or review as permitted under the terms of the UK Copyright, Designs and Patents Act, 1988, this publication may not be reproduced, stored or transmitted, in any form or by any means, without the prior permission in writing of The Royal Society of Chemistry, or in the case of reprographic reproduction only in accordance with the terms of the licences issued by the Copyright Licensing Agency in the UK, or in accordance with the terms of the licences issued by the appropriate Reproduction Rights Organization outside the UK. Enquiries concerning reproduction outside the terms stated here should be sent to The Royal Society of Chemistry at the address printed on this page.

Published for SCI by The Royal Society of Chemistry,
Thomas Graham House, Science Park, Milton Road,
Cambridge CB4 4WF, UK

For further information visit the RSC web site at www.rsc.org

Preface

RM315
P75
1999
CHEM

The chapters in this book represent the majority of the presentations made at the Neurotox '98 conference held at St Catherine's College, Oxford in July 1998. This was the fifth conference in the series, the first being held at York in 1979 and, like this one, conceived and organised by the Physicochemical & Biophysical Panel of the Pesticides Group of the Society of Chemical Industry. The aim of all of the Neurotox meetings has been to increase the communications between those scientists working on pure invertebrate neurobiology and those working on its principal practical application, pest control. In his opening address to the York meeting, Dr Charles Potter spelt out the advantages of such increased communication and the belief was that an increased knowledge of the structure, physiology, pharmacology and genetics of pest organisms would lead to a more rational approach to the design of pesticides and a better understanding of resistance.

This belief continued to be the basis of the next two meetings at Bath and Nottingham and it was strengthened by advances in insect molecular neurobiology, new studies on natural products and a better understanding of the mechanisms of resistance. It was with great enthusiasm, then, that the fourth meeting was held at Southampton in 1991 but the participants were quickly brought face to face with the realities of pesticide science by the opening address from Günther Voss and Rainer Neumann from the Agro Division of Ciba-Geigy. They presented a very different picture from the one presented by Charles Potter twelve years earlier. In their view more industrial R&D resources would be put into new and alternative pest control technologies than into neuroactive pesticides because these would have to comply with the needs of the market and society and could not be "designed" by neuroscience. The number of neurotargets suitable for pest control opportunities was also much smaller than anticipated by academic research. Despite this pessimistic start the 1991 Southampton Conference was considered to be very successful and the participants left the meeting full of excitement and optimism for the future of invertebrate neurobiology and its impact on pest control.

However, seven years elapsed before the next Neurotox conference but advances both in academia concerned with genome science and in industry concerned with combinatorial chemistry and genetic modification led to this meeting being approached with general enthusiasm. One again there was a full exchange of ideas and knowledge between academics and industrial scientists with participants coming from fifteen different countries and twelve major agrochemical companies. Progress in molecular biology and the use of natural products, particularly toxins, showed how our knowledge of the invertebrate nervous system and target sites within it had advanced during the last decade of the century. Although much of the conference was concerned with *Drosophila melanogaster* and *Caenorhabditis elegans* an increasing number of scientists were working on pest species and using new approaches. Once again the meeting ended in optimism and with a view that the future was looking bright for collaborations between academics and industrial pesticide scientists. The contents of this book show why Neurotox '98 was considered to be such a success and why the participants were already looking ahead to the next meeting.

D J Beadle
Oxford, April 99

Contents

Ion Channels and Receptors as Targets

Leslie L. Iversen

DEPARTMENT OF PHARMACOLOGY, UNIVERSITY OF OXFORD, MANSFIELD ROAD,
OXFORD OX1 3QT, UK

1. INTRODUCTION

With the exception of the organophosphate and carbamate acetylcholinesterase inhibitors, the majority of neuroactive insecticides act on ion channels or receptors that control ion channels. The known targets are quite limited, with sodium channels and GABA-controlled chloride channels as the main ones. However, there is a great diversity of ion channels and receptors and more are being discovered in the current wave of new information emerging from molecular genetics. The application of these techniques to classical mammalian pharmacology has revealed the existence of an unexpectedly large number of genes encoding ion channels and receptors[1].
In mammals we know of 5 different voltage-sensitive calcium channels, 14 different potassium channels (voltage sensitive, calcium sensitive and ligand-gated varieties) and 6 distinct voltage-sensitive sodium channels[1]. Several of these are composed of more than one type of protein sub-unit, each encoded by a separate gene.

Cell surface receptors similarly exist in many different varieties. During the past decade great strides have been made in the application of molecular genetics to receptor studies, mainly in the mammalian nervous system. This has resulted in the understanding that receptors of both the G-protein coupled and ligand-gated ion channel types are encoded for by large gene families[1]. For example, pharmacologists used to think of two adrenoceptors recognising noradrenaline and adrenaline, the α and β classes, now nine different subtypes of adrenoceptor are recognised. Nearly 40 different G-protein coupled receptors exist just for the monoamines acetylcholine, histamine, noradrenaline and dopamine (Table 1). Among ligand gated ion channels the GABA-A receptor comprises three different sub-units, and each of these is encoded by multiple genes, giving a total of 14 genes and the possibility of constructing thousands of different GABA-A receptors through different combinations of such sub-units. The mammalian glutamate receptor family is equally complex, with more than 16 genes encoding the different sub-units already recognised.

Table 1 - Multiple G-protein coupled receptors for monoamines

Monoamine	Number of receptor genes
Noradrenaline	9
Dopamine	5
Serotonin	14
Acetylcholine	5

As more is known about the families of genes encoding ion channels and receptors in insects a similar diversity will be revealed - and indeed such information is already available for some of the gene families. This should offer new opportunities for the rational development of new insecticides with improved efficacy and safety. A detailed knowledge of the molecular pharmacology should allow the choice of insect targets that are either not expressed at all in mammals, or least resemble their mammalian counterparts.

2. ION CHANNELS

Voltage-sensitive sodium channels represent a key target for many existing insecticides, including the pyrethroids[2]. Little is known, however, about the number of sodium channels or their molecular pharmacology, and few of the relevant genes have yet been cloned. In other areas genetics studies have revealed an extraordinary diversity of ion channels in invertebrates. For example, genome sequencing of the nematode worm *Caenorhabditis elegans* is now essentially complete. The worm sequencing project has already revealed large numbers of new ion channel and receptor subunits[3]. These include at least 80 different potassium channel sub-units, a remarkable number considering that the worm possesses only 302 neurones in its nervous system! Many of the newly discovered potassium channel sub-units had not been described previously, and they are expressed in a highly selective manner in the nervous system - with some genes expressed in only a few neurones and in at least one case only in a single neurone. In addition to the unexpected multiplicity of genes encoding ion channels further diversity is introduced by alternative mRNA splicing and by RNA editing.

Insect calcium channels offer another interesting target, some of the potent spider venom ω-agatoxins act on calcium channels that are associated with neurotransmitter release and can, for example cause muscular paralysis by blocking glutamate release at the insect neuromuscular junction.

3. INSECT GABA RECEPTORS

The inhibitory neurotransmitter GABA plays a key role in the neural control of insect muscle. Each muscle fibre is innervated by both an excitatory and by an inhibitory motor nerve, using L-glutamate and GABA respectively as their neurotransmitter substances. Thus, in insects the inhibitory control of muscle is carried out to a large extent at the periphery, and is not confined to the CNS as in vertebrates. This makes the GABA receptor a particularly attractive target, and indeed many of the currently known insecticides act as antagonists at this receptor. These include Type II pyrethroids, lindane, dieldrin and other cyclodienes, and hexachlorocyclohexane[2]. The insect GABA receptor, like the mammalian GABA-A receptor, controls a chloride ion channel - which when activated inhibits the target cell by stabilising the membrane potential at the chloride equilibrium potential. Insect GABA receptors resemble mammalian GABA-A receptors in their sensitivity to the convulsant picrotoxin, but unlike mammalian receptors the insect receptors are insensitive to the convulsant alkaloid bicuculline. Until recently little was known about the detailed molecular pharmacology of the insect GABA receptor but that has now changed, with the identification of unique protein sub-units, which differ quite markedly from the mammalian GABA-A sub-units. Three insect genes encode sub-units known as RDL (resistance to dieldrin), GRD (GABA and glycine like receptor of Drosophila) and LCCH3 (ligand-gated chloride channel homologue 3) (for review see[4]). The improved knowledge of the molecular architecture of the insect GABA receptor should permit accelerated progress in screening for new drugs that selectively target this receptor. Presently available drugs show selectivity between insect and mammalian GABA receptors but this therapeutic window could probably be improved. Dieldrin, for example, discriminates between mammalian and insect GABA receptors by less than 2 orders of magnitude, and its relative safety in mammals relies also on other factors (more rapid metabolism, etc.)[2].

4. THE INSECT GLUTAMATE RECEPTOR

As explained above, L-glutamate plays a key role as the excitatory neurotransmitter released by motor nerves innervating insect muscle. It thus represents an attractive target, but this so far has been little exploited. Rather little is known about the molecular pharmacology of insect glutamate receptors, and to what extent this parallels the families of mammalian glutamate receptors that have been described. There is also a lack of useful pharmacological tools, although some of the polyamine spider venom toxins have been found to act as potent antagonists at insect glutamate receptors - and this may account for the paralysing actions.

One significant advance has been made, however, in defining a novel family of glutamate receptors in insect muscle that are coupled to the opening of chloride channels, rather than the cation channels normally associated with excitatory glutamate receptors. These were first described in neuropharmacological experiments in the 1970's[5], and more recently the receptor has been cloned from *C.elegans* and from *Drosophila*[6]. The pharmacological significance of these discoveries is that the glutamate-gated chloride channel seems to represent a key target for the avermectin class of macrocyclic lactones, which have proved to be highly successful as pesticides, with a good therapeutic window and a low incidence of resistance. The glutamate-gated chloride channel is a good example of a near ideal target, as these receptors do not appear to have any vertebrate counterparts. However, avermectin also targets the insect GABA-gated chloride channel to some extent, and this may contribute to some mammalian neurotoxicity, so there is still room for improvement here in designing more selective agents.

5. OTHER TARGETS

Another way of focusing on targets likely to yield an attractive therapeutic window of safety would be to study receptor mechanisms associated with chemical mediators that are commonly used in insects but not found in mammals. Good examples of this are the insect monoamine neurotransmitters tyramine and octopamine. These are monophenolic phenylethylamine derivatives equivalent to the mammalian catecholamines dopamine and noradrenaline - insects lack the enzyme tyrosine hydroxylase needed to synthesise the catechol group. Octopamine and tyramine play a number of physiological roles, particularly in the co-ordination of insect flight and considerable progress has been made in recent years in defining their pharmacology - with a family of receptors identified and cloned[7,8]. Some of these are located peripherally (for example, on muscle) other are on neurones. There are receptors that exhibit preference for tyramine while others prefer octopamine. Few agonist or antagonist drugs are yet available, although the tricyclic antidepressant mianserin and an analogue of this, maroxepine, act as nanomolar affinity antagonists at one of the neuronal octopamine receptors[7], and phenyliminimidazoline and amono-oxazoline insecticides (e.g. AC-6) act as agonists at some octopamine receptors.

Other options are to target the numerous neuropeptides and neuroendocrine peptides and their receptors found in insects, for example the tetrapeptide FMRFamide.

REFERENCES

1. S.P.H.Alexander and J.A.Peters (1997) Receptor and Ion Channel Nomenclature Supplement, 8th Edition, *Trends in Pharmacol.Sci.,* **18**
2. T.Narahashi (1996) *Pharmacol.Toxicol.* **78**: 1-14
3. Editorial (1998) *Nature Neuroscience*, **1**: 169-170
4. A.M.Hosie, K.Aronstein, D.B.Sattelle, and R.H. Ffrench-Constant (1997) *Trends in Neuroscience*, **20**: 578-583
5. T.J.Lea and P.N.R.Ushwerwood (1973) *Comp.Gen.Pharmacol.* **4**: 333-363
6. D.F.Cully, P.S.Paress, K.K.Liu, J.M.Schaeffer and J.P. Arena (1996) *J.Biol.Chem.,* **271**:20187-20191
7. T.Roeder and J.A.Nathanson (1993) *Neurochem.Res.***18**:921-925
8. C.C.Gerhardt, R.A.Bakker, G.J.Piek, R.J.Planta, J.E.Leysen and H. Van-Heerikhuizen (1997) *Mol. Pharmacol.* **51**:293-300

Opportunities for Neurotoxic Compounds as Crop Protectants

D.K. Lawrence and S.J. Dunbar

ZENECA AGROCHEMICALS, JEALOTT'S HILL RESEARCH STATION, BRACKNELL RG42 6ET, UK

1 INTRODUCTION

In the introductory talk at Neurotox '91, Günther Vos administered a dose of realism by pointing out the gap between neuroscience and the practical realities of the insecticide market.[1] The three key points were these:

- The negative perception of neuroactive insecticides, whether real or perceived, was forcing attention to "softer" modes-of-action and alternative methods of pest control.
- Most of the features required for a commercial product – safety, performance, selectivity, manufacturing costs and patents – cannot be "designed" by neuroscience.
- The number of neurotargets capable of providing acceptable and economic pest control is smaller than anticipated by academic research.

Although few, if any, at the meeting predicted it, the period from then to now has been one of unprecedented change in technology. Firstly, combinatorial chemistry has revolutionised the way the pharmaceutical industry screens for new drugs, and the approach has spilled over into the agricultural arena. Then genome science has transformed our ability to identify target sites for drug intervention, and has provided a huge leap in the information on the basic machinery of biological organisms. Finally, the ambition to modify crop plants to dramatically improve their ability to resist pests has become a commercial reality. The aim of this paper is, therefore, to review the changes in both the marketplace and the enabling technology since 1991, highlighting the opportunities for neuroscience.

2 THE INSECT CONTROL MARKET

2.1 The need

World population continues to grow, albeit at a slightly slower rate than was predicted in 1991, squeezing agriculture between the demand for increased production and using farmland for housing. Urbanisation has proceeded apace, reducing the number of farm workers. It is widely accepted that sometime since 1991 we have passed the point where current agricultural production could supply the WHO recommended minimum dietary intake to the whole world. In effect, this means that those of us who live in the developed world are able to maintain our (excessive) food intake only because someone elsewhere is starving. Many of us find it hard to see the continuing pressure, especially in the EU, for extensification and a return to labour intensive organic farming practices as sustainable – though this is precisely the slogan used to advocate them.

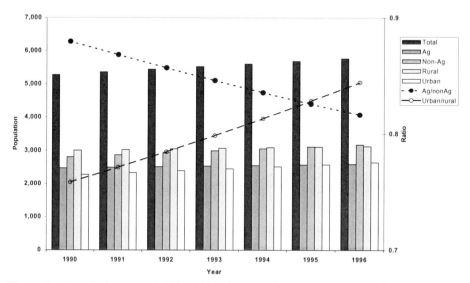

Figure 1   *Population growth 1990-1996, showing shift away from agriculture and rural communities*[2]

On the face of it, then, the need for agricultural insecticides is greater than it has ever been. The public health situation is even clearer, however. Several life-threatening diseases spread by insect vectors remain endemic in large parts of the world. These include yellow fever, river sickness, sleeping sickness and most importantly, malaria. The fight against these diseases seemed close to won in the 1950's when the widespread use of compounds such as DDT reduced the incidence of malaria from millions a year to tens of thousands of cases.

However, the environmental persistence of DDT led to a ban on its use, and the present situation according to the World Health Organisation is worsening.[3] In 1997, some degree of malaria risk exists in 100 countries, the great majority of which (92%) include the malignant form of the disease caused by *Plasmodium falciparum*. Over 40% of the world population live in areas with malaria risk, with 300-500 million clinical cases annually. Of those affected, 1.5-2.7 million die each year. As many as one million children under five years of age die from malaria alone or in combination with other diseases. To date, the major cause of the reversal has been the decline in the control of the mosquito vector, though the removal of DDT and the more conservative use of less persistent compounds to avoid environmental pollution. The threat for the future is that increased resistance to antimalarial drugs, and the spread of the disease through increased travel and global warming will exacerbate the problem further. Malaria has already reappeared in Eastern European countries such as Armenia, Azerbaijan, Tajikistan, and Uzbekistan,[3] and it is predicted that in the next decade it could reach such areas as Southern Europe and Australia.

Surely there can be no doubt that there will continue to be a need for chemical insecticides for the foreseeable future? As the effectiveness of existing compounds is eroded by the development of resistance in the target pests, this inevitably means a continued need to find new molecules. The challenge is to ensure that these new insecticides are as effective as the organochlorines, but are lacking the environmental consequences, so that they can be used sustainably.

2.2 Chemical insecticides

The vision in 1991 was that, at least until 1995, the insecticide market would remain dominated by compounds acting at acetylcholinesterase and voltage-gated sodium channels, principally organophosphates and pyrethroids respectively. New toxophores were seen as likely to be targeted towards narrow-spectrum compounds compatible with integrated pest management strategies. There was an implicit assumption that IPM-compatible compounds would probably not be neuroactive, and that their commercial value would be small. The reality, as shown in the table below, has turned out to be subtly different.

Table 1   *Insecticide sales*

Target site			US $m sales			
	1972	*1988*	*1995 forecast[1]*	*1995 actual[4]*	*1996[5]*	*Example products*
GABA-activated ion channels	1,580	500	350	360	380	cyclodienes, **Fipronil**
Sodium channels	0	1,150	1,500	1,695	1,935	DDT, pyrethroids
Acetylcholine esterase	1,375	2,325	2,520	3,295	3,305	organophosphates
	885	1,400	1,400	1,520	1,505	carbamates
Acetylcholine receptor	0	0	?	270	460	Nitromethylenes **Spinosad**
All others	175	700	1,330	1,620	1,300	

This table illustrates several points. It is clear that the great majority of the world's agricultural insecticides still act at a very small set of neuronal target sites. However, an old site, the GABA-activated ion channel has been given new life by the launch of Fipronil, one of a new class of insecticides which do not suffer from the environmental problems of the older compounds, though cross-resistance remains a risk.[6] In addition, a new mode-of-action has appeared which contains the world's largest selling insecticide in value terms, imidacloprid. The target site, the nicotinic acetylcholine receptor, had been widely predicted as having the potential to provide commercial products. Although the nitromethylenes had been around for some time, none of the previous analogues had combined the other essential properties that make up a successful product. These examples both illustrate that there was nothing wrong with the predictions on the target sites, just that the right molecule had not been made.

Apart from imidacloprid, perhaps the most interesting new neuroactive insecticide is the natural product 'Spinosad'. The interest is that it seems to have a novel mode-of-action, and is to date, the only commercial manifestation of the widespread interest in new natural products illustrated by the coverage at Neurotox '91. Whilst the detailed mechanism remains to be determined, there is compelling electrophysiological evidence that it potentiates, rather than inhibits, the activity of acetylcholine acting on nicotinic acetylcholine receptors in the central nervous system.[7] It is not yet clear how important a product it will become, mainly because it is a complex natural product which has to be made by fermentation, but it offers the exciting prospect that simpler synthetic molecules with the same mode-of-action may be found.

What the table does not show is that the trend towards niche products for IPM has not been sustained, for two reasons. Firstly, the economics did not make sense, given that it costs at least $30m to develop even a narrow-spectrum, non-neurotoxic insecticide. In addition, it has been shown that even broad-spectrum, neuroactive compounds can be used in IPM programmes, by controlling rates and timing to avoid harming beneficial insects. For example, ZENECA's potent pyrethroid Karate®, can be used as a component in IPM programmes.[8,9] Furthermore, biological control has still not produced cost-effective robust performance, even when the organism has been genetically modified. The main problem is getting sufficiently rapid kill to avoid crop damage, especially with later instars.

More worrying, though, is that the overall rate of introduction of new insecticides has continued to decline. Whilst some of this is probably due to commercial pressures restricting the development of niche products, it seems to be as much about a slowing of the invention rate. Over the next decade it is likely that many organophosphate insecticides will increasingly be withdrawn, through concerns on their environmental and human toxicity. In the USA in particular, this is expected to happen sooner rather than later, due to the introduction of the Food Quality Protection Act, which sets even greater

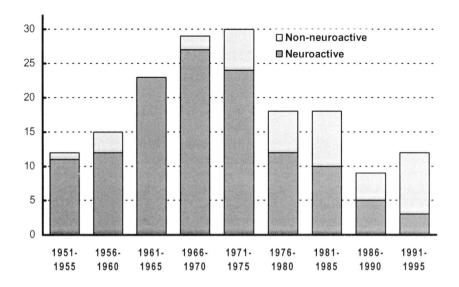

Figure 2 *Numbers of commercial insecticides and acaricides introduced through 1995*[10]

safety margins between the levels shown to cause harm and the maximum levels permitted in food. This Act considers residue levels not just for a single compound or crop, but for the accumulation of all compounds with the same human effect in all food sources. This has a particular effect on widely used classes such as the organophosphates, and the EPA has given notice that this class will be a priority for scrutiny. This will both remove a set of valuable compounds, but will increase the usage of other classes to replace them. To date, the battle to manage resistance to the other major class, the pyrethroids, has been largely successful in the developed world. However, over-use and poorly managed use in less developed agriculture has shown how serious resistance can develop, so efforts to maintain the effectiveness of the remaining weapons in the armoury will become even more important.

2.3   Genetically-modified plants

Probably the greatest change to the insect control market since 1991 has been the arrival of plants genetically-modified to give levels of insect resistance far beyond those achieved through conventional plant breeding. The possibility of achieving this was certainly recognised then, but few would have predicted the scale of the impact. Work of this type has been going on since the early 1980's, either around the toxin genes from the soil organism *Bacillus thuringiensis*, lectins or inhibitors of proteases involved in insect digestion.

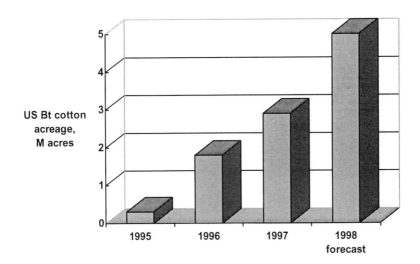

Figure 3   *Graph showing rapid expansion of US acreage planted with Bt cotton*[11] *(total acreage ca. 15m acres)*

One reason for doubting the efficacy of this approach is that it appears to be flying in the face of all that makes neuroactive insecticides so desirable. They are fast acting and typically are effective through direct contact. The insect therefore does not even have to start feeding on the plant before it can be controlled, but even it is already feeding, it rapidly stops, even where death occurs hours or even days later. When applied as a spray, the *Bacillus thuringiensis* toxins (Bt's) were only active when ingested, and were slow acting, so significant damage to the crop continued after application. On the face of it, putting the gene into a plant might have been expected to make things worse – and generally this was the prevailing view held by agrochemical companies. However, as we now know, Bt works *much* better when the gene is incorporated into the plant. Even a single mouthful probably contains a lethal dose, and feeding stops much more rapidly than after spray application.

To date, the performance of genes such as protease inhibitors and lectins has been less impressive than Bt.[12] So perhaps there is more in common with neuroactive toxins, and some of the learning may remain relevant? The target sites for the Cry toxins are receptors in the brush border membranes of the insect mid-gut, resulting in the formation of pores across the membrane.[13] Whilst this does not make Bt a neurotoxin, these pores appear to have much in common with ion channels in insect nerves, in terms of structure, though they are ungated. It has been reported[14] that the *Androctonus* scorpion toxin – a potent inhibitor of sodium channels – has oral activity. However, this observation remains unconfirmed, and introduction of a *Buthus* scorpion toxin into tobacco did not increase insect resistance,[15] and it seems inherently unlikely that a proteinaceous neurotoxin will be able to provide commercial insect-resistant plants. Apart from the scientific problems of retaining adequate stability in the insect gut, and achieving efficient, rapid uptake, would it ever be possible to persuade the public that eating a potent neurotoxin was safe, whatever the facts?

Several big questions remain over the future of insect resistant crops. Will it be possible to manage the onset of resistance to even the same extent as has been achieved with chemical insecticides? Pyrethroid resistance is managed largely through the strict observance of pyrethroid-free windows in the spray regime, but with the current generation of engineered crops, selection pressure is present throughout the growing season, and the resistance management strategy is based on keeping insect-susceptible refugia. How easy will it be to discover new genes, which provide high-level insect control? Much less effort has gone into searching for genes than chemicals, though at the time of writing the balance must be closer. The evidence to date suggests that success may be equally hard, with few leads and none so far reduced to practice. Two relatively new areas may offer some promise. Firstly, a group at CSIRO has introduced a DNA copy of an insect RNA virus[16] into a plant and has shown insecticidal activity, though there are obvious environmental consequences to be considered before commercialisation could be considered. More recently, the sequences of a novel toxin from the nematicidal bacterium *Photorhabdus luminescens*[18] have been cloned[19] and shown to act on a range of insects, though again there are formidable obstacles to be overcome before this can reach the market. Furthermore, all of the commercial plant constructs control only phytophagous insects, primarily Lepidoptera and Coleoptera. Whilst coincidentally these are major pest classes, there has been much less progress with achieving control of sucking pests, and arguably there are greater theoretical problems, at least with the insect toxin approach.

2.4   Prognosis

All the evidence points to a continuing need for insect control in agriculture and in public health. The rate of discovery of new classes of insecticide has declined, and the rate of deregistration of older compounds, especially organophosphates, looks set to increase.

Given that resistance advances relentlessly, the battle is on to discover new toxophores with a currently-acceptable environmental profile before the performance of current compounds degrades enough to affect crop yields. The arrival of genetically modified crops has brought a valuable new weapon in the fight against insect pests, but here too the prognosis is that the battle to invent faster than insects develop resistance will be a hard one. Hopefully, the combination of highly potent insecticides with resistant crops will help slow resistance to both, whilst also reducing the environmental burden, and even providing better insect control as has been shown with a combination of Karate® sprayed on Bt cotton.[9,20]

3   TECHNOLOGY

Since Neurotox '91, the approach to drug discovery in the pharmaceutical industry has dramatically changed, and to a lesser extent the same changes have happened in the agrochemical industry. The revolution is technology-driven, by the combination of advances in genome science, ultra high throughput automated screening and combinatorial chemical synthesis.

3.1   Genome science and drug targets

Whilst in the agrochemical area we have had the luxury of being able to screen directly for the target effect, usually the death of a pest, the drug industry has had to screen compounds on *in vitro* model systems. A key rate limiting step was the number of disease models available, each depending on painstaking analysis of disease biology. In fact, the same was true in agriculture though it was less of a problem, with the only sure way to validate an insecticide target being to develop a commercial product acting through it. Genome science has totally transformed the development of disease models. New target sites can be identified by cloning genes mapping to regions of the genome linked to susceptibility to particular diseases, building on the advances in large-scale sequencing, and array technology to analyse gene expression. A whole new industry has sprung up, led by Human Genome Systems and Incyte, initially to provide contract services, and in the longer term to develop proprietary drugs. The result is that drug companies now have probably more target sites than they can handle, despite the fact that the precise function of many of the sites remains uncertain.

Despite the fact that the *Caenorhabditis elegans* and *Drosophila melanogaster* were two of the first eukaryotes to which genome science was applied, there seems to have been much less progress in identifying target sites for nematicides and insecticides. At the time of writing, the *C. elegans* Genome Sequencing Consortium were reporting progress at 1411 sequences (41,278,830 bases) from St. Louis, and 1330 sequences (38,433,732 bases) from Cambridge, totalling 79,712,562 bases or an estimated 79% of the genome.[21] The expectation is that no more than half of the genes will have a known or postulated function.

Although there is a need for new, environmentally friendly nematicides, and the number of validated target sites is small, there seems to be very little work seeking new ones, and most of that is focused on human parasites, not agriculture. *Drosophila* is much further behind, at around 10% of the genome, and relative to some of the other representative genomes, such as human, *C. elegans*, *Arabidopsis* and rice, seems to be slowing. Arguably this is because the use of genome science, combined with a large library of detailed mutants, has led to the identification of a family of genes which are critical control points in development of limbs and organs. The work has provided a huge boost to understanding of cell-to-cell signalling, as analogous genes have been found in a wide range of other higher organisms.

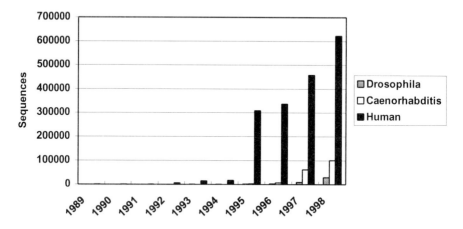

Figure 4   *A comparison of the numbers of sequences submitted to Genebase for C. elegans, D. melanogaster and H. sapiens.*

The power of this approach can be illustrated in the research of ffrench-Constant and his colleagues in which resistance to Dieldrin has been genetically characterised and mapped.[22] Extending this to the invention end of agrochemical research in which a new compound's target site is identified and characterised from a genetic starting point is now a reality. This will not only enable novel chemicals to be developed, but will allow us to better understand such properties as resistance to the current insecticide portfolio. Pharmaceutical interest in cell signalling has uncovered a wide range of drug targets for diseases as diverse as cancer and viral infection. Research in intracellular cell signalling pioneered by Berridge and co-workers[23] has highlighted the opportunities available in invertebrates and it is reasonable to assume that these too will represent new and exciting targets for insecticide attack. However the invertebrate field does have an advantage over the pharmaceutical one in that the genes responsible for cell signalling are amenable to genetic manipulation, so it has become possible to identify and isolate the genes responsible for whole pathways in *Drosophila*. For example, Rubin and his colleagues at Berkley[24] have made enormous strides in understanding the genetic codes underlying the Ras signalling pathway in *Drosophila*. The significance of this technology has been realised by companies such as Exelixis, the major genomics company working on insects, which is focused on using the homology between *Drosophila* and human control sequences to identify new drug targets. We already know that many of the genes involved in cell signalling are lethal and it is probable that, as we investigate further, novel target sites for insecticides will be revealed. Whilst to our knowledge much less work is being done to identify new target sites for neuroactive agrochemicals using *Drosophila*, very recently Exelixis and Bayer have announced an alliance to identify target sites for crop protection.[25] Even less is being done on species other than Diptera, although there are good pragmatic and scientific reasons for expecting significant differences between flies and major economic pests such as Lepidoptera and Coleoptera. It is hard not to take the view that a great scientific opportunity, with real commercial potential, is largely passing us by.

3.2 Rational design

The goal of being able to rationally design insecticides has been discussed at every Neurotox. However, unlike the situation in the pharmaceutical industry, reducing ideas into the reality of agrochemical design has not yet been achieved. Perhaps this will change dramatically, as new technologies converge. Computing power is enabling the scientist to make real time calculations on protein movements. Developments in spectroscopy and X-ray crystallography mean that accessing protein structural information is becoming much easier, although crystallisation itself seems still to be an "art". Genomics is allowing us to isolate genes for candidate target proteins in reasonable timeframes, and express them in systems for subsequent use in crystallisation and biochemical studies. It will be a challenge to apply these technologies to multi-subunit, membrane-bound neuronal proteins, but as knowledge about the binding sites of neurotransmitters increases, it may be possible to utilise smaller portions of these large proteins as models. Progress in this area has indeed been made on potassium channels.[26] Work at the Weizmann Institute in Israel[27] has demonstrated the power of this approach for a soluble protein, the acetylcholinesterase enzyme in both invertebrates and vertebrates. It will be exciting to see how the invention of new agrochemicals is transformed in the future from the old "spray and pray" approach into more design-oriented methodologies. However, for many of our well known membrane bound multi-subunit targets the task remains daunting, and we anticipate that initial progress in this area will mostly be made in the realm of new soluble targets such as cell signalling pathways.

3.3 Ultra high throughput automated screening

Simply having a growing list of potential target sites would not be much use, without the ability to look for compounds that interact with them. In parallel with the advance of genomics, there has been a similar advance in assay miniaturisation and automation, again primarily driven by pharmaceutical companies who have no choice but to use *in vitro* disease models for primary screening. In 1991, most pharmaceutical companies were screening perhaps 200,000 compounds a year through tens of tests. Today, both the throughput and number of tests has increased dramatically, with talk of testing up to a million compounds in a week, a few assays at a time. At the same time, genomics is identifying hundreds of potential new target sites a week. To achieve this throughput, new test methods have been developed. Microtitre plates have gone from 96-well to 384-well, and even 1536-well. New array technologies allow binding to proteins anchored to solid supports to be measured, using ink-jet technology to dispense the nanovolumes of reagent. New assays, such as scintillation proximity and a range of fluorescence technologies, such as Homogeneous Time Resolved Fluorescence (HTRF), Fluorescence Correlation Spectroscopy, Fluorescence Polarisation and Fluorescence Imaging Plate Readers (FLIPR) have been refined, which allow changes to be measured in extremely low-volume samples. Amongst the many assays run, are ones looking for inhibitors of various members of the family of seven transmembrane helix receptors, which are commonly G-protein coupled, or linked to some other reporter system.[28]

It is not just biochemical assays that have been transformed. "On-chip" technology is now in widespread use to study gene expression levels, using immobilised arrays of DNA and tissue RNA, and this is one of the cornerstones of the functional analysis of new genes isolated through genome projects.[29] Moreover, it is now possible to measure physical parameters, such as lipid solubility, "on a chip" and fully automatically, and microfluidics is opening the possibility of chromatographic separation on microchips.[30]

Inevitably, the costs of entry, preference for *in vivo* screens and innate conservatism have slowed the impact in the agrochemical arena. In 1991, most agrochemical companies were probably screening 10-20,000 compounds a year, mostly on whole organism screens, with a few companies still running no routine high throughput *in vitro* screens. Today, most are running at ten times this rate, with ambition to move towards 1,000,000 a year. At this throughput, *in vitro* screens play a much larger role. Given the small number of validated and novel insecticide targets, if we were operating to the drug company model many agrochemical companies would be screening against them *in vitro* in ultra high throughput assays. However, this may be harder to achieve. Many of our neuronal target sites are ligand-gated ion channels rather than G-protein coupled receptors, and to date there has been very little success in generating functional assays suitable for high-throughput screening. It is not only harder to detect a change in the ion flux, but there has been much less progress in getting functional expression of multiple sub-unit ion channels in engineered cell lines, although progress has been made with GABA-gated ion channels in insects[31], and the avermectin receptor[32]. Although technologies exist using calcium reporter systems, such as fluorescent dyes and laser based measuring methodologies including FLIPR[33], real challenges remain in reducing these to practice with a multi-subunit insect receptor protein such as the nicotinic acetylcholine receptor. Addressing targets such as voltage gated potassium channels may be more tractable and the pioneering work on insects through the *Drosophila* shaker K$^+$ channel story[34] may provide a model for pursuing ion channels through *in vitro* screening, although their suitability as target sites may need proving. ZENECA is one of several companies that has put significant effort into screening both ligand- and voltage-gated ion channels, but with only limited success – at least, as far as any one is prepared to reveal!

Even if we could solve the basic technology problem, we still would struggle to run assays on the channels from the target pests, as rarely has the right genes been cloned from these species. Whilst this may not be a fundamental problem at the initial screening stage, it hardly fits with the environmental thrust to find compounds which selectively control pest species, and not beneficial ones.

3.4 Combinatorial chemistry

The picture of modern drug screening, as described above, is one of testing massive numbers of compounds against an increasing range of *in vitro* target sites. If it were not for another technology change, this would not be sustainable. The total number of organic chemicals individually characterised since the subject started is probably around eight million, based on scanning journals and assuming that companies have substantial collections which are not in the literature, but that the collections of competitors will contain substantial overlap. Physical samples of most of these materials no longer exist, so there are probably few, if any companies, with a collection of more than one million samples in any amount. Even if the same collection were re-used on every assay, this number would rapidly become limiting, especially in agriculture where almost certainly the compounds would already have been tested in a whole organism screen.

However, A major spin-off from assay miniaturisation has been that the sample size required to test a compound has fallen dramatically, from a few ten's of milligrammes even in the drug field, to microgrammes or less. In contrast, in 1991 a screen on whole insects still required up to 100mg, depending on the range of species and the instar tested. The small amount of sample required, means that chemists have been able to devise new ways of synthesising small amounts of very large numbers of compounds, using combinatorial methods. Most of these techniques involve setting up a large number of starting materials, usually bound to a solid support, and subjecting each to a selection of reactions which add another structural unit, giving rise to a large number of molecules with related, but different structures.

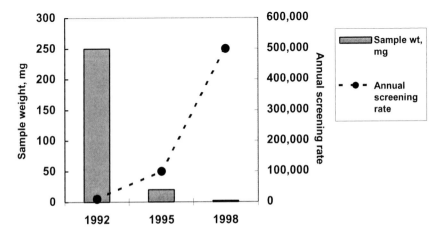

Figure 5   *Schematic showing how sample size has reduced as automation and new screening methods allow higher throughput testing.*

The Affymax technique, for example, involves binding a starter unit to a silicon chip, in a discrete array of 4096 spots. The spatial control is obtained using a laser and photo-etched masks of the type used to etch solid state circuits, combined with photochemical reaction chemistry triggered by the laser. After the starter unit has been attached at each array position, additional structural units can be added at chosen array points by treating with chemical reagent, and illuminating the chosen array elements. By repeating this with different mask and reagents, the end result is effectively a miniature set of reagent bottles containing 4096 different chemical compounds. The assays are performed by looking for binding of fluorescently labelled target sites, which obviously limits the types of sites one can study. However, there are several alternative techniques, each imposing different constraints of the assays which can be performed, and the technology continues to develop. The range of options is too large to describe here, but there are several good reviews available. [35,36,37]

4   OPPORTUNITIES AND CHALLENGES

Our thesis is that the need for new methods of insect control is greater than ever, both in agriculture and public health. This would be no more than a pious hope, if it were not for the fact that there have unprecedented advances in science, which provide the opportunity to make the hope a reality in the first decade of the new millennium. However, we see a gap developing between the advances made in the medical area and the application of the same methods to insects, nematodes and molluscs. Whilst we in the industry are struggling to bridge this gap in our own work, the scale and pace of the change is far too large for us to do this on our own. Even if one takes the view that the industry should fund all the basic science it needs, the fact that systems such as *C. elegans* and *Drosophila* are being so widely used to inform about mammalian systems, shows that there is a wealth of fundamental science to be explored using invertebrate systems.

We suggest therefore, that the challenge to the academic invertebrate world is to use technology to increase understanding of the ways invertebrate neuronal systems function, in order to identify potential target sites for safer and more effective chemical and genetic insect control, and to develop methods to study them. We offer these as ideas for consideration:

- Genome analysis to characterise the key components of invertebrate nervous systems, and the variation across species, *e.g.* between pests, beneficial insects and mammals. Most obviously this includes the pharmacologically well-characterised ion channels, since even now we do not understand the organisation of the acetylcholine receptor – which mediates the activity of the bulk of the world's insecticides.

- Functional analysis methods, in which the function of these key components can be manipulated, and their effect on insect behaviour and viability tested. In the plant field especially, rapid techniques to generate full or partial gene knockouts and additions are developing rapidly. The *Drosophila* mutants and p-element system offer an excellent base, but are relatively slow and *Drosophila* is a poor model for the economically important growth stage of many of the most serious pest species.

- New work focused on the insect gut, *e.g.* the ion channels and receptors of the brush border membranes, to identify new targets for insect control using genetically modified plants.

- Development of functional assays, both *in vitro* and *in vivo*, as tools to gain understanding of the regulation of individual systems and the whole neuronal system, and to enable high throughput screening.

- Exploitation of new chemical technology, to help translate the potential activity from a complex, expensive natural product into simpler structures, which could be, used as commercial products. This would include the most recent techniques such as chemical evolution.

The corresponding challenge to us in the industry would be to use this information to develop new chemical pesticides and genes, targeted at the sites which could give more effective control of the pest species, whilst at the same time have less effect on the environment, including closely-related beneficial species. As was pointed out at Neurotox '91, there are many other factors than activity at a good target site which need to be right to have a commercial product. If the academic challenge were matched, the onus would then be on us to use the new screening and synthesis technologies to combine all of these properties in novel structures which also have high activity at desirable target sites. Given the existing developments in screening for physical properties, and the increased knowledge genome science is bringing to differential metabolism, this is a challenge which at least ZENECA feels able to take on.

References

1. G. Vos and R. Neumann, in 'Neurotox '91: molecular basis of drug and pesticide action', Editor I. Duce, Elsevier Applied Science, 1992.
2. FAOSTAT online database, *http://www.fao.org.*
3. WHO Division of Control of Tropical Diseases, *http://www.who.org/ctd.*
4. Product update, Wood Mackenzie Agrochemical Service, 1996.
5. Product update, Wood Mackenzie Agrochemical Service, 1997.
6. J.R. Bloomquist, *Archives of Insect Biochemistry and Physiology,* **26**, 69, 1994.
7. V.L. Salgado, G.B. Watson and J.J. Sheets, *Proceedings of the Beltwide Cotton Conference 1997,* 1082, 1997.
8. E.D. Pilling and T. J. Kedwards, Effects of Lambda-cyhalothrin on Natural Enemies of Rice Insect Pests, *Proceedings of the Brighton Crop Protection Conference, UK, 1996,* 361, 1996.
9. J.F.H. Cole, E.D. Pilling, R. Boykin and J.R. Ruberson, *Proceedings of the Beltwide Cotton Conference 1997,* 1118, 1997.
10. Pesticide Manual, 11th Edition, Editor C.D.S Tomlin, BCPC, 1997.
11. Monsanto.
12. T.H. Schuler, G.M. Poppy, B.R. Kerry and I. Denholm, *Trends in Biotechnology,* **16**, 168, 1998.
13. B.A. Frederici, *Archives of Insect Biochemistry and Physiology,* **22**, 357, 1993.
14. E. Zlotkin, L. Fishman and J.P. Shapiro, *Archives of Insect Biochemistry and Physiology,* **21**, 41, 1992.
15. S-Z. Pang, S.M. Oberhaus, J.L Ramussen, D.C. Knipple, J.R Bloomquist, D.H. Dean, K.D. Bowman and J.C. Sanford, *Gene,* **116**, 165, 1992.
16. T.L. Hanzlik, S.J. Dorrian, K.N. Johnson, E.M. Brooks and K.H.J. Gordon, *Journal of General Virology,* **76**, 799, 1995.
17. R. Service, *Science,* **271**, 145, 1996.
18. E. Stackenbrandt, S. Forst, B. Dowds and M. Boemare, *Annual Review of Microbiology,* **51** 47, 1997.
19. Patent application WO 98/08932, Dow Elanco/Wisconsin Alumini Research Foundation.
20. J. Mink, S. Harrison and S. Martin, *Proceedings of the Beltwide Cotton Conference 1997,* **2**, 898, 1997.
21. *C. elegans* Genome Sequencing Progress, *http://www.acusd.edu/~cloer/worm-countdown.html.*
22. R.H. ffrench-Constant, T.A. Rocheleau, J.C. Steichen and A.E. Chalmers, *Nature,* **383**, 449, 1993.
23. M.J. Berridge, *Journal of Experimental Biology,* **200**, 315, 1997.
24. F.D. Karim, H.C. Chang, M. Therrien, D.A. Wassarman, T. Laverty and G.M. Rubin, *Genetics,* **143**, 315, 1996.

25. Exelixis Pharmaceuticals and Bayer AG sign genetics research alliance, *http://www.exelixis.com/text/news/releases/98news/05_22.htm*, 1998.
26. M.K. Schott, C. Antz, R. Frank, J.P. Ruppersberg and H.R. Kalbitzer *European Biophysics Journal*, **27**, 99, 1998.
27. I. Silman, M. Harel, P. Axelsen, M. Raves and J.L. Sussman *Transactions of the Biochemical Society*, **22**, 12, 1994.
28. M.H. Pausch, *Trends in Biotechnology*, **15**, 487, 1997.
29. J.D. Hoheisel, *Trends in Biotechnology*, **15**, 465, 1997.
30. L.J. Licklider, M.T. Davis and T.J. Lee, *Proceedings of the 214ᵗʰ American Chemical Society*, **214**, ANYL 94, 1997.
31. L.A. Smith, M. Amar, R.J. Harvey, M.G. Darlison, F.G.P. Earley, D.J. Beadle, L.A. King and I. Bermudez, *Journal of Receptor and Signal Transduction Research*, **15**, 33, 1995.
32. D.F. Cully, H. Wilkinson, D.K. Vassilatis, A. Etter and J.P. Arena, *Parasitology*, **113**, S191, 1996.
33. FLIPR - Molecular Devices, *http://www.moldev.com*.
34. L.Y. Jan and Y.N. Yan, *Journal of Physiology*, **505**, 267, 1997.
35. H. Maehr, *Bioorganic and Medicinal Chemistry*, **5**, 473, 1997.
36. F. Balkenhohl, C. Vondembusschehunnefeld, A. Lansky and C. Zechel, *Angewande Chemie, International Edition*, **35**, 2289, 1996.
37. J. Szostak (Editor), *Chemical Reviews*, **97**, 347, 1997.

Ion Channels and Receptors

Ion Channels as Targets for Insecticides: Past, Present and Future

Toshio Narahashi, Gary L. Aistrup, Tomoko Ikeda, Keiichi Nagata, Jin-Ho Song and Hideharu Tatebayashi

DEPARTMENT OF MOLECULAR PHARMACOLOGY AND BIOLOGICAL CHEMISTRY, NORTHWESTERN UNIVERSITY MEDICAL SCHOOL, 303 EAST CHICAGO AVENUE, CHICAGO, IL 60611, USA

1. INTRODUCTION

After nearly half a century of extensive studies by a number of investigators, it has now become abundantly clear that neuronal ion channels are the major target sites of many insecticides. With the exception of organophosphate and carbamate insecticides, the target sites of most other insecticides are limited to three types of ion channels, i.e. voltage-gated sodium channels, γ-aminobutyric acid (GABA) receptor channels, and neuronal nicotinic acetylcholine (ACh) receptor channels. The reasons for such limitation are not completely clear. One possible reason would be that slight functional alterations of any of the three types of channels could lead to severe sensorimotor disruptions. Another intriguing aspect of these three types of ion channels is that they are all present in both insects and mammals. This is somewhat surprising because the selective toxicity in insects and mammals is an important character as a useful insecticide. As described later, most recent experiments utilizing patch clamp technologies are throwing light on this mystery.

The present paper gives the highlights of insecticide toxicology of ion channels based primarily on the results obtained in our laboratory. Comprehensive reviews of the mechanisms of neurotoxic action of insecticides have been published.[1-11] Readers are encouraged to consult them for details and complete literature. First, a brief historical development of the study of the actions of DDT and pyrethroids on voltage-gated sodium channels is given, since this study, together with a variety of technological developments, has led us to the significance of ion channels as the target site for insecticide actions. A series of studies of pyrethroid actions on sodium channels have developed a new concept of toxicity amplification from channels to animals, clarified the mechanism underlying the negative temperature dependence of pyrethroid action that remained mysterious until recently, and accounted for the mechanism of selective toxicity of pyrethroids in mammals and insects.

GABA$_A$ receptor channels are also an important target site of some insecticides including cyclodienes, hexachlorocyclohexane (HCH), and fipronil. Since it is anticipated that certain newer GABAergic agents may be developed into useful insecticides, some of the recent developments along this line will be described. Neuronal nicotinic ACh receptor channels are by no means new as the target of insecticide as exemplified by nicotine, a classical insecticide. Recent studies of nitromethylene heterocycles revive and document the significance of the ACh receptor channels as a target for developing newer insecticides.

1.1 Historical Developments of Insecticide Toxicology of Ion Channels

The insecticide toxicology of ion channels began when DDT and pyrethrins/pyrethroids were discovered to cause hyperexcitation of the nervous system.

1.1.1 Repetitive discharge and after-potential produced by DDT and pyrethroids. DDT was discovered to initiate repetitive discharges in insect nerves in extracellular recording experiments conducted from mid-1940s to mid-1950s.[1] However, it was not until 1952 that a clue for the ion channel mechanism was obtained.[5,12] Postsynaptic responses as evoked by a presynaptic stimulus in the cockroach ganglion consisted of the initial compound action potentials followed by a few after-discharges of individual neurons (Figure 1A). DDT greatly increased the initial compound postsynaptic responses which decayed slowly. It was not clear whether the slow decay was due to the summation of repetitive action potentials or due to changes in the action potential from individual neurons. However, close inspection

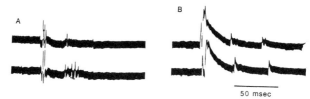

Figure 1 *Postsynaptic responses recorded extracellularly from the abdominal nerve cord of the cockroach as evoked by a presynaptic stimulus applied to the cercal nerve. A. Control. B. After application of 28 µM DDT. Depolarizing after-potential of individual nerve fibers is greatly prolonged. From Yamasaki and Ishii (Narahashi).[12]*

of after-discharges revealed that the action potential arising from individual nerve fibers also exhibited a slow decay phase (Figure 1B). The increase in depolarizing after-potential was later demonstrated more clearly by intracellular recording of action potentials from both insect and other crustacean nerves.[13-15] The pyrethroid allethrin exerted the same effect as DDT.[16,17] As soon as the depolarizing after-potential reached the threshold membrane potential for excitation, repetitive discharges are produced (Figure 2).[13,16-18] Thus, the next question was how DDT and pyrethroids increased the depolarizing after-potential. Voltage clamp experiments gave a definitive answer.

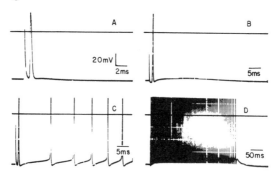

Figure 2 *Repetitive discharges induced by a single stimulus in a crayfish giant axon exposed to 10 µM (+)-trans tetramethrin. A. Control. B. 5 min after application of tetramethrin. C and D. 10 min after application. From Lund and Narahashi.[18]*

1.1.2 Modification of sodium currents by DDT and pyrethroids. Voltage clamp experiments using lobster, crayfish and squid giant axons have clearly demonstrated that both DDT and pyrethroids greatly prolong the sodium current during a depolarizing voltage step and the sodium tail current upon termination of the depolarizing step (Figure 3).[14,15,18-21] The classical voltage clamp experiments allowed us to record whole-cell ionic currents flowing through a number of open channels, but did not provide insight into changes that occurred in each ion channel. Thus, single-channel patch clamp experiments were performed.

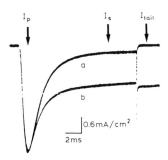

Figure 3 *Membrane sodium currents in a squid giant axon before (a) and during (b) internal perfusion with 1 μM (+)-trans allethrin. Sodium current associated with a step depolarization from -100 mV to -20 mV. In the control record (a), the peak sodium current (I_p) is followed by a small slow sodium current (I_s) during a depolarizing pulse, and the tail current (I_{tail}) associated with step repolarization decays quickly. In the presence of allethrin (b), I_p remains unchanged while I_s is greatly increased in amplitude. I_{tail} is also increased in amplitude and decays very slowly. From Narahashi and Lund.[22]*

Pyrethroids were found to substantially prolong the open time of individual sodium channels (Figure 4).[23-25] It is also important to note that some sodium channels modified by the pyrethroids open with a long delay and are kept open even after termination of a depolarizing voltage step (Figure 4). This and other experiments such as gating current measurement have led to the conclusion that pyrethroids slow the kinetics of both opening and closing of sodium channel.[25-27]

2. UNIQUE FEATURES OF PYRETHROIDS

As briefly outlined above, the pyrethroids modulate the function of sodium channels in several ways: to prolong the open time from the normal value of a few milliseconds to as long as several seconds; to slow the kinetics of both activation and inactivation gates; to shift the activation voltage in the hyperpolarizing direction; and to shift the steady-state inactivation curve in the hyperpolarizing direction. Based on these characteristics, some unique features of pyrethroid action have been unveiled.

2.1 Toxicity Amplification from Ion Channel to Animal

Since pyrethroids cause hyperexcitation in nerves and animals through modification of sodium channels, a question arises as to how many sodium channels need to be modified to elicit hyperexcitation. We made preliminary calculations based on the data available in 1982, and came up with very small percentages, ranging from 0.05% to 0.2%, that are required for nerve hyperexcitation.[28] We have now been able to estimate the percentage of sodium channel modification more precisely using two new protocols.[29-31]

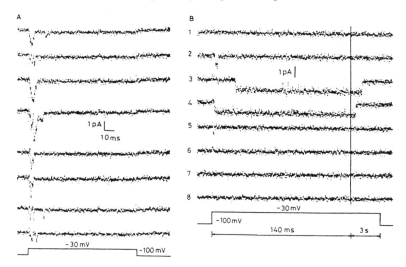

Figure 4 *Effects of deltamethrin on single sodium channel currents. A. Currents from an N1E 115 neuroblastoma cell before drug treatment in response to 140 ms depolarizing steps from a holding potential of -100 to -30 mV with a 3 s interpulse interval. B. Currents after exposure to 10 μM detramethrin. The membrane patch was depolarized for 3140 ms from a holding potential of -100 to -30 mV. The interpulse interval was 3 s. The time scale changes during the voltage step as indicated in the Figure. From Chinn and Narahashi.[25]*

2.1.1 Whole-cell current protocol. Rat dorsal root ganglion (DRG) neurons are endowed with tetrodotoxin-sensitive (TTX-S) and tetrodotoxin-resistant (TTX-R) sodium channels.[32,33] In addition to TTX sensitivity, these two types of sodium channels exhibit several differential characteristics: 1) both activation and inactivation kinetics are faster in TTX-S than in TTX-R sodium channels; 2) both activation and inactivation voltages are at more negative levels in TTX-S than in TTX-R sodium channels; 3) single-channel conductance is larger in TTX-S (6.3 - 10.7 pS) than in TTX-R (3.4 - 6.3 pS) sodium channels;[31,34] and 4) the sensitivity to chemicals other than TTX is different. TTX-S channels are more sensitive to lidocaine, riluzole, and phenytoin than TTX-R channels,[33,35,36] whereas the opposite is found for pyrethroids,[29,37,38] batrachotoxin (unpublished data) and grayanotoxins (I. Seyama, personal communication). Rat cerebellar Purkinje neurons are sensitive to TTX, but show relatively low sensitivity to pyrethroids.[30]

Following exposure to the pyrethroid tetramethrin, TTX-S and TTX-R sodium channels of DRG neurons and TTX-S sodium channels of cerebellar Purkinje neurons generate a large and slowly decaying tail sodium current upon cessation of a depolarizing pulse. The peak sodium current during the depolarizing pulse is not greatly affected. Since single sodium channel conductance is not changed by pyrethroids,[23,25] it is possible to calculate the conductance of peak sodium current which is unmodified by pyrethroids and the conductance of tail sodium current which is modified by pyrethroids. Thus from the ratio of the conductance during tail current to that during peak current, the percentage of the modified sodium channels (M) can be calculated according to the following equation:[29]

$$M = \{[I_{tail}/(E_h - E_{Na})]/[I_{Na}/(E_t - E_{Na})]\} \times 100$$

where I_{tail} is the initial amplitude of tail current upon repolarization to E_h, I_{Na} is the peak current during the depolarizing pulse to E_t, and E_{Na} is the sodium equilibrium potential. An example of such an experiment with a cerebellar Purkinje neuron is shown in Figure 5A, and the concentration-response relationship for the percentage of sodium channel modification by tetramethrin is shown in Figure 5B. Comparison of the concentration-response relationships in Purkinje neuron TTX-S channels, and in DRG TTX-S and TTX-R channels is given in Table 1. The percentages of sodium channel modification thus obtained can be related to the threshold concentration of tetramethrin to evoke repetitive excitation. It was found that tetramethrin produced repetitive after-discharges in Purkinje neurons at a concentration of 100 nM which modified only 0.62% of the sodium channels (Table 1, Figure 5B). Thus, toxicity is greatly amplified from channels to the whole nerve and then to animals through the threshold phenomenon. This accounts for the potent insecticidal action of pyrethroids.

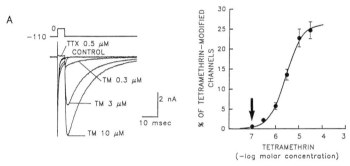

Figure 5 *Concentration-dependent effect of tetramethrin on TTX-S sodium currents. A. Currents were evoked by a 5-msec step depolarization to 0 mV from a holding potential of -110 mV under control conditions and in the presence of tetramethrin (0.3 μM, 3 μM and 10 μM). TTX (0.5 μM) completely blocked both the peak current and tetramethrin-induced tail current. B. The concentration-response relationship for the percentage of channel modification. Each point indicates the mean ± S.E.M. (n=6). Arrow indicates the threshold concentration to evoke repetitive after-discharges. From Song and Narahashi.[30]*

Table 1 *Percentage of the Fraction of Sodium Channels Modified by Tetramethrin*

Tetramethrin Concentration μM	Cerebellar Purkinje Neuron TTX-S %	Dorsal Root Ganglion Neuron TTX-S %	TTX-R %
0.01			1.31 ± 0.28
0.03		0	5.15 ± 0.30
0.1	0.62 ± 0.15	0.24 ± 0.10	15.35 ± 0.79
0.3	2.19 ± 0.36	1.25 ± 0.13	35.48 ± 2.70
1	5.75 ± 0.87	3.53 ± 0.66	57.82 ± 2.29
3	13.58 ± 1.35	7.70 ± 1.20	74.85 ± 1.23
10	22.77 ± 2.26	12.03 ± 1.89	81.20 ± 1.57
30	24.73 ± 2.11		

(From Tatebayashi and Narahashi,[29] Song and Narahashi[30])

2.1.2 Single-channel current protocol. The percentage of sodium channel modification caused by pyrethroids was also estimated from single-channel experiments.[31]   The open time distribution is expressed by a single exponential function in controls, whereas it is composed of two exponential functions in the presence of tetramethrin, a shorter time constant close to the value of the control, and a longer time constant representing the tetramethrin-modified channels. Thus, the percentage of the longer time constant represents that of modified channels.   This value for TTX-S channels at 10 μM tetramethrin concentration (38%) is somewhat larger than that obtained by the whole-cell current method (12%, Table 1). However, the two values for TTX-R channels agree at 85% by the single-channel method and 81% (Table 1) by the whole-cell method. This discrepancy may be ascribed to some errors involved in the methods.[30,31]

2.2 Temperature Dependence of Pyrethroid Action

It has long been known that DDT and pyrethroids exhibit negative temperature dependence of insecticidal action.[1,3,5] The negative temperature dependence is ascribed largely to the nerve sensitivity to these insecticides which is increased by lowering the temperature. However, the mechanism underlying this phenomenon remained unclear. We have finally found reasonable explanations.[30]

In rat cerebellar Purkinje neurons, the potency of tetramethrin to evoke repetitive activity increases with lowering the temperature. The sodium tail current represents the activity of tetramethrin-modified channels and was analyzed as a function of temperature. Although, the peak amplitude of tail current did not change much by lowering the temperature from 35°C to 20°C, its rising and falling phases became considerably slow at lower temperatures resulting in a prolongation of tail current (Figure 6). The percentage of channel modification increased somewhat and the time constant of tail current decay increased drastically upon lowering the temperature.   However, the ratio of tail current area (charge transfer) to peak current area also increased drastically upon lowering the temperature. The charge transfer during the tail current is deemed directly responsible for large tail current produced by tetramethrin-modified sodium channel.   Thus, the negative temperature dependence of pyrethroid action can be accounted for in terms of slowing of the tail current kinetics upon lowering the temperature.

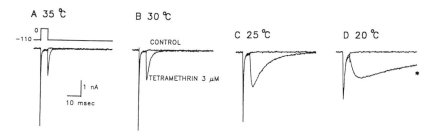

Figure 6 *Temperature-dependent effect of 3 μM tetramethrin on sodium currents recorded from a rat cerebellar Purkinje cell. The currents were evoked by a 5-msec step depolarization to 0 mV from a holding potential of -110 mV at various temperatures. The currents before and during application of tetramethrin are superimposed. *, Current recording is terminated before the tail current returns to the base-line. From Song and Narahashi.*[30]

2.3 Selective Toxicity

One of the important characteristics for a chemical to be useful insecticide is selective toxicity between insects and mammals. For many insecticides, the selective toxicity could be explained on the basis of selective detoxication. A classic example is malathion which is shown to be detoxified differentially due to different metabolizing enzymes involved in insects and mammals.[39] By contrast, pyrethroids have been found to show selective toxicity due primarily to their direct action on the sodium channel.[30]

Table 2 summarizes the results of analyses. The Q_{10} value for the nerve sensitivity to tetramethrin was estimated to be 5 based on electrophysiology experiments. Since there is approximately 10°C difference between insects and mammals this factor plays an important role. The difference in the intrinsic sensitivity of sodium channels to tetramethrin between insects and mammals was 10-fold. The rate of recovery from *in vitro* tetramethrin action after washout was 5 times faster in mammals than in insects. The difference in enzymatic degradation of tetramethrin between insects and mammals was estimated to be 3-fold. The larger the body size, the more chance is expected for tetramethrin to be detoxified before reaching the target site. This difference is assumed as 3-fold. Multiplying all these differences, we obtain an overall difference of 2250, which is in the same order of magnitude as LD_{50} differences between insects and mammals for tetramethrin. Thus, it is concluded that the major factor contributing to the negative temperature dependence of insecticidal action of tetramethrin is the sensitivity of nerve sodium channels.

Table 2 *Factors Contributing Selective Toxicity of Pyrethroids*

Selectivity Factor	Mammals	Insects	Differences
Potency on nerve			
Due to temperature dependence	Low (37°C)	High (25°C)	5
Due to intrinsic sensitivity	Low	High	10
Recovery	Fast	Slow	5
Detoxication rate			
Due to enzymatic action	High	Low	3
Due to body size	High	Low	3

Overall difference = 2250.
(From Song and Narahashi[30])

3. NEURONAL NICOTINIC ACh RECEPTOR CHANNELS

Whereas muscle nicotinic ACh receptors have been studied for a long time for their physiology and pharmacology, studies of neuronal nicotinic ACh receptors have received attention only recently. In the field of insecticide toxicology, the significance of neuronal nicotinic ACh receptors has been recognized since the development of nitromethylene heterocyclic insecticides such as imidacloprid. Binding studies have shown that these insecticides act on the nicotinic ACh receptors.[40-42] However, there have been some controversies as to whether nitromethylene heterocycles behave as antagonists or as agonists.[40,41,43-49] Thus, we have performed detailed patch clamp experiments using both whole-cell and single-channel recording techniques.[50-52] Single-channel analyses have also revealed significant differences between imidacloprid and cartap which were not obvious from whole-cell recording experiments.[51]

3.1 Imidacloprid

3.1.1 Whole-cell currents. Clonal rat phaeochromocytoma (PC12) cells generate nicotinic ACh receptor currents. Imidacloprid suppressed carbachol-induced whole-cell currents reversibly in a concentration-dependent manner.[52] Imidacloprid by itself generated currents, but the efficacy was much smaller than that of carbachol. Thus, imidacloprid appears to have both agonist and antagonist actions.

3.1.2 Single-channel currents. Single-channel currents were recorded from PC12 cells using the cell-attached variation of patch clamp techniques. Single-channel currents evoked by 10 μM ACh comprised main conductance currents and subconductance currents, corresponding to conductances of 25 pS and 10 pS, respectively (Figures 7A and 8A).[50-52] Imidacloprid at 10 μM also generated single-channel currents, but they were mostly in the subconductance state (Figures 7B and 8B). Thus, when 10 μM ACh and 10 μM imidacloprid were co-applied, both main conductance and subconductance state currents were observed (Figure 7C).

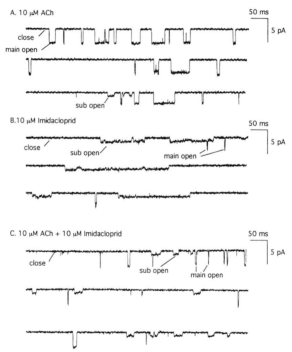

Figure 7 *Single-channel currents activated by 10 μM ACh, 10 μM imidacloprid, and co-application of 10 μM ACh and 10 μM imidacloprid to cell-attached membrane patches clamped at a membrane potential 40 mV more positive than the resting potential. A. Currents induced by 10 μM ACh occurred during brief isolated openings or longer openings interrupted by a few short closures or gaps. Main conductance state currents were observed more frequently than subconductance state currents. B. Currents induced by 10 μM imidacloprid. Subconductance state currents were more frequently observed than main conductance state currents. C. Co-application of 10 μM imidacloprid. Main conductance and subconductance state currents were induced, and channel openings were shortened. From Nagata et al.[52]*

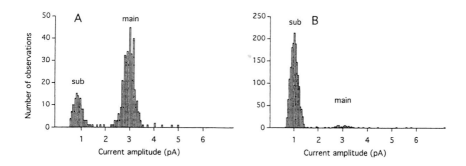

Figure 8   *A. Amplitude histogram of single-channel currents generated by 10 μM ACh in a PC12 cell. Two conductance states are clearly observed. B. Amplitude histogram of single-channel currents induced by 10 μM imidacloprid in a PC12 cell. Two conductance states are clearly observed. From Nagata et al.[50]*

Analyses of open time distribution of main conductance state currents revealed some differences between currents induced by ACh and by imidacloprid. The open time in ACh-induced currents had three components, with time constants of 0.7, 9.9 and 42.3 ms. Imidacloprid-induced currents also had three components, but the time constants were shorter than those in ACh except for the shortest one, i.e. 0.7, 2.7 and 11.5 ms. With co-application of ACh and imidacloprid, the open time distribution mimicked that of imidacloprid with time constants of 0.9, 4.2 and 12.1 ms. The difference in burst duration distribution among ACh, imidacloprid, and ACh plus imidacloprid resembled those in open time distribution. In ACh, the time constants were 0.6, 11.1 and 71.9 ms. In imidacloprid, the time constants were 0.9, 3.8 and 12.2 ms, which were mimicked by those in ACh plus imidacloprid with time constants of 0.8, 3.0 and 12.5 ms.

These data clearly indicate that imidacloprid has both multiple agonist and antagonist effects on the neuronal nicotinic ACh receptor channels.

3.2 Cartap

Cartap and nereistoxin are known to block muscle and neuronal nicotinic ACh receptors.[53-56] Although both cartap and imidacloprid block nicotinic ACh receptors, single-channel experiments revealed significant differences between them in terms of their blocking mechanisms.[51] One important difference was that unlike imidacloprid, cartap did not open any channels by itself. Another difference was that the co-application of ACh and cartap caused channel openings in bursts which were not observed with the co-application of ACh and imidacloprid. This study is among many by which significant differences in blocking mechanism are disclosed only by single-channel experiments.

4. GABA$_A$ RECEPTOR CHANNELS

Lindane and dieldrin were demonstrated many years ago to facilitate synaptic transmission in inducing prolonged after-discharges in cockroach ganglia.[57,58] However, it was not until the early 1980s that their inhibitory actions on the GABA receptor was shown through ^{36}Cl$^-$ flux and [^{35}S]TBPS binding experiments.[59,60] Patch clamp experiments have directly demonstrated lindane inhibition of GABA-induced currents.[61]

4.1 Dieldrin Modulation of GABA$_A$ Receptor Channels

Contrary to our initial prediction that dieldrin would simply suppress GABA$_A$ receptors thereby causing hyperexcitation of animals, a dual effect of potentiation and suppression was discovered by whole-cell patch clamp experiments using rat DRG neurons (Figure 9).[62] These two effects are different in nature for several reasons: first, potentiation occurs quickly upon co-application of dieldrin and GABA, while suppression takes place slowly during repeated co-applications or a prolonged co-application; second, the EC$_{50}$ for potentiation is 5 nM, whereas the IC$_{50}$ for suppression is 92 nM; and third, potentiation requires the γ2S subunit, whereas suppression occurs without the γ2S subunit.[63] Therefore, these two effects are exerted by the entirely different mechanisms.

Whole-cell current competition experiments demonstrated that dieldrin and picrotoxin shared a common binding site, presumably located in the chloride channel.[62] Our recent single-channel analyses have clearly shown that both dieldrin and picrotoxinin modulate the channel in the same manner by prolonging the mean closed time and decreasing the channel open probability (T. Ikeda, K. Nagata, T. Shono and T. Narahashi, unpublished data).

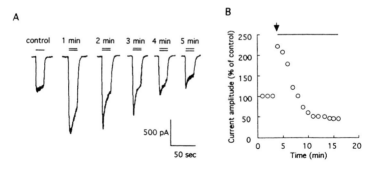

Figure 9 *Effects of dieldrin on GABA-induced chloride currents. A. Current records in response to 20-sec application of 10 µM GABA (solid bar) and to co-application of 10 µM GABA and 1 µM dieldrin (dotted bar) at the time indicated after taking control record. The peak amplitude of current is greatly enhanced but gradually decreases during repeated co-applications. Desensitization of current is accelerated. B. Time course of the changes in peak current amplitude before and during repeated co-applications (dotted line). From Nagata and Narahashi.*[62]

4.2 Anisatin Modulation of GABA$_A$ Receptor Channels

Sikimi plant, *Illicium anisatium*, contains toxic substances which exhibit insecticidal activity. Extracts from Sikimi blocks GABA-induced currents in rat DRG neurons.[64]

Anisatin is a toxic, insecticidally active component of Sikimi plant. Repeated co-applications of GABA and anisatin suppressed GABA-induced whole-cell currents with an EC$_{50}$ of 1.1 µM (T. Ikeda, Y. Ozoe, E. Okuyama, K. Nagata, H. Honda, T. Shono and T. Narahashi, unpublished data). No recovery of currents was observed after washout with anisatin-free solution. However, pre-application of anisatin through the bath had no effect on GABA-induced currents. The decay phase of currents was accelerated by anisatin. These results indicate that anisatin suppression of GABA-induced currents requires opening of the channels and is use dependent. Picrotoxinin attenuated anisatin suppression indicating that anisatin bound to the picrotoxinin site that is closely associated with the chloride channel. At the single-channel level, anisatin did not alter the open time but prolonged the closed time. The burst duration was reduced and channel openings per burst were decreased indicating that anisatin decreased the probability of openings.

Acknowledgements

The authors thank Julia Irizarry for secretarial assistance. The author's work described in this paper was supported by a grant from the National Institutes of Health NS14143.

References

1. T. Narahashi, 'Advances in Insect Physiology', Academic Press, London and New York, 1971, **8**, 1.
2. T. Narahashi 'Insecticide Biochemistry and Physiology', Plenum Press, New York, 1976, 327.
3. T. Narahashi, *Neurotoxicology*, 1985, **6**(2), 3.
4. T. Narahashi, 'Neurotox '88. Molecular Basis of Drug and Pesticide Action', Elsevier Amsterdam, 1988, 269-288.
5. T. Narahashi, 'Insecticide Action: From Molecule to Organism', Plenum Press, New York, 1989, 55.
6. T. Narahashi, *Trends Pharmacol. Sci.,* 1992, **13**, 236.
7. T. Narahashi, *Pharmacology and Toxicology.* 1996, **78,** 1.
8. T. Narahashi, J.M. Frey, K.S. Ginsburg, K. Nagata, M.L. Roy and H. Tatebayashi, 'Molecular Action of Insecticides on Ion Channels', Amer. Chem. Soc., Washington, D.C., 1995, 26.
9. G.S.F. Ruigt, 'Comprehensive Insect Physiology, Biochemistry and Pharmacology', Pergamon Press, Oxford, 1984, **12**, 183.
10. D.M. Soderlund and J.R. Bloomquist, *Annu. Rev. Entomol.*, 1989, **34**, 77.
11. H.P.M. Vijverberg and J. van den Bercken, *Crit. Rev. Toxicol.*, 1990, **21**(2), 105.
12. T. Yamasaki and T. Ishii (Narahashi). *Oyo-Kontyu (J. Nippon Soc. Appl. Entom.)* 1952, **8**, 111.
13. T. Narahashi and T.Yamasaki, *J. Physiol.,* 1960, **152,** 122.
14. T. Narahashi and H.G. Haas, *Science*, 1967, **157,** 1438.
15. T. Narahashi and H.G. Haas, *J. Gen. Physiol.,* 1968, **51**, 177.
16. T. Narahashi, *J. Cell. Comp. Physiol.,* 1962, **59**, 61.
17. T. Narahashi, *J. Cell. Comp. Physiol.,* 1962, **59**, 67.
18. A.E. Lund and T. Narahashi, *Neurotoxicology*, 1981, **2**, 213.
19. A.E. Lund and T. Narahashi, *Neuroscience,* 1981, **6**, 2253.
20. A.E. Lund and T. Narahashi, *J. Pharmacol. Exp. Ther.*, 1981, **219**, 464.
21. T. Narahashi and N.C. Anderson, 1967, *Toxicol. Appl. Pharmacol.,* **10**, 529.
22. T. Narahashi and A.E. Lund, 'Insect Neurobiology and Pesticide Action (Neurotox. 79)', Soc. Chem. Industry, London, 1980, 497.
23. D. Yamamoto, F.N. Quandt and T. Narahashi, *Brain Res.*, 1983, **274**, 344.

24. S.F. Holloway, T. Narahashi, V.L. Salgado and C.H. Wu, *Pflügers Arch.*, 1989, **414**, 613.
25. K. Chinn and T. Narahashi, *J. Physiol.*, 1986, **380**, 191.
26. V.L. Salgado and T. Narahashi, *Mol. Pharmacol.*, 1993, **43**, 626.
27. H.P.M. Vijverberg, J.M. van der Zalm and J. van den Bercken, *Nature*, 1982, **295**, 601.
28. A.E. Lund and T. Narahashi, *Neurotoxicology,* 1982, **3**, 11.
29. H. Tatebayashi and T. Narahashi, *J. Pharmacol. Exp. Ther.*, 1994, **270**, 595.
30. J.-H. Song and T. Narahashi, *J. Pharmacol. Exp. Ther.* 1996, **277**, 445.
31. J.-H. Song and T. Narahashi, *Brain Res.,* 1996, **712**, 258.
32. P.G. Kostyuk, N.S. Veselovsky and Y. Tsyndrenko, *Neuroscience*, 1981, **6**, 2423.
33. M.L. Roy and T. Narahashi, *J. Neurosci.*, 1992, **12**, 2104.
34. M.L. Roy, E. Reuveny and T. Narahashi, *Brain Res.,* 1994, **650**, 341.
35. J.-H. Song, K. Nagata, C.-S. Huang, J.Z. Yeh and T. Narahashi, *NeuroReport.*, 1996, **7**, 3031.
36. J.-H. Song, C.-S. Huang, K. Nagata, J.Z. Yeh and T. Narahashi, *J. Pharmacol. Exp. Ther.,* 1997, **282,** 707.
37. K.S. Ginsburg and T. Narahashi, *Brain Res,* 1993, **627**, 239.
38. I.V. Tabarean and T. Narahashi, *J. Pharmacol. Exp. Ther.,* 1998, **24**, 958.
39. R.D. O'Brien, 'Insecticides Action and Metabolism', Academic Press, New York, 1967, 253.
40. D. Bai, S.C.R. Lummis, W. Leicht, H. Breer and D.B. Sattelle, *Pestic. Sci.,* 1991, **33**, 197.
41. D.B. Sattelle, S.D. Buckingham, K.A. Wafford, S.M. Sherby, N.M. Bakry, A.T. Eldefrawi, M.E. Eldefrawi and T.E. May, *Proc. Roy. Soc. Lond. B.*, 1989, **237**, 501.
42. M.Y. Liu and J.E. Casida, *Pestic. Biochem. Physiol.*, 1993, **46**, 40.
43. S. Sone, K. Nagata, S. Tsuboi and T. Shono, *J. Pestic. Sci.,* 1994, **19**, 69.
44. J.A. Benson, 'Progress and Prospects in Insect Control', British Crops Protection Council, Farnham, UK, 1989, 59.
45. J.A. Benson, *J. Exp. Biol.*, 1992, **170**, 203.
46. H. Cheung, B.S. Clarke and D.J. Beadle, *Pestic. Sci.*, 1992, **34**, 187.
47. C.A. Leech, P. Jewess, J. Marshall and D.B. Sattelle, *FEBS Lett.*, 1991, **290**, 90.
48. R. Zwart, M. Oortgiesen and H.P. Vijverberg, *Eur. J. Pharmacol.,* 1992, **228,** 165.
49. R. Zwart, M. Oortgiesen and H.P. Vijverberg, *Pestic. Biochem. Physiol.*, 1994, **48**, 202.
50. K. Nagata, G.L. Aistrup, J.-H. Song and T. Narahashi, *NeuroReport,* 1996, **7**, 1025.
51. K. Nagata, Y. Iwanaga, T. Shono and T. Narahashi, *Pestic. Biochem. Physiol.*, 1997, **59**, 119.
52. K. Nagata, J.-H. Song, T. Shono and T. Narahashi, *J. Pharmacol. Exp. Ther.*, 1998, **285**, 731.
53. S. Chiba, Y. Saji, Y. Takeo, T. Yui and Y. Aramaki, *Japan. J. Pharmacol.,* 1967, **17**, 491.
54. T. Deguchi, T. Narahashi and H.G. Haas, *Pestic. Biochem. Physiol.*, 1971, **1**, 196.
55. D.B. Sattelle, I.D. Harrow, J.A. David, M. Pelhate and J.J. Callec, *J. Exp. Biol.*, 1985, **118**, 37.
56. S.M. Sherby, A.T. Eldefrawi, J.A. Davis, D.B. Sattelle and M.E. Eldefrawi, *Arch. Insect Biochem. Physiol.,* 1986, **3**, 431.
57. T. Yamasaki and T. Ishii (Narahashi), *Botyu-Kagaku (Scientific Insect Control)*, 1954, **19**, 106.
58. T. Yamasaki and T. Narahashi, *Botyu-Kagaku (Scientific Insect Control)*, 1958, **23**, 47.

59. S.M. Ghiasuddin and F. Matsumura, *Comp. Biochem. Physiol.,* 1982, **73C**, 141.
60. F. Matsumura and S.M. Ghiasuddin, *J. Environ. Sci. Health,* 1983, **B18**, 1.
61. N. Ogata, S.M. Vogel and T. Narahashi, *FASEB J.*, 1988, **2**, 2895.
62. K. Nagata and T. Narahashi, *J. Pharmacol. Exp. Ther.*, 1994, **269**, 164.
63. K. Nagata, B.J. Hamilton, D.B. Carter and T. Narahashi, *Brain Res.*, 1994, **645**, 19.
64. T. Ikeda, , K. Nagata, H. Honda, T. Shono and T. Narahashi, *Pesticide Sci.*, 1998, **52**, 337.

Neurotoxic Insecticides as Target Site Radioligands and Photoaffinity Probes

John E. Casida and Gary B. Quistad

ENVIRONMENTAL CHEMISTRY AND TOXICOLOGY LABORATORY, DEPARTMENT OF
ENVIRONMENTAL SCIENCE, POLICY AND MANAGEMENT, UNIVERSITY OF CALIFORNIA,
BERKELEY, CA 94720, USA

1   INTRODUCTION

Neuroactive insecticides are the first line of defense against insects attacking crops and transmitting diseases of man and livestock.[1]   The dominant position of neuroactive chemicals results from a combination of potency, rapid action, sublethal effects on pest behavior, and sometimes selectivity and safety.   Research on neuroactive insecticides has two goals: define the mechanisms for current compounds to prolong their effectiveness and ensure their safety; discover new compounds, ideally with a novel target.   There are only a few biochemical targets involved (a "finite number" of practical targets)[2] and selection of populations for resistant strains has eroded the effectiveness of commercial neuroactive insecticides and new ones falling into the cross-resistance pattern.

Interaction of an insecticide with its target involves ligand association and dissociation from its binding site.   Radioligand binding assays allow screening at the target to optimize the insecticide structure or to seek new and unusual compounds acting at the same site or a coupled region.   This target is stripped of its outlying defenses of membrane barriers and detoxification and therefore a high potency may be a false positive relative to organismal effects.   The radioligand can be a pharmacological probe, a toxicant, or the insecticide itself.

2   PRINCIPLES

2.1 Probe Selection and Design

This review emphasizes using the neurotoxic insecticide *per se* or a close analog as the target site radioligand and photoaffinity probe.   The closer the structure of the probe is to that of the actual insecticide the higher the relevance.   However, sometimes an analog is better since potency is only one factor in the selection of an insecticide for development, i.e. economic, environmental and safety issues are also involved.   The binding must be specific for the target protein and usually with an affinity constant (K_d) of 0.1-50 nM. Ligands which are soluble in water at 10-5000 nM or higher are preferred.   Radioligands of high specific activity are normally required, *e.g.* labeled with ^3H, ^{32}P, ^{35}S or ^{125}I, for quantitation at normal receptor levels.   Fluorescent probes can sometimes be used, thereby avoiding problems of radioactivity experiments.

The target source is usually nerve membranes used directly or following detergent solubilization. Most assays are made by filtration techniques and typically require specific binding of 500-5000 dpm per filter, involving 10-1000 μg membrane protein per assay. Hundreds or thousands of assays may be necessary so the membranes must be readily available, *e.g.* bovine brain, rat brain or housefly (*Musca*) heads (or *Drosophila* heads when background information on gene sequences is required). Studies with agricultural pests are preferred but field collection or mass rearing is a major limiting factor. The alternative is to use cloned and expressed targets which is now possible with individual subunits or subunit combinations for many receptors. The use of a radioligand with similar affinity for insects and mammals allows selective toxicity studies relative to ligand displacement.

2.2 Probe Validation

The radioligand (or fluorescent) probe is validated first as to specific, saturable and high-affinity binding, second by pharmacological profile, and then as to toxicological relevance based on structure-activity relationships and *ex vivo* inhibition assays on brain or other nerve tissue from poisoned animals. Establishing the pharmacological profile is a critical step, *e.g.* the inhibition of binding by γ-aminobutyric acid (GABA) or acetylcholine (ACh) as natural ligands. The toxicological relevance can be established with a series of 10-40 unlabeled analogs or related compounds of varying potency, comparing their inhibition of radioligand binding (IC_{50}) and effective concentration (EC_{50}) for a toxicologically-relevant endpoint, *e.g.* topical knockdown or LD_{50} (alone or with synergist) or neurophysiological effect. If the *in vitro* binding data faithfully predict the tissue or organismal effect, there is good evidence for relevance. Compounds that do not correlate (outlyers) are evaluated for possible detoxification or activation (more or less potent in the receptor than in the functional assay). The K_d is often lower for insect than mammalian brain because insecticide development focuses on compounds with higher insecticidal activity than toxicity to mammals. The finding that resistant pest strains have lower affinity target sites than susceptible strains supports the relevance of the radioligand probe assays.

2.3 Covalent Affinity Probes and Localizing the Binding Site

The simplest, most common and most specific covalent derivative for insecticides is formed by phosphorylation of acetylcholinesterase at its serine hydroxyl functional site. Analogous carbamoylation reactions are involved with methylcarbamate insecticides. More general derivatizing agents can be used as chemical affinity probes for other targets, *e.g.* isothiocyanate or alkyl halide for thiol groups. The most commonly-used photo-affinity substituents are arylazides, aryltrifluoromethyldiazirines and benzophenones. One distinct advantage of a radiolabeled chemical affinity or photoaffinity probe is that a stable covalent attachment permits isolation of the labeled protein without loss of the tag. This allows the labeled protein to be purified to constant specific activity or homogeneity for identification by antibody recognition, high resolution mass spectrometry, or sequence determination after selective proteolysis. It also allows overcoming binding artifacts from liposolubility since electrophoretic separation has far more resolving power than a mere filtration assay. The receptor can be fractionated and then labeled (to define the most relevant parts or subunits) or labeled then fractionated (so that the initial attachment is created in the native target form); importantly, the binding site is often between subunits rather than within a subunit.

The two primary methods for elucidating the structure of receptor active sites or topography are site-directed 1) radioligand binding and photoaffinity labeling, and 2) mutagenesis. Photoaffinity labeling remains a reliable method which should be considered complementary to (rather than in competition with) site-directed mutagenesis.[3] Photoaffinity labeling has two major advantages: 1) direct chemical derivatization of amino acids at the target site, and 2) minimizing misinterpretations from functional alterations of the receptor-ligand binding relative to allosteric conformational changes in protein structure at distant sites which may occur from point mutagenesis. Designing a photoaffinity probe for an insecticide is much more difficult than designing a radioligand since it must meet five requirements: 1) high affinity and specific binding; 2) ease of radiosynthesis; 3) suitable photoreactive substituent near the central or structurally-specific part of the molecule; 4) photoreactive and labeled positions that do not cleave apart on receptor isolation and sequencing; and 5) no photoproducts that interfere with binding or give spurious attachment. It is fully as important to establish the binding isotherms and pharmacological profiles for a photoaffinity probe as for a radioligand. Ultimately, the specific target region is defined by sequencing followed by site-directed mutagenesis. Once defined, the binding site localization is generally applicable to a large set of related compounds (and potentially several classes of apparently unrelated chemicals).

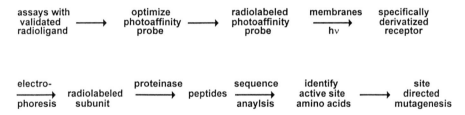

3　PROGRESS

3.1 Acetylcholine Receptor

3.1.1 Nicotinic. The nicotinic AChR (nAChR) is of current interest for two reasons. First, it is the target of the latest class of major insecticides, exemplified by imidacloprid (IMI). Second, the insecticides themselves can be used as the radioligands. [³H]IMI was synthesized[4] and shown to bind with high affinity (K_d 1 nM) to the nAChR agonist site in housefly head membranes.[5,6] Assays with [³H]IMI ultimately resulted in a novel nicotinoid-agarose affinity column for purification of *Drosophila* and *Musca* nAChRs.[7] [³H]Acetamiprid and other insecticidal analogs (CH-IMI, NMI) also were used to characterize insect nAChRs.[8,9] A novel [¹²⁵I]nicotinoid photoaffinity probe bound with high affinity (IC_{50} 8 nM for [³H]IMI binding) in *Drosophila* head membranes and upon irradiation radiolabeled primarily a 66-kDa protein and secondarily a 61-kDa subunit at a specific site, possibly at the interface between the 66 and 61 kDa subunits; this binding is inhibited by cholinergic ligands including (-)-nicotine and α-bungarotoxin, consistent with the insecticide-binding subunit of the nAChR.[10,11]

IMI   desnitro-IMI   CH - IMI   acetamiprid

NMI   photoaffinity probe   nithiazine

The chloropyridyl or chlorothiazolyl moiety is an important structural feature for high insecticidal activity and nAChR potency. The radioligands above (except desnitro-IMI) have much lower affinity for mammalian brain as compared to insect sites, consistent with the apparent safety of this class of insecticides for mammals. However, considerable species specificity is involved. The potent mammalian analgesic epibatidine (an nAChR agonist with a chloropyridyl moiety) binds with high affinity (K_d 6 nM) to American cockroach nerve homogenates using [^{3}H]($\pm$)-epibatidine, but not to house fly head membranes, suggesting species-specific binding sites.[12] The metabolites may also have a different target specificity than the parent insecticides. Thus, the metabolite desnitro-IMI is less active than IMI on the insect nAChR but much more potent on the mammalian brain nAChR, suggesting possible metabolic activation in mammals.[13]

Photoaffinity probes based on insecticidal components in wasp venom (philanthotoxins) radiolabeled the α subunit from the *Torpedo* nAChR when the 43-kDa cytosolic protein was present but photolinked to all five subunits (α, α', β, γ, δ) in its absence.[14] Extensive synthesis of philanthotoxin analogs based on structure-activity relationships has provided candidate photoaffinity probes for future studies.[15]

3.1.2 Muscarinic. Although muscarinic ACh receptors are important components of the insect central nervous system, no commercial insecticides utilize this site as a primary target for intoxication[16] and some of the muscarinic agents are highly toxic to mammals. Nithiazine partially blocks these receptors in rat brain but only at millimolar concentrations.[17] [^{3}H]Quinuclidinyl benzilate has been a useful nonselective radioligand for brain membranes from several insects[18] and its displacement by known mammalian muscarinic receptor agonists correlates to their insecticidal/acaricidal activity.[19]

3.2 GABA Receptor

Four major insecticides (and closely related compounds) act at the GABA receptor blocker or activator site to close or open the chloride channel.

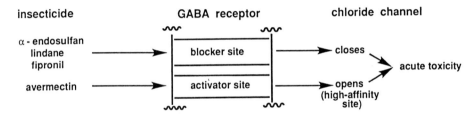

insecticide   GABA receptor   chloride channel

α - endosulfan
lindane   ──────▶   blocker site   ─────▶ closes
fipronil   acute toxicity
avermectin   ──────▶   activator site   ─────▶ opens
                                                         (high-affinity
                                                           site)

3.2.1 Blocker Site. The blocker site for insecticides has been characterized with four progressively-improved heterocyclic radioligands, i.e. [³H]dihydropicrotoxinin, [³⁵S]TBPS, [³H]TBOB and [³H]EBOB. Picrotoxinin (from the fishberry plant, used as an insecticide 125 years ago) has an isopropenyl group allowing catalytic tritiation to [³H]dihydropicrotoxinin, the first important radioligand for the noncompetitive blocker site.[20] This radioligand was adequate to clearly suggest but not firmly establish the GABA-gated chloride channel as a target for cyclodiene insecticides[21] and resistance associated with lower binding site affinity.[22] A major advance in radioligands was based on the discovery of very toxic 2,6,7-trioxabicyclooctanes and adapting the orthophosphorus compounds (TBPS) and orthocarboxylates (TBOB and EBOB) to study the GABA receptor. Investigations with [³⁵S]TBPS confirmed and expanded the evidence for the polychlorocycloalkanes (PCCAs) acting at the chloride channel in mammals[23,24] and this was supported by studies with [³H]TBOB[25] and most convincingly with [³H]EBOB.[26] PCCAs differ from the heterocyclic blockers (trioxabicyclooctanes, dithianes) whose mammalian receptor affinities correlate with their association rates whereas the potency of PCCAs is limited by dissociation rates.[27] TBPS and EBOB act at different sites in houseflies with different cross resistance phenomena.[28] [³H]EBOB in houseflies detects the common binding site or domain for seven different classes of chloride channel blockers[29] which is coupled to the avermectin site, establishing that it also resides in the GABA-gated chloride channel.[30] Low affinity [³H]EBOB binding correlates with the alanine → serine mutation conferring resistance in *Rdl Drosophila* to these multiple classes of insecticides.[31] The heterocyclic radioligands are also useful for localizing GABA receptors in various brain regions as determined by incubation of [³⁵S]TBPS, [³H]TBOB and [³H]EBOB with rodent and human brain slices (comparing total and nonspecific sites) and autoradiography to visualize the specific binding sites.[32-34]

dihydropicrotoxinin   TBOB

TBPS   EBOB

There have been many candidate trioxabicyclooctane- and dithiane-derived photoaffinity probes for the noncompetitive blocker site, but no one of them has been combined with radiolabeling and appropriate biochemical studies to validate the probe and define this site.[35-38] It is difficult to combine high affinity with suitable photoreactivity and an additional goal is to find a probe suitable for both mammals and insects. IC$_{50}$ values (nM) are given below for several of the candidate photoaffinity probes in bovine brain with [³H]TBOB (top two lines) or [³H]EBOB (bottom two lines) assays.

The PCCAs are a continuing challenge to develop and use as radioligands. There are two "success" stories, [³H]α-endosulfan[39] and [³H]BIDN.[40] The binding of [³H]α-endosulfan in housefly head membranes is plagued by high nonspecific binding and it competes specifically with the PCCAs. [³H]BIDN also labels the PCCA site and both ligands are not displaced by picrotoxinin, TBPS and EBOB. It is not clear if the ability to detect only PCCAs with [³H]PCCAs and to the detect the PCCAs, fipronil types and several groups of heterocyclics with the heterocyclic probes means they act at different sites. The best candidates for further study, because of potency, solubility and toxicological relevance, are [³H]α-endosulfan, [³H]lindane and a [³H]fipronil-type compound, but insecticides targeted at the blocker site other than the fipronil series are currently not favored for further development.

3.2.2 Activator Site. [³H]Avermectin and its dihydro analog [³H]ivermectin are potent pesticides that are used directly as radioligands. The activator or avermectin site is readily examined in membranes of mammalian brain,[41,42] rat cerebellar granule neurons,[43] *Musca* and *Drosophila* heads[30] and whole nematodes (*Caenorhabditis elegans*)[44,45] with minor but critical modifications to the standard filtration technique to accommodate the low water solubility and tendency for nonspecific adsorption to surfaces. The binding of [³H]avermectin or [³H]ivermectin in houseflies[30] and nematodes[45] is displaced by analogs in proportion to their biological activity, establishing toxicological relevance. Photoaffinity labeling of the *Drosophila* and *Caenorhabditis* receptors has been achieved using a 4'-azido-2'-hydroxy-3'-iodobenzoyl derivative with a long spacer unit, giving radiolabeled proteins (45 kDa for *Drosophila*; 8, 47 and 53 kDa for *Caenorhabditis*), not isolated or further characterized.[45] Analogs without the dioleandrosyl moiety are sometimes more selective but they are not reported as radioligands. No other compounds combine simple structure and high potency at this site.

photoaffinity probe

avermectin B₁ₐ

3.3 Sodium Channel

It is generally accepted that the pyrethroids and DDT act at the same site which is second only to AChE in importance as an insecticide target. It is located in the voltage-sensitive sodium channel. This target is not defined with the insecticide itself as a radioligand but instead is interpreted from investigations with other sodium channel radioligands and from electrophysiological studies and molecular biology approaches.[46] [^{35}S]TBPS binding is inhibited by pyrethroids with appropriate stereospecificity but at 5 μM which is excessive for a high-affinity site.[47] DDT analogs are borderline in potency for use as radioligands and their liposolubility is too high for establishing binding kinetics. The potency of some pyrethroids is such that they should act at 0.01-1 nM at the insect site and at least below 10 nM in mammals. Narahashi's calculation[48] that < 0.1% of the sodium channel population needs to be modified for initiation of repetitive discharges and poisoning is somewhat discouraging for the case of establishing binding kinetics relative to physiological changes. It is becoming increasingly clear that success will depend on a high affinity and high specific activity radioligand and a nerve preparation or expressed receptor from a sensitive species and even then photoaffinity labeling may be required to validate the target. The progress is considered below.

NRDC 157 (*1R, cis*)

X = H, Y = Z = ³H
(αS, Z, 1R, 3R)
cyhalothrin

X = Z = ³H, Y = F
(αS, Z, 1R, 3R)
fluorocyhalothrin

(*R,S*)- descyano-azidofenvalerate

kadethrin analog

RU 58487

The first attempt to directly study pyrethroid binding utilized labeled tetramethrin with rat brain homogenate.[49] A number of [³H]pyrethroids have been used in attempts to characterize the pyrethroid binding site, but they were compromised by poor specific binding (*e.g.* 3% for [³H]NRDC 157), a major problem for very hydrophobic compounds.[50,51] (αS,Z,1R,3R)-Cyhalothrin and fluorocyhalothrin (among the most potent of all insecticides) were radiosynthesized at high specific activity (55 Ci/mmol) as optimized [³H]radioligands.[52] Unfortunately, they exhibited the usual difficulty of nonspecific binding to rodent brain and insect neuronal membranes and they are no longer available because of radiolysis. Racemic [3H]descyanoazidofenvalerate as a photoaffinity probe labels an unknown 36-kDa protein in rat brain rather than the sodium channel subunits, but inhibition of radioligand binding by analogs occurred incompletely, at high (μM) levels and did not correlate to biopotency or expected stereochemistry.[53] A photoreactive trifluoromethyldiazirine .analog of kadethrin mimics the nerve effects induced by conventional pyrethroids and is a candidate probe for photoaffinity labeling after radiosynthesis.[54] [3H]RU58487 has fairly high affinity (K_d 58 nM) as a radioligand using rat brain membrane preparations, and 75% specific binding is attained using nonionic detergent (0.05% Triton X-100) with a 40% enhancement from the allosteric interactions of α-scorpion toxin at site 3 (but not by other toxins at sites 2 and 5).[55] Irradiation of bound [3H]RU58487 photolabels a 240-kDa protein corresponding to the sodium channel α-subunit, immunoprecipitated by peptide-induced antibodies. Although the toxicological relevance remains to be established by structure-activity studies, this may be the first direct detection of a high affinity pyrethroid receptor site in the sodium channel.

Veratridine has been used for more than 50 years as a component in the insecticide sabadilla and it can be structurally modified for enhanced activity but the binding site in insects has not been examined with structurally-related radioligand probes. The dihydropyrazoles and *N*-alkylamides, both potent insecticides, bind to distinct sites different from that of the pyrethroids to modify sodium channel function.[46] Even though they have attained adequate potency, there are no reports on their successful use as radioligands.

3.4 Other Receptors

3.4.1 Octopamine. Octopamine receptors are very important and widely distributed in insects and therefore are a target for selective pest control. Current insecticides with this site of action are minor although chlordimeform was once prominent prior to removal from the market in the late 1970s because of carcinogenicity. [3H]Octopamine binds to firefly light organ membranes (K_d 1 nM for high-affinity site and 60 nM for more abundant but lower-affinity site)[56] but desmethylchlordimeform, an activated metabolite, is even better than octopamine in reducing [3H]octopamine binding at the receptor.[56] [3H]NC-5Z is an octopamine agonist which as a photoaffinity probe binds irreversibly to membranes from the firefly light organ as well as those from a variety of other insect tissues.[57] [3H]NC-5Z binds with high affinity (K_d 2.5 nM) and photolabels the class 3 octopamine receptor in nerve tissue from the desert locust, *Schistocerca gregaria*; electrophoresis of solubilized membranes gave a single radiolabeled protein (53 kDa).[58]

[3H]octopamine

R = CH3, chlordimeform
R = H, desmethylchlordimeform

[3H]NC-5Z

3.4.2 Glutamate. The ionotropic excitatory glutamate receptor in insects is an attractive target for insecticides but so far without commercial success.[16,59] [^{125}I]Philanthotoxin-343 was evaluated as a radioligand probe for the glutamate receptor in rat brain synaptic membranes, but most of the toxin binding sites were insensitive to displacement by glutamate and all drugs known to bind at this receptor.[60] Photolabile analogs of philanthotoxin are bioactive in locust muscle preparations.[61]

4 PROSPECTS

4.1 Radioligands to Screen for Insecticide Action

[^{3}H]EBOB, [^{3}H]IMI, [^{3}H]ryanodine (see below) and other radioligands have been used to screen large numbers of synthetic compounds and biological extracts for candidate insecticide leads. An increasing array of validated radioligands will facilitate future insecticide discovery and optimization. In addition, each new type of insecticide that is discovered potentially serves as the basis for a radioligand for screening and mode of action research. A great variety of insecticidal compounds of unknown mode of action may ultimately yield useful radioligands.

Insecticides acting as respiratory inhibitors and at calcium release channels may have important effects in the nervous system. NADH:ubiquinone oxidoreductase has been examined with [^{3}H]dihydrorotenone as a radioligand and photoaffinity probe and with an arylazido analog of rotenone.[62-64] More recent studies on this oxidoreductase involve [^{3}H]fenazaquin as a radioligand and ^{3}H-labeled trifluoromethyldiazirinyl-fenazaquin and -pyridaben as photoaffinity ligands.[65-67] The carbodiimide metabolite and photoproduct of diafenthiuron serves as a chemical affinity probe for ATP synthase.[68,69] The calcium release channel is conveniently assayed with [^{3}H]ryanodine which binds with higher affinity and is occluded in the active site.[70,71]

4.2 Binding Site Versus Bioactivation and Detoxification

Toxicants that act quickly, are readily transported, and are slowly metabolized often give excellent correlation of binding site data with toxicity, *e.g.* bicyclophosphates.[72] When the insecticide is readily metabolized, a high correlation of potency at the receptor with toxicity is only achieved by blocking the metabolism, such as with piperonyl butoxide for a variety of chloride channel blockers[72] and *O*-propyl *O*-propynyl phenylphosphonate for nicotinoid insecticides.[73] Compounds that fall outside of the correlation region for binding versus toxicity may be activated or detoxified. The ideal is to couple the metabolic system (usually P450) with the target site assay but this requires a radioligand resistant to metabolism.[24]

5 CONCLUSIONS

Important advances in understanding receptors and ion channels have come from binding site studies with radioligands based on insecticides. Probe selection or design has the option of using the insecticide itself or an optimized analog, generally labeled with ^{3}H, ^{32}P, ^{35}S or ^{125}I. When binding sites are similar in insects and mammals, often the same radioligand can be used, but successful mapping mandates high affinity of the probe for the target. Probe validation is based on: 1) specific and saturable binding, 2) suitable pharmacological profile and 3) correlation of structure-activity relationships for binding site interaction and biological function. Validated radioligands allow high-throughput screens of candidate insecticides and studies of target site selectivity and pest resistance from target site insensitivity. Localizing the binding site requires overcoming nonspecific binding artifacts (a major problem with liposoluble insecticides) and optimizing the source of receptor or channel and conditions for solubilization and fractionation. Photoaffinity probes, incorporating a photoactivatable derivatizing moiety into the optimized radioligand, are used to define: 1) subunit involvement, 2) the locus within (or between) subunits or domains, and 3) the amino acid derivatized. Neurotoxic insecticide radioligands and photoaffinity probes have been most important for ACh and GABA receptors. The nAChR differs greatly between insects and mammals as revealed by studies with labeled nicotine, IMI, desnitro-IMI, epibatidine and α-bungarotoxin. The GABA receptor blocker site, assayed with [^{3}H]EBOB (preferred) or labeled TBOB, TBPS, BIDN or dihydropicrotoxinin, shows marked similarity for insects and mammals but still allows major target site selectivity. The GABA receptor activator site, probed with [^{3}H]avermectin, is generally similar in insects and mammals. Pyrethroid action is poorly understood as to the specific binding site although there is recent progress with [^{3}H]pyrethroids. No information is currently available from radioactive dihydropyrazoles or *N*-alkylamides as to their specific binding sites in the sodium channel. Assays are available for octopamine and glutamate receptor targets, but new insecticides of suitable properties are not. An increasing array of validated radioligands will facilitate future insecticide discovery and optimization.

Acknowledgment. The project described was supported by Grants P01 ES00049, R01 ES08762 and R01 ES08424 from the National Institute of Environmental Health Sciences (NIEHS), NIH, and its contents are solely the responsibility of the authors and do not necessarily represent the official views of the NIEHS, NIH.

References

1. C.D.S. Tomlin, Ed., 'The Pesticide Manual, Eleventh Edition,' British Crop Protection Council, Farnham, UK, 1997.
2. J.E. Casida, In 'Pesticides and Alternatives: Innovative Chemical and Biological Approaches to Pest Control', J.E. Casida, Ed., pp 11-22, Elsevier, Amsterdam, 1990.
3. F. Kotzyba-Hibert, I. Kapfer and M. Goeldner, *Angew. Chem. Int. Ed. Engl.*, 1995, **34**, 1296.
4. B. Latli and J.E. Casida, *J. Labelled Compd. Radiopharm.*, 1992, **31**, 609.
5. M.-Y. Liu and J.E. Casida, *Pestic. Biochem. Physiol.*, 1993, **46**, 40.
6. M.-Y. Liu, B. Latli and J.E. Casida, *Pestic. Biochem. Physiol.*, 1995, **52**, 170.
7. M. Tomizawa, B. Latli and J.E. Casida, *J. Neurochem.*, 1996, **67**, 1669.
8. B. Latli, C. Than, H. Morimoto, P.G. Williams and J.E. Casida, *J. Labelled Compd. Radiopharm.*, 1996, **38**, 971.
9. M.-Y. Liu, B. Latli and J.E. Casida, *Pestic. Biochem. Physiol.*, 1994, **50**, 171.
10. B. Latli, M. Tomizawa and J.E. Casida, *Bioconj. Chem.*, 1997, **8**, 7.
11. M. Tomizawa and J.E. Casida, *Neurosci. Lett.*, 1997, **237**, 61.
12. N. Orr, A.J. Shaffner and G.B. Watson, *Pestic. Biochem. Physiol.*, 1997, **58**, 183.
13. S.L. Chao and J.E. Casida, *Pestic. Biochem. Physiol.*, 1997, **58**, 77.
14. S.-K. Choi, A.G. Kalivretenos, P.N.R. Usherwood and K. Nakanishi, *Chem. & Biol.* 1995, **2**, 23.

15. K. Nakanishi, X. Huang, H. Jiang, Y. Liu, K. Fang, D. Huang, S.-K. Choi, E. Katz and M. Eldefrawi, *Bioorg. Med. Chem.* 1997, **5**, 1969.
16. J.A. Benson, In 'Neurotox '91-Molecular Basis of Drug and Pesticide Action,' I.R. Duce, Ed., pp 57-70, Elsevier Applied Science, London, 1991.
17. D.B. Sattelle, S.D. Buckingham, K.A. Wafford, S.M. Sherby, N.M. Bakry, A.T. Eldefrawi, M.E. Eldefrawi and T.E. May, *Proc. Royal Soc. London, Ser. B. Biol. Sci.*, 1989, **237**, 501.
18. E.A. Abdallah, M.E. Eldefrawi and A.T. Eldefrawi, *Arch. Insect Biochem. Physiol.*, 1991, **17**, 107.
19. M.R. Dick, J.E. Dripps and N. Orr, *Pestic. Sci.*, 1997, **49**, 268.
20. M.K. Ticku, M. Ban and R.W. Olsen, *Mol. Pharmacol.*, 1978, **14**, 391.
21. F. Matsumura and S.M. Ghiasuddin, *J. Environ. Sci. Health*, 1983, **B18**, 1.
22. K. Tanaka and F. Matsumura, In 'Membrane Receptors and Enzymes as Targets of Insecticidal Action', J.M. Clark and F. Matsumura, Eds., pp 33-49, Plenum, New York, 1986.
23. R.F. Squires, J.E. Casida, M. Richardson and E. Saederup, *Mol. Pharmacol.*, 1983, **23**, 326.
24. L.J. Lawrence and J.E. Casida, *Life Sci.*, 1984, **35**, 171.
25. L.J. Lawrence, C.J. Palmer, K.W. Gee, X. Wang, H.I. Yamamura and J.E. Casida, *J. Neurochem.*, 1985, **45**, 798.
26. L.M. Cole and J.E. Casida, *Pestic. Biochem. Physiol.*, 1992, **44**, 1.
27. J.E. Hawkinson and J.E. Casida, *Mol. Pharmacol.*, 1992, **42**, 1069.
28. Y. Deng, C.J. Palmer and J.E. Casida, *Pestic. Biochem. Physiol.*, 1993, **47**, 98.
29. Y. Deng, C.J. Palmer and J.E. Casida, *Pestic. Biochem. Physiol.*, 1991, **41**, 60.
30. Y. Deng and J.E. Casida, *Pestic. Biochem. Physiol.*, 1992, **43**, 116.
31. L.M. Cole, R.T. Roush and J.E. Casida, *Life Sci.*, 1995, **56**, 757.
32. E.R. Korpi and H. Lüddens, *Mol. Pharmacol.*, 1993, **44**, 87.
33. S.Y. Sakurai, A. Kume, D.E. Burdette and R.L. Albin, *J. Pharmacol. Exp. Ther.*, 1994, **270**, 362.
34. A. Kume and R.L. Albin, *Eur. J. Pharmacol.*, 1994, **263**, 163.
35. J.E. Hawkinson, M.P. Goeldner, C.J. Palmer and J.E. Casida, *J. Receptor Res.*, 1991, **11**, 391.
36. I. Kapfer, J.E. Hawkinson, J.E. Casida and M.P. Goeldner, *J. Med. Chem.*, 1994, **37**, 133.
37. Q.X. Li and J.E. Casida, *Biorg. Med. Chem.*, 1995, **3**, 1667.
38. Q.X. Li and J.E. Casida, *Biorg. Med. Chem.*, 1995, **3**, 1675.
39. L.M. Cole, M.A. Saleh and J.E. Casida, *Pestic. Sci.*, 1994, **42**, 59.
40. J.J. Rauh, E. Benner, M.E. Schnee, D. Cordova, C.W. Holyoke, M.H. Howard, D. Bai, S.D. Buckingham, M.L. Hutton, A. Hamon, R.T. Roush and D.B. Sattelle, *Br. J. Pharmacol.*, 1997, **121**, 1496.
41. S.-S. Pong and C.C. Wang, *Neuropharmacol.*, 1980, **19**, 311.
42. G. Drexler and W. Sieghart, *Eur. J. Pharmacol.*, 1984, **99**, 269.
43. J. Huang and J.E. Casida, *J. Pharmacol. Exp. Ther.*, 1997, **281**, 261.
44. J.M. Schaeffer and H.W. Haines, *Biochem. Pharmcol.*, 1989, **38**, 2329.
45. S.P. Rohrer and J.P Arena, *ACS Symp. Ser.*, 1995, **591**, 264.
46. D.M. Soderlund and D.C. Knipple, *ACS Symp. Ser.* 1995, **591**, 97.
47. L.J. Lawrence and J.E. Casida, *Science*, 1983, **221**, 1399.
48. T. Narahashi, *Trends Pharmacol. Sci.*, 1992, **13**, 236.
49. F. Matsumura and M. Hayashi, *Residue Rev.*, 1969, **25**, 265.

50. D.M. Soderlund, S.M. Ghiasuddin and D.W. Helmuth, *Life Sci.* 1983, **33**, 261.
51. A. Lombet, C. Mourre and M. Lazdunski, *Brain Res.* 1988, **459**, 44.
52. B. Latli, L.J. Greenfield and J.E. Casida, *J. Labelled Cmpd. Radiopharm.* 1993, **33**, 613.
53. D.P. Rossignol, *Pestic. Biochem. Physiol.* 1991, **41**, 103.
54. K. Matsuda, K. Iharada, K. Komai, H. Okimoto, T. Ueno and K. Nishimura, *J. Pestic. Sci.*, 1996, **21**, 179.
55. V.L. Trainer, J.C. McPhee, H. Boutelet-Bochan, C. Baker, T. Scheuer, D. Babin, J.-P. DeMoute, D. Guedin and W. A. Catterall, *Mol. Pharmacol.* 1997, **51**, 651.
56. H. Hashemzadeh, R.M. Hollingworth and A. Voliva, *Life Sci.* 1985, **37**, 433.
57. J.A. Nathanson, *Mol. Pharmacol.* 1989, **35**, 34.
58. T. Roeder and J.A. Nathanson, *J. Neurochem.* 1994, **63**, 1516.
59. D.M. Soderlund, In 'Eighth International Congress of Pesticide Chemistry, Options 2000', N.N. Ragsdale, P.C. Kearney, J.R. Plimmer, Eds., pp 309-319, American Chemical Society, Washington, D.C., 1995.
60. R.A. Goodnow Jr., R. Bukownik, K. Nakanishi, P.N. Usherwood, A.T. Eldefrawi, N.A. Anis and M.E. Eldefrawi, *J. Med. Chem.* 1991, **34**, 2389.
61. H.L. Sudan, C.J. Kerry, I.R. Mellor, S.-K. Choi, D. Huang, K. Nakanishi and P.N. Usherwood, *Invertebrate Neurosci.* 1995, **1**, 159.
62. F.G.P. Earley and C.I. Ragan, *Biochem. J.*, 1984, **224**, 525.
63. F.G.P. Earley, S.D. Patel, C.I. Ragan and G. Attardi, *FEBS Lett.*, 1987, **219**, 108.
64. P.J. Jewess, *Biochem. Soc. Trans.*, 1994, **22**, 247.
65. B. Latli, E. Wood and J.E. Casida, *Chem. Res. Toxicol.*, 1996, **9**, 445.
66. E. Wood, B. Latli and J.E. Casida, *Pestic. Biochem. Physiol.*, 1996, **54**, 135.
67. B. Latli, H. Morimoto, P.G. Williams and J.E. Casida, *J. Labelled Compd. Radiopharm.*, 1998, **41**, 191.
68. J.R. Knox, R.F. Toia and J.E. Casida, *J. Agric. Food Chem.*, 1992, **40**, 909.
69. F.J. Ruder and H. Kayser, *Pestic. Biochem. Physiol.*, 1992, **42**, 248.
70. I.N. Pessah, A.L. Waterhouse and J.E. Casida, *Biochem. Biophys. Res. Commun.*, 1985, **128**, 449.
71. E. Lehmberg and J.E. Casida, *Pestic. Biochem. Physiol.*, 1994, **48**, 145.
72. C.J. Palmer and J.E. Casida, *ACS Symp. Ser.*, 1987, **356**, 71.
73. M.-Y. Liu, J. Lanford and J.E. Casida, *Pestic. Biochem. Physiol.*, 1993, **46**, 200.

Expression of Cloned House Fly Sodium Channels in *Xenopus* Oocytes: Action of Pyrethroids and Analysis of Resistance-Associated Mutations

D.M. Soderlund, T.J. Smith, S.H. Lee, P.J. Ingles and D.C. Knipple

DEPARTMENT OF ENTOMOLOGY, NEW YORK STATE AGRICULTURAL EXPERIMENT STATION, CORNELL UNIVERSITY, GENEVA, NY 14456, USA

1 INTRODUCTION

Voltage-sensitive sodium channels mediate the transient sodium conductance of excitable cell membranes that is associated with the propagation of action potentials.[1] The central importance of sodium channels in nerve function is revealed by the diverse array of naturally-occuring neurotoxins acting on the sodium channel that are employed by a variety of organisms as chemical weapons of defense or predation.[2] Sodium channels are also the principal site of action of widely-used diphenylethane (e.g., DDT) and pyrethroid insecticides, as well as other classes of experimental insecticides (e.g., dihydropyrazoles) that may contribute to the chemical control of insect pests in the future.[3, 4] Genetic linkage studies implicate insect sodium channel genes as the likely sites of mutations conferring knockdown resistance to DDT and pyrethroids, exemplified by the *kdr* and *super-kdr* traits in the house fly (*Musca domestica*) and phenotypically similar traits in other insect species.[5]

Most of the functional and pharmacological properties of sodium channels are conferred by the α subunit, a large pseudotetrameric protein having the structural hallmarks of the voltage-gated cation channel gene superfamily.[6, 7] The α subunit contains structural domains that form the ion pore and also contains the binding domains for most sodium channel-directed neurotoxins and insecticides. In mammals, sodium channel α subunit isoforms with varied patterns of expression and distinct biophysical properties and pharmacological profiles are encoded by a multi-gene family.[8] In addition, sodium channels of vertebrate brain and skeletal muscle are heteromultimers composed of an α subunit and smaller auxiliary subunits, β_1 and β_2.[7, 9] Coexpression of brain and skeletal muscle sodium channel α subunit isoforms with the β_1 and β_2 subunits results in channels with kinetic properties more typical of the native sodium channels found in these tissues.[7,9] In contrast to the situation in vertebrates, insects appear to employ a single sodium channel α subunit gene, first identified as the *para* locus of *Drosophila melanogaster*,[10] and generate a diversity of α subunit structures from this gene by alternative exon usage.[11-13] A second genetic locus in *D. melanogaster*, designated *tipE*, encodes a smaller protein with two transmembrane domains that appears to function as a sodium channel auxiliary subunit in a manner analogous to the role of the mammalian β_1 subunit, enhancing the level of expression and accelerating the kinetics of *D. melanogaster para* sodium channels in *Xenopus laevis* oocytes.[14, 15]

The importance of insect sodium channels as sites of insecticide action and their inferred significance as the likely site of mutations conferring knockdown resistance to diphenylethane and pyrethroid insecticides in the house fly and other pest species have provided the impetus for the molecular cloning and functional expression of house fly sodium channels. The ultimate goal of these studies has been the unambiguous identification of the mutations causing knockdown resistance. This chapter reviews recent progress in these areas from the perspective of the contributions made by our research programs.

2 MOLECULAR CLONING AND FUNCTIONAL EXPRESSION

Elucidation of the sequence of the *para* sodium channel gene of *D. melanogaster*[10] provided a point of entry for the isolation of segments of the orthologous genes from the house fly and other insect species using the polymerase chain reaction (PCR).[16, 17] The entire coding sequence of the *para*-orthologous voltage-sensitive sodium channel gene of the house fly (designated *Vssc1*) was obtained by using PCR with first-strand cDNA prepared from adult house fly head mRNA as the template to amplify overlapping cDNA fragments[18] or by using hybridization probes derived from *para* or *Vssc1* sequences in the iterative screening of adult house fly head cDNA libraries.[19] Comparisons based on the sequences of *Vssc1* alleles of the insecticide-susceptible NAIDM[18] or Cooper[19] house fly strains show that the inferred amino acid sequence of the *Vssc1* gene product is ~90% identical to the the the amino acid sequence of the $a^+b^-c^-d^+e^-f^-h^+i^+$ splice variant of *para*. Neither strategy employed for cloning the *Vssc1* cDNA identified other *Vssc1* splice variants among adult head cDNAs, but subsequent studies using cDNAs from different house fly developmental stages and adult anatomical regions identified 9 sites of alternative splicing, which permit the generation of 512 possible structural variants from the *Vssc1* gene (S. H. Lee, D. C. Knipple and D.M. Soderlund, unpublished).

A full-length cDNA clone for the wildtype *Vssc1* coding sequence was assembled from two large partial cDNAs that were amplified from fly head first strand cDNA.[20] Injection of cRNA synthesized *in vitro* from this *Vssc1* cDNA template into *Xenopus* oocytes resulted in the expression of sodium channels in the oocyte membrane that were detected by eletrophysiological analysis.[20, 21] Injection of *Vssc1* cRNA alone produced sodium currents carried by monomeric Vssc1 channels that were clearly detected by two-electrode voltage clamp analysis (Table 1). However, co-injection with *D. melanogaster* *tipE* cRNA increased the magnitude of expressed currents approximately two-fold (Table 1), presumably due to the expression of heteromultimeric sodium channels, which we designate Vssc1/tipE channels. Currents carried by both Vssc1 and Vssc1/tipE channels were sensitive to inhibition by sub-micromolar concentrations of tetrodotoxin (TTX), with half-maximal inhibition of sodium currents carried by Vssc1/tipE channels at a concentration of 2.4 nM TTX.[21] The TTX sensitivity of Vssc1/tipE sodium channels is similar to that of rat brain sodium channels expressed in oocytes[22] but is approximately 10-fold less than that of *D. melanogaster* para/tipE channels expressed in this system.[15]

In addition to enhancing the level of expression of Vssc1 sodium channels in oocytes, coexpression with the tipE protein also modified the voltage dependence and inactivation kinetics of the resulting Vssc1/tipE channels. Vssc1 channels exhibited half-maximal activation at -23 mV and half-maximal steady-state inactivation at -36 mV (T. J. Smith and D. M. Soderlund, unpublished). Coexpression with tipE shifted the half-maximal activation of Vssc1/tipE channels to -19 mV but did not affect the voltage dependence of steady-state inactivation of Vssc1/tipE channels.[20, 21] The voltage dependence of activation and inactivation of Vssc1 and Vssc1/tipE sodium channels in oocytes differ somewhat from those of *D. melanogaster* para and para/tipE channels assayed under comparable conditions.[15] Half-maximal activation of Vssc1 channels is shifted by ~11 mV in the direction of hyperpolarization when compared to para channels; however, coexpression with tipE shifts the voltage dependence of these channels in opposite directions so that the resulting para/tipE and Vssc1/tipE channels exhibit very similar values for half-maximal activation. Also, both para and para/tipE channels inactivate at more hyperpolarized potentials than Vssc1 and Vssc1/tipE channels. Coexpression of Vssc1 with tipE also produces an approximately two-fold increase in the rate of decay of the peak transient sodium current when compared to Vssc1 channels; the mean first-order decay constants obtained upon depolarizations to -10 mV were 6.4 ms for Vssc1 channels and 3.9 ms for Vssc1/tipE channels (T. J. Smith and D. M. Soderlund, unpublished).

Table 1 *Expression of Wildtype and Specifically Mutated House Fly Vssc1*
Voltage-Sensitive Sodium Channels in Xenopus Oocytes[a]

Vssc1 Variant	Oocytes Assayed	Percent With Currents	Mean Peak Current, nA
Wildtype (-tipE)	34	29	295
Wildtype (+tipE)	60	33	613
L1014F (+tipE)	21	62	1144
M918T/L1014F (+tipE)	102	24	196
M918T (+tipE)	151	6	79

[a]*Data from Lee et al.* [31]

3 ACTIONS OF PYRETHROIDS

We used cismethrin and [1R,*cis*,αS]-cypermethrin, pyrethroids that produce Type I or Type II effects, respectively, on invertebrate nerve preparations,[23] to characterize the actions of pyrethroids on Vssc1/tipE sodium channels expressed in oocytes.[20, 21] Figure 1 illustrates the two distinct effects of cismethrin (40 μM) on sodium currents measured in a voltage-clamped oocyte expressing Vssc1/tipE sodium channels during and after a 50-msec step depolarization from -100 to -10 mV. First, cismethrin caused a sustained current during the depolarizing pulse that activates more slowly than the peak transient current and does not inactivate during a 50-msec depolarization. Second, cismethrin induced a biphasic tail current comprised of a rising phase during the first ~150 msec following depolarization and a falling phase, beginning ~200 msec after repolarization, that decays with a first-order time constant (τ_{tail}) of ~650 msec. These effects are qualitatively similar to the effects of permethrin, another Type I pyrethroid, on para/tipE sodium channels expressed in oocytes.[15] Application of trains of depolarizing pulses did not produce any further modification of the sodium current by cismethrin. The shape and kinetics of the cismethrin-modified current imply that the modification of Vssc1/tipE sodium channels by cismethrin occurs in the closed state and that modified channels activate, inactivate, and deactivate more slowly than unmodified channels.

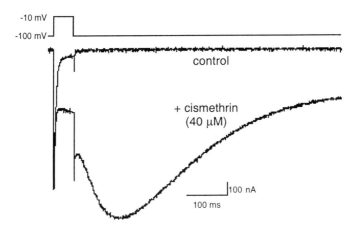

Figure 1 *Net sodium current trace recorded using the indicated depolarization protocol from an oocyte expressing Vssc1/tipE sodium channels before and 5 min after exposure to cismethrin; redrawn from Smith et al.*[21]

The amplitude of the cismethrin-modified current measured at the end of a 50-msec depolarizing pulse, normalized to the amplitude of the peak transient current measured in the same oocyte prior to cismethrin exposure, was used as a quantitative index of the extent of sodium channel modification by different concentrations of cismethrin. Fitting concentration - effect data from such experiments to the Hill equation yielded a concentration of cismethrin producing half-maximal effect ($K_{0.5}$ value) of 29 μM.[20] Statistically significant cismethrin-modified currents were observed at a threshold cismethrin concentration of 0.02 μM.[20]

In addition to these effects on channel kinetics, cismethrin also altered the voltage dependence of Vssc1/tipE channels expressed in oocytes. The effects of cismethrin were determined by comparing the voltage dependence of activation and steady-state inactivation of the current measured in cismethrin-treated oocytes at the end of a 50 msec depolarization, which is carried exclusively by cismethrin-modified channels, to the same parameters measured for the peak transient sodium current in the same oocyte prior to cismethrin exposure. Half-maximal activation of the cismethrin-modified current was shifted by ~ 7mV to more negative potentials when compared to the unmodified current, whereas half-maximal steady-state inactivation was shifted by ~ 4mV to more negative potentials.[21] The cismethrin-dependent shift in the activation curve increases the probability that cismethrin-modified channels will open at subthreshold membrane potentials, thereby contributing to the nerve hyperexcitation caused by this compound.

The principal effect of cypermethrin on Vssc1/tipE sodium channels expressed in oocytes was the induction of an extremely persistent tail current that decayed with a first-order time constant of ~40 sec.[21] The action of cypermethrin was use-dependent, requiring approximately 10 depolarizing pulses to produce modified currents that were distinguishable from control currents. Modified currents increased in amplitude with repeated depolarization (Figure 2) for up to at least 10,000 pulses.[21] Unlike cismethrin, cypermethrin did not cause a conspicuous slowly-activating modified current during a 50-msec depolarizing pulse and also did not induce a biphasic tail current. These results imply that modification of Vssc1/tipE channels by cypermethrin occurs principally in the open state and that modified channels remain open for long periods. The use dependence and extreme persistence of the cypermethrin modified current prevented detailed studies of the sensitivity of Vssc1/tipE channels to cypermethrin or the effects of this compound on the voltage dependence of these channels.

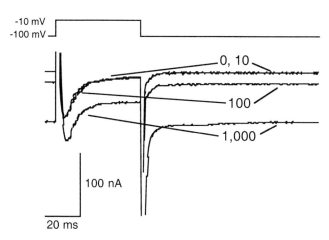

Figure 2 *Net sodium current traces recorded using the indicated depolarization protocol from an oocyte expressing Vssc1/tipE sodium channels 5 min after exposure to cypermethrin (40 μM) and following the indicated number of depolarizing prepulses; redrawn from Smith et al.[21]*

4 MUTATIONS ASSOCIATED WITH KNOCKDOWN RESISTANCE

To test the hypothesis that the *kdr* trait in the house fly resulted from a mutation of a sodium channel structural gene, we identified a restriction fragment length polymorphism (RFLP) in the *Vssc1* gene that reliably identified pyrethroid-susceptible (NAIDM strain) and *kdr* (538ge strain) fly populations. Using a diagnostic PCR/RFLP assay on individual house fly genomic DNA preparations coupled with a rapid paralysis bioassay for the unambiguous detection of individual progeny from genetic crosses that were homozygous for the *kdr* trait, we demonstrated that the *Vssc1* gene and the *kdr* resistance trait were tightly linked at a resolution of approximately 1 map unit.[24] Similarly, Williamson and co-workers[25] identified another RFLP in the *Vssc1* gene and employed this marker to demonstrate equally tight linkage between the *Vssc1* gene and the *super-kdr* trait.

Williamson and colleagues[19] also determined the complete sequences of *Vssc1* cDNAs from three house fly strains (exemplifying the susceptible, *kdr*, and *super-kdr* phenotypes), as well as partial *Vssc1* sequences of one additional *kdr* strain and 6 additional *super-kdr* strains, and identified mutations at two sites that were consistently associated with resistance. All of the resistant strains contained a replacement of leucine at amino acid sequence position 1014 by phenylalanine (designated L1014F), whereas the *super-kdr* strains also contained a replacement of methionine at position 918 by threonine (M918T) (Figure 3). The leucine residue corresponding to L1014 of *Vssc1* is also replaced by phenylalanine in *Vssc1*-orthologous sodium channel gene sequences of pyrethroid-resistant strains of *Blattella germanica*,[26, 27] *Haematobia irritans*,[28] *Anopheles gambiae*,[29] and *Plutella xylostella*,[30] whereas amino acid substitutions corresponding to the M918T/L1014F double mutation have been documented to date only in *super-kdr* house fly strains[19] and a strain of *H. irritans* that exhibits a high level of pyrethroid resistance.[28]

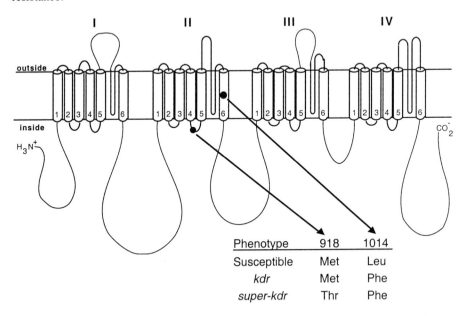

Phenotype	918	1014
Susceptible	Met	Leu
kdr	Met	Phe
super-kdr	Thr	Phe

Figure 3 *Diagram of the Vssc1 gene product as an extended polypeptide chain showing the four internally homologous segments (I-IV), the six transmembrane domains within each segment (1-6) and the location and identity of amino acid substitutions associated with the kdr and super-kdr resistance traits; based on data of Williamson et al.[19]*

5 FUNCTIONAL ANALYSIS OF RESISTANCE-ASSOCIATED MUTATIONS

To assess the effects of resistance-associated mutations on the properties and pyrethroid sensitivity of house fly sodium channels, we constructed three specifically mutated *Vssc1* cDNAs by site-directed mutagenesis of the wildtype *Vssc1* cDNA: one containing the L1014F mutation associated with *kdr*, a second containing the M918T/L1014F double mutation associated with *super-kdr*, and a third containing the M918T single mutation.[20, 31] These cDNAs were employed as templates for the synthesis of cRNA, which was injected together with *D. melanogaster tipE* cRNA into oocytes. The resulting specifically mutated Vssc1/tipE sodium channels were detected and characterized by eletrophysiological analysis using two-electrode voltage clamp.[20, 31]

We observed substantial differences between the wildtype and three specifically mutated variants of the Vssc1/tipE sodium channel in both the proportion of injected and surviving oocytes that expressed detectable sodium currents and the magnitude of the sodium currents that were expressed (Table 1). Channels mutated to contain the L1014F substitution (here designated L1014F channels) were expressed in a higher proportion of injected oocytes than wildtype channels, and the mean amplitude of the expressed peak transient current was almost two-fold greater. In contrast, the proportion of oocytes expressing M918T/L1014F channels was lower than that observed for wildtype channels, and the mean amplitude of the peak transient current was reduced to less than half of that observed for wildtype channels. The most severe effects on expression were found with M918T channels. Of the 151 injected oocytes that were assayed only 6% expressed detectable sodium currents. Moreover, the mean amplitude of these currents was not only substantially less than that found for wildtype Vssc1/tipE channels but also less than that observed for wildtype channels in the absence of tipE.

We also compared the voltage dependence of activation and steady-state inactivation of wildtype and specifically mutated Vssc1/tipE channels. The L1014F mutation shifted the midpoint potential for the activation ~7 mV in the direction of depolarization,[20, 31] whereas the M918T mutation, either alone or in combination with the L1014F mutation, had no effect on the voltage dependence of activation.[31] The small shift in the voltage dependence of activation of L1014F channels could contribute to the expression of pyrethroid resistance by reducing the probability of channel opening at normal resting potentials and during depolarization, effects that would partially counteract the ability of pyrethroids to increase channel open times. None of the specifically mutated channels exhibited alterations in voltage dependence of steady-state inactivation.[20, 31]

To assess the effects of resistance-associated mutations on the pyrethroid sensitivity of Vssc1/tipE sodium channels expressed in oocytes, we used the normalized amplitude of the cismethrin-induced currents at the end of a 50-ms depolarizing pulse as an index of the extent of sodium channel modification following exposure to a range of cismethrin concentrations. Plots of current amplitude against cismethrin concentration yielded an extrapolated $K_{0.5}$ value of 1227 µM for the L1014F channel assuming a maximal current amplitude equal to that obtained with wildtype channels.[20] This result suggests that the L1014F mutation confers a 40-fold reduction in the sensitivity of Vssc1/tipE sodium channels to cismethrin. We also determined that the threshold concentration of cismethrin required to produce statistically significant modification of sodium currents in oocytes expressing the L1014F variant was 0.2 µM. By this criterion, the L1014F mutation confers a 10-fold reduction in sensitivity to cismethrin. In addition to its effect on the sensitivity of Vssc1/tipE channels to cismethrin, the L1014F mutation also altered the kinetic properties of the cismethrin-modified channel. With the L1014F variant, the τ_{tail} value was decreased by a factor of 4.6-fold when compared to the wildtype variant. Thus, the L1014F mutation reduces the duration of the pyrethroid-modified current, an effect that would contribute to the phenotypic expression of resistance at the level of neuronal excitability. In contrast to the results obtained with the L1014F variant, assays with the M918T/L1014F and M918T variants did not detect any modification of sodium currents during or after a depolarizing pulse by cismethrin at concentrations up to 500 µM, the highest nominal concentration attainable in these assays.[31]

The persistent and use-dependent effects of cypermethrin on Vssc1/tipE sodium channels (see Figure 2) rendered the use of this compound to assess the pyrethroid sensitivity of Vssc1 variants more problematic. Nevertheless, assays with the wildtype and three specifically mutated channel variants confirmed the same pattern of sensitivity that was observed with cismethrin. With the L1014F variant, higher cypermethrin concentrations were required to produce modified current amplitudes equivalent to those obtained with the wildtype variant at lower concentrations (Figure 4). Moreover, the decay of the cypermethrin-induced tail current was greatly accelerated (τ_{tail} values of ~42 and 0.8 s for the wildtype and L1014F variant, respectively).[32] Like cismethrin, cypermethrin also did not produce any detectable modification of currents in oocytes expressing the M918T/L1014F and M918T variants at concentrations that caused large modified currents in oocytes expressing the wildtype and L1014F variants.[31]

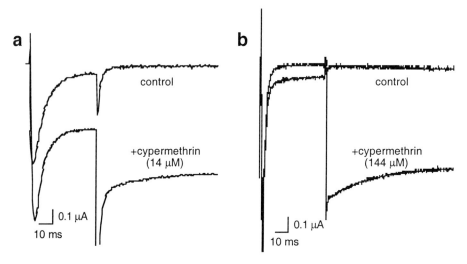

Figure 4 *(a) Net sodium current traces recorded during and after a 50-ms depolarization from -100 to -10 mV from an oocyte expressing the wildtype variant of the Vssc1/tipE sodium channel before and 5 min after bath application of 14 µM cypermethrin; (b) Net sodium current traces recorded during and after a 50-ms depolarization from -100 to -10 mV from an oocyte expressing the L1014F variant of the Vssc1/tipE sodium channel before and 5 min after bath application of 144 µM cypermethrin; redrawn from Smith.[32]*

6 CONCLUSIONS

We have reconstituted functional house fly sodium channels in *Xenopus* oocytes by the expression of the house fly Vssc1 sodium channel α subunit protein either alone or in combination with the *D. melanogaster* tipE sodium channel auxiliary subunit protein. The Vssc1 protein by itself is sufficient to form functional voltage-sensitive sodium channels in *Xenopus* oocytes. However, coexpression with the tipE protein not only increases the amplitude of expressed sodium currents but also shifts the voltage-dependence of activation and accelerates the inactivation of those currents. These results imply that the Vssc1 and tipE proteins coassemble to form a heteromultimeric sodium channel complex, in which the tipE protein functions in a manner analogous to the β_1 subunit of vertebrate sodium channels. Our results with Vssc1/tipE sodium channels parallel those obtained with *D. melanogaster* para/tipE channels[14, 15] and imply the existence of an ortholog of the *tipE* gene in the house fly. We have recently isolated a novel cDNA from house fly heads that encodes a protein with >70% amino acid sequence identity to the tipE protein; moreover, this gene product enhances Vssc1 sodium channel expression in oocytes in a manner identical to tipE (S. H. Lee, T. J. Smith and D. M. Soderlund, unpublished). The functional role of tipE in insect sodium channel expression has been investigated in combination with only two splice variants of para[15] and a single splice variant of Vssc1 and only in *Xenopus* oocytes. Therefore, it is not known whether all splice variants of para-orthologous insect sodium channels are candidates for coassembly with tipE or tipE-like proteins in oocytes and whether such coassembly also occurs in insect neurons.

The actions of cismethrin and cypermethrin on Vssc1/tipE sodium channels expressed in oocytes are consistent with the actions of Type I and and Type II pyrethroids on sodium channels in a variety of vertebrate and invertebrate nerve preparations.[33] Cismethrin binds to one or more closed states of the Vssc1/tipE sodium channel and slows the kinetics of at least three sodium channel gating events observed under voltage clamp conditions: the opening of the activation gate, resulting in the slow onset of the cismethrin-dependent current during depolarization; the closing of the inactivation gate, resulting in the slow decay of the cismethrin-modified current during depolarization; and the closing of the activation gate following repolarization (termed deactivation), resulting in the slowly-decaying tail current. The combination of these effects results in a prolongation of the sodium current flowing after a depolarizing pulse that is consistent with the neuroexcitatory actions of this compound and other Type I pyrethroids on invertebrate nerve.[23] Cismethrin also shifts the voltage dependence of activation of Vssc1/tipE sodium channels to more hyperpolarized potentials, an effect that would enhance neuronal excitation by increasing the probability of sodium channel opening at nerve membrane potentials that are normally below the threshold for action potential generation.

In contrast to cismethrin, cypermethrin appears to bind preferentially to the activated state of Vssc1/tipE sodium channels, as shown by the clear use dependence of the development of the cypermethrin-modified current. Once bound, cypermethrin selectively prolongs sodium channel deactivation without significantly affecting inactivation; this conclusion is based on the induction of cypermethrin-induced tail currents using conditioning pulse protocols that result in little or no detectable modification of the sodium current measured during depolarization (see Figure 2). Finally, the effect of cypermethrin on deactivation is much more persistent than the effect of cismethrin, so that sodium currents continue to flow minutes after repolarization from the final pulse of a series of depolarizing pulses. The use dependence and persistence of the effects caused by cypermethrin on Vssc1/tipE sodium channels are therefore consistent with the use-dependent depolarizing block of action potentials observed for this compound and other Type II compounds in invertebrate nerve preparations.[23] These effects of cypermethrin also place technical limitations on experiments to assess the effects of this compound on the voltage dependence of Vssc1/tipE sodium channels in oocytes.

The L1014F mutation associated with the *kdr* trait of the house fly alters three independent aspects of the action of pyrethroids on Vssc1/tipE sodium channels. First, this mutation reduces the apparent affinity of these channels for cismethrin by at least 10-fold (based on threshold concentrations for the modification of sodium currents by cismethrin) and perhaps as much as 40-fold (based on $K_{0.5}$ values for the induction of cismethrin-dependent currents). A more limited data set suggests that the L1014F mutation also reduces the apparent affinity for cypermethrin by approximately 10-fold, based on the normalized amplitude of the tail current as an index of the extent of channel modification by this compound (see Figure 4). Second, the L1014F mutation alters the kinetic properties of the pyrethroid-modified channel. This effect is most clearly evident in the acceleration of the decay of cismethrin- and cypermethrin-induced tail currents in oocytes expressing L1014F channels. Third, the L1014F mutation shifts the voltage dependence of activation of Vssc1/tipE channels in the direction of depolarization, which would reduce sensitivity to pyrethroids by raising the threshold for depolarization. The combination of these three effects is sufficient to account for the reduction in neuronal sensitivity to pyrethroids observed in *kdr* insects. Our results therefore provide functional confirmation that the L1014F mutation is the cause of the *kdr* trait.

The M918T/L1014F double mutation associated with the *super-kdr* trait renders Vssc1/tipE sodium channels expressed in oocytes completely insensitive to the action of both cismethrin and cypermethrin at the highest concentrations of these compounds attainable in this assay system. This finding is not consistent with structure-toxicity data for the action of pyrethroids on susceptible and *super-kdr* house flies,[34] which predict that M918T/L1014F channels should be substantially more resistant to cypermethrin than cismethrin. If the complete insensitivity to pyrethroids of M918T/L1014F channels expressed in oocytes mirrors that of sodium channels in the nervous system of *super-kdr* insects, then pyrethroid intoxication in these insects may well involve a target site other than the Vssc1 sodium channel.[33] Structure-toxicity studies of pyrethroids on *super-kdr* insects have typically employed insecticidally active isomers or mixtures of isomers and therefore have not considered the stereochemistry of pyrethroid intoxication in these strains.[34-36] It would be of interest to determine whether the stereochemical requirements for pyrethroid intoxication in susceptible insects, which reflect the stereochemical requirements for pyrethroid action on sodium channels,[3, 33] are conserved in *super-kdr* strains. The lack of conservation of these structure-activity relationships would lend further credence to the hypothesis that the *super-kdr* resistance trait causes a change in the primary site of action for pyrethroids.

The properties of Vssc1/tipE sodium channels containing the M918T single mutation provide insight into the origin of the *super-kdr* allele. The M918T substitution, either as a single mutation or in combination with the L1014F mutation, severely impaired the expression of functional Vssc1/tipE sodium channels in oocytes. The M918T single mutation also appeared to confer complete insensitivity to both cismethrin and cypermethrin, as was observed previously for the M918T/L1014F double mutation. If the impaired function of M918T channels in oocytes faithfully reflects the properties of such channels in insect neurons, then this mutation is likely to be deleterious where it occurs in nature. This interpretation is consistent with the absolute conservation of Met in amino acid sequence positions corresponding to M918 of the Vssc1 protein in sodium channel sequences from insecticide-susceptible strains of 13 insect species.[10, 18, 19, 26-29, 37, 38] The reduced but nevertheless more efficient expression of M918T/L1014F channels in oocytes suggests that the L1014F mutation partially rescues the functional deficiency of the the M918T mutation, an interpretation consistent with the observation that the M918T substitution has only been found in resistant insects in combination with the L1014F substitution.[19, 28] Taken together, these results imply that the *super-kdr* allele of *Vssc1* in the house fly arose from the *kdr* allele by selection of a second-site mutation (M918T) that confers even greater resistance to pyrethroids. Additional evidence for the sequential selection of the *kdr* and *super-kdr* traits comes from RFLP analyses of the *Vssc1* locus in susceptible, *kdr*, and *super-kdr* house fly strains, which document strong conservation of a single RFLP pattern in all resistant strains but extensive polymorphism in susceptible strains.[39]

References

1. B. Hille, 'Ionic Channels of Excitable Membranes,' second edn., Sinauer, Sunderland, MA, 1992, p. 607.
2. W. A. Catterall, *Physiol. Rev.*, 1992, **72**, S15.
3. D. M. Soderlund and J. R. Bloomquist, *Annu. Rev. Entomol.*, 1989, **34**, 77.
4. J. R. Bloomquist, *Annu. Rev. Entomol.*, 1996, **41**, 163.
5. D. M. Soderlund, in 'Molecular Mechanisms of Resistance to Agrochemicals,' ed. V. Sjut, Springer, Berlin, 1997, p. 21.
6. R. G. Kallen, S. A. Cohen and R. L. Barchi, *Mol. Neurobiol.*, 1993, **7**, 383.
7. W. A. Catterall, *Annu. Rev. Biochem.*, 1995, **64**, 493.
8. G. Mandel, *J. Membrane Biol.*, 1992, **125**, 193.
9. L. L. Isom, K. S. DeJongh and W. A. Catterall, *Neuron*, 1994, **12**, 1183.
10. K. Loughney, R. Kreber and B. Ganetzky, *Cell*, 1989, **58**, 1143.
11. J. R. Thackeray and B. Ganetzky, *J. Neurosci.*, 1994, **14**, 2569.
12. J. R. Thackeray and B. Ganetzky, *Genetics*, 1995, **141**, 203.
13. D. K. O'Dowd, J. R. Gee and M. A. Smith, *J. Neurosci.*, 1995, **15**, 4005.

14. G. Feng, P. Deak, M. Chopra and L. M. Hall, *Cell*, 1995, **82**, 1001.
15. J. W. Warmke, R. A. G. Reenan, P. Wang, S. Qian, J. P. Arena, J. Wang, D. Wunderler, K. Liu, G. J. Kaczorowski, L. H. T. Van der Ploeg, B. Ganetzky and C. J. Cohen, *J. Gen. Physiol.*, 1997, **110**, 119.
16. D. C. Knipple, L. L. Payne and D. M. Soderlund, *Arch. Insect Biochem. Physiol.*, 1991, **16**, 45.
17. K. E. Doyle and D. C. Knipple, *Insect Biochem.*, 1991, **21**, 689.
18. P. J. Ingles, P. M. Adams, D. C. Knipple and D. M. Soderlund, *Insect Biochem. Mol. Biol.*, 1996, **26**, 319.
19. M. S. Williamson, D. Martinez-Torres, C. A. Hick and A. L. Devonshire, *Mol. Gen. Genet.*, 1996, **252**, 51.
20. T. J. Smith, S. H. Lee, P. J. Ingles, D. C. Knipple and D. M. Soderlund, *Insect Biochem. Mol. Biol.*, 1997, **27**, 807.
21. T. J. Smith, P. J. Ingles and D. M. Soderlund, *Arch. Insect Biochem. Physiol.*, 1998, **38**, 126.
22. K. J. Kontis and A. L. Goldin, *Mol. Pharmacol.*, 1993, **43**, 635.
23. A. E. Lund and T. Narahashi, *Pestic. Biochem. Physiol.*, 1983, **20**, 203.
24. D. C. Knipple, K. E. Doyle, P. A. Marsella-Herrick and D. M. Soderlund, *Proc. Natl. Acad. Sci. USA*, 1994, **91**, 2483.
25. M. S. Williamson, I. Denholm, C. A. Bell and A. L. Devonshire, *Mol. Gen. Genet.*, 1993, **240**, 17.
26. M. Miyazaki, K. Ohyama, D. Y. Dunlap and F. Matsumura, *Mol. Gen. Genet.*, 1996, **252**, 61.
27. K. Dong, *Insect Biochem. Mol. Biol.*, 1997, **27**, 93.
28. F. D. Guerrero, R. C. Jamroz, D. Kammlah and S. E. Kunz, *Insect Biochem. Mol. Biol.*, 1997, **27**, 745.
29. D. Martinez-Torres, F. Chandre, M. S. Williamson, F. Darriet, J. B. Bergé, A. L. Devonshire, P. Guillet, N. Pasteur and D. Pauron, *Insect Mol. Biol.*, 1998, **7**, 179.
30. T. H. Schuler, D. Martinez-Torres, A. J. Thompson, I. Denholm, A. L. Devonshire, I. R. Duce and M. S. Williamson, *Pestic. Biochem. Physiol.*, 1998, **59**, 169.
31. S. H. Lee, T. J. Smith, D. C. Knipple and D. M. Soderlund, *Insect Biochem. Mol. Biol.*, submitted.
32. T. J. Smith, Ph.D. dissertation, Cornell University, 1998.
33. J. R. Bloomquist, in 'Reviews in Pesticide Toxicology,' eds. M. Roe and R. J. Kuhr, Toxicology Communications, Raleigh, NC, 1993, p. 181.
34. A. W. Farnham, A. W. A. Murray, R. M. Sawicki, I. Denholm and J. C. White, *Pestic. Sci.*, 1987, **19**, 209.
35. R. M. Sawicki, *Nature*, 1978, **275**, 443.
36. A. W. Farnham and B. P. S. Khambay, *Pestic. Sci.*, 1995, **44**, 269.
37. Y. Park and M. F. J. Taylor, *Insect Biochem. Mol. Biol.*, 1997, **27**, 9.
38. D. Martinez-Torres, A. L. Devonshire and M. S. Williamson, *Pestic. Sci.*, 1997, **51**, 265.
39. M. S. Williamson, C. A. Bell, I. Denholm and A. L. Devonshire, in 'Molecular Action and Pharmacology of Insecticides on Ion Channels,' ed. J. M. Clark, American Chemical Society, Washington, DC, 1995, p. 86.

Calcium Channels in Insects

I.R. Duce, T.R. Khan, A.C. Green, A.J. Thompson, S.P.M. Warburton
and J. Wong

SCHOOL OF BIOLOGICAL SCIENCES, UNIVERSITY OF NOTTINGHAM, UNIVERSITY PARK,
NOTTINGHAM NG7 2RD, UK

1 INTRODUCTION

Calcium ions are known to be centrally involved in a wide range of cellular functions. In excitable cells they are intimately involved in functions such as: secretion, intracellular movement, neurotransmitter release, muscular contraction, enzyme activity, membrane potential, control of other ion channels and ultimately cell toxicity and death. It is thus apparent that careful regulation of intracellular calcium concentration is vital, and that manipulation of these processes might provide potent methodology for perturbing such functions for therapeutic or disruptive purposes.

2 [^{45}Ca^{++}] ENTRY INTO LOCUST SKELETAL MUSCLES VIA GLUTAMATE-GATED AND VOLTAGE GATED ION CHANNELS

The excitatory amino acid L-glutamate acts on depolarising junctional and extrajunctional receptors in locust skeletal muscle to gate non-specific cationic channels which are permeable to Na$^+$, K$^+$, and Ca^{++}[1,2]. Normally these quisqualate sensitive L-glutamate receptors desensitise rapidly in the presence of agonists, however this desensitisation can be blocked by preincubation in the lectin Concanavalin A (ConA). Incubation of locust muscle in L-glutamate has been shown to cause muscle cytotoxicity following ConA treatment, and this toxic response to glutamate has been shown to be calcium dependent. It has been proposed that the damage to muscle cells is caused by the entry of Ca^{++} through glutamate-receptor gated channels when they are prevented from desensitising and this system has been proposed as a model for excitotoxicity[3]. δ-Philanthotoxin (PTX-433) is a toxin from the venom of the digger wasp *Philanthus triangulum* which has been shown to block L-glutamate gated ion channels in a number of systems including locust skeletal muscle[4,5].

It has also been shown that insect skeletal muscles possess voltage-gated Ca^{++}

channels (VGCC) [6-10] whose pharmacology is broadly similar to vertebrate L-type Ca^{++} channels[11] and can be blocked by phenylalkylamines such as verapamil and dihydropyridines such as nifedipine. We have therefore carried out experiments to examine the influx of $[^{45}Ca^{++}]$ through glutamate-gated and voltage-gated channels in locust skeletal muscle and to investigate the pharmacological differences between them.

2.1 Method

Metathoracic legs of female locusts (*Schistocerca gregaria*) were dissected to expose the *extensor tibiae* muscle. Muscles were incubated in standard locust saline containing (mM): NaCl (180); KCl (10); CaCl₂ (1); HEPES (10); pH 6.8; for 10 minutes followed by a further 30 mins in saline with or without ConA (1μM). Channel blockers, PhTX or nifedipine, were included in the preincubation for 20 minutes.

Muscles were incubated for 3 minutes in saline containing 0.037MBq/ml $[^{45}Ca^{++}]$ and depolarised by addition of L-glutamate (100pM-10mM) or by elevating $[K^+]_o$ to 50mM, contralateral legs served as unstimulated controls.

After various times (optimum 15 minutes) muscles were washed (x3) with ice cold saline and finally with ethanol. Ethanol was discarded and the muscle was detached and allowed to dry overnight. The dry weight of the muscle was determined. Muscles were solubilised in 350ml Triton X100 1%v/v for 3-4 hrs, before addition of 4ml of aqueous scintillation fluid. Levels of $[^{45}Ca^{++}]$ were determined by liquid scintillation counting and results were expressed as cpm/mg dry muscle weight.

2.2 Pharmacology of $[^{45}Ca^{++}]$ Entry into Locust Skeletal Muscle

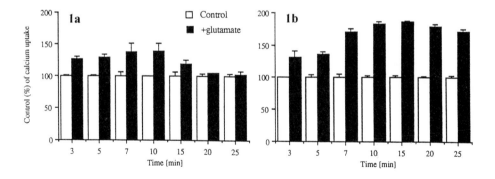

Figure 1 *Time course of $[^{45}Ca^{++}]$ uptake following addition of L-glutamate 100μM. In the absence of ConA* **(Figure 1a)** *uptake peaks at 40% above control levels. Preincubation in 1μM ConA* **(Figure 1b)** *results in a higher level of uptake (87% above control) which persists for up to 25 minutes. Each bar represents mean ± SEM of at least six experiments.*

L-glutamate produced a dose dependent and time dependent increase in $[^{45}Ca^{++}]$ entry into the muscle. $[^{45}Ca^{++}]$ entry was maximally stimulated by 100μM glutamate and peaked after 10-15 minutes (Figure 1). Preincubation in ConA increased both the time course and amount of $[^{45}Ca^{++}]$ entry.

Preincubation in PhTX-343 did not affect basal uptake but reduced L-glutamate (100μM) induced uptake dose dependently with an IC_{50} of approximately 10 nM. (Figure 2)

Elevated $[K^+]_o$ (50mM) induced an influx of $[^{45}Ca^{++}]$ of similar magnitude to that produced by L-glutamate however this process was unaffected by preincubation in ConA. The dihydropyridine calcium channel blocker nifedipine reduced $[^{45}Ca^{++}]$ entry in a dose dependent fashion with an IC_{50} of approximately 50 nM (Figure 3). In contrast to the results described above PhTX-343 has little effect on elevated $[K^+]_o$ induced $[^{45}Ca^{++}]$ entry and nifedipine does not block $[^{45}Ca^{++}]$ movement through L-glutamate gated channels (Fig 4).

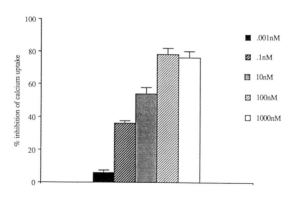

Figure 2 *PhTX-343 inhibited L-glutamate (100μM) induced $[^{45}Ca^{++}]$ uptake dose dependently. Each bar represents mean ±SEM of at least six experiments for a particular dose of PhTX-343.*

It is thus apparent that $[^{45}Ca^{++}]$ can enter locust muscles through both voltage and ligand gated ion channels, and the use of pharmacological tools can enable these two ionic fluxes to be isolated. Presumably during normal function excitability is regulated by both of these mechanisms, but their pharmacological distinctiveness may provide opportunities to target them individually as a potential control strategy.

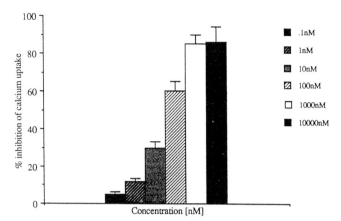

Figure 3 *Dose inhibition relationship for the action of nifedipine on elevated $[K^+]_o$ induced $[^{45}Ca^{++}]$ uptake by locust muscle. Each point represents mean ± SEM of at least six experiments.*

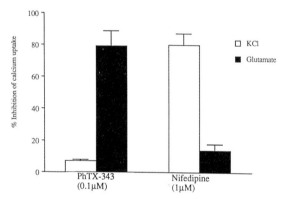

Figure 4 *PhTX-343 and Nifedipine inhibit $[^{45}Ca^{++}]$ uptake induced by L-glutamate (100µM) and elevated $[K^+]_o$ (50mM) respectively. Each point represents mean ± SEM of at least six experiments.*

3. INTERACTIONS OF HOUSEFLY NEURONAL CALCIUM CHANNELS WITH DELTAMETHRIN

VGCC are known to be widespread in the nervous systems of invertebrates[10] and whilst their properties resemble those of the well-characterised calcium channel sub-types identified in vertebrate preparations[12] functional differences have also been described[10]. Cloning studies have now enabled the molecular structure of vertebrate VGCC to be extensively characterised. They consist of a number of subunits, with the α_1–subunit being identified as the component responsible for forming the voltage gated pore. The α_1–subunit consists of a peptide with 24 membrane spanning   helices arranged in four repeating domains reminiscent of the structure of the α_1–subunit of the voltage-gated sodium channel. The α_1–subunits have been cloned and sequenced from a number of vertebrate VGCC[12], and more recently from the insects *Musca domestica* (Md1α)[13] and *Drosophila melanogaster* (Dmca1D)[14]. Comparisons of sequence homologies between insect VGCC α_1–subunits and those of mammals have suggested that the insect channels are most similar to L-type calcium channels.

It is firmly established that the pyrethroid insecticides act on insect voltage-gated sodium channels[15] to modify their gating properties. In view of the molecular similarities between voltage-gated sodium and calcium channels, a series of experiments was carried out to see if there was any interaction between the type II pyrethroid deltamethrin and housefly neuron calcium currents.

3.1 Method

Adult houseflies (Musca. domestica) were anaesthetised with CO_2, decapitated and the thoracic ganglia were transferred to ice cold sterile Ca^{++}/Mg^{++}-free dipteran saline containing (mM): NaCl (135), KCl (2.5), $NaH_2PO_3.H_2O$ (0.4), $NaHCO_3$ (1.25), Glucose (0.5), HEPES (5.0) pH 7.2 . 10-15 ganglia, were cut to disrupt the neural sheath, placed in 1ml centrifuge-tube and washed three times in saline. Following treatment with a mixture of 0.5mg/ml collagenase and 2mg/ml dispase for 10 minutes at $37^{\circ}C$, the ganglia were washed three times and transferred to a laminar air-flow cabinet. Ganglia were washed a further three times and slowly introduced into modified Schneider's medium (85% Schneider's Drosophila medium (Gibco GBL), 15% foetal bovine serum (FBS), 100 units/ml penicillin, 100mg/ml streptomycin and 50mg/ml insulin pH 7.2) by gentle repeated washes into a final volume of 1ml. Ganglia were gently triturated through a flame polished Pasteur pipette and allowed to settle to the bottom of the centrifuge-tube. The overlying supernatant was transferred to sterile poly-D-lysine coated 55mm Falcon dishes. Ganglia were resuspended and the procedure repeated twice. Cultures were incubated in a polystyrene container at room temperature for up to 36 hours.

Isolated neurons were bathed in saline containing (mM); NaCl (140), KCl (3), $MgCl_2$ (4), $CaCl_2$ (1), HEPES (5), potassium channel blockers tetraethyl ammonium chloride (TEA-Cl, 30) and 4-aminopyridine (1), pH 7.2. Cationic currents were measured using the whole-cell configuration of the patch clamp. Unpolished patch-electrodes (2-3MΩ) were filled with solution containing (mM); CsCl (70), CsF (70), EGTA, (1.1), $MgCl_2$ (2), $CaCl_2$ (0.1), adjusted to pH 7.2 with CsOH.

Neurons were maintained at a holding potential of -100mV and currents were evoked by depolarising steps to a test potential between -70mV and +60mV. Experiments were performed at room temperature and analysed on-line. Potentials were corrected for liquid junction potentials, leak currents and capacitive currents. For each cell voltage-protocols were performed in triplicate and the average used for further analysis. Voltage-dependence of activation was measured using the same method but results were normalised relative to the maximum current for each cell.

3.2 Properties of Voltage-Activated Currents

Three classes of voltage-gated current were evoked when cell membranes were step depolarised from a holding potential of -100mV to potentials between -70mV and +60mV. These currents exhibited properties characteristic of calcium currents and sodium currents and were studied following pharmacological isolation (figure 5; Table 1) with either 10mM CoCl₂ (sodium current, figure 5a) or 1mM tetrodotoxin (calcium current, figure 5b).

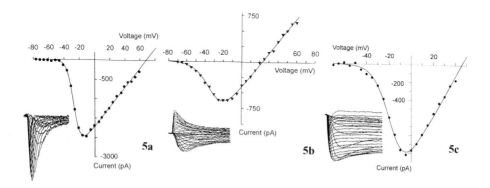

Figure 5 *Current-voltage (I/V) relationships for voltage-activated currents recorded in neurons cultured from the thoracic ganglia of M. domestica (Cooper). Data points represent the mean of triplicate experiments performed in the same cell. Curves were fitted with a Boltzmann function. Inset shows the family of currents used to construct the I/V curve.* **Figure 5a** *In the presence of 10mM CoCl₂, this current has properties consistent with a voltage-activated sodium current (Table 1).* **Figure 5b** *In the presence of 1μM TTX, this smaller current has properties consistent with a low-voltage activated calcium current (Table 1).* **Figure 5c** *shows a high-voltage activated calcium current which is blocked by CoCl₂, unaffected by TTX and is particularly sensitive to Cd⁺⁺ ions, (EC₅₀ 2.4μM)*

In some cells a further current (figure 5c) could be isolated which had somewhat different biophysical properties from the calcium current described above (figure 5b). It activated at -50 to -40 mV and reached a peak of activation at around -10 mV. The current was sensitive to divalent cations with EC_{50} values of 2.44μM for Cd^{++}, 762μM for Ni^{++} and 321μM for Co^{++}. At present a full pharmacological characterisation of these calcium currents has not been carried out; however the clear difference in activation voltage and the sensitivity of the second current to Cd^{++} suggest that the designation of low-voltage activated (LVA) (figure 1b) and high-voltage activated (HVA) (figure 1c) are appropriate.

Table 1 *Properties of Voltage-gated Channels from Fly Neurons*

Property	LVA Calcium current Figure 1b	Sodium Current Figure 1a
Onset of activation	-70 to -60mV (3)	-40 to -35mV (17)
Peak of activation	-35 to -30mV (3)	-10 to -5mV (17)
Time to max. peak I	5.03 ± 0.59ms (3)	2.61 ± 0.17ms (17)
Onset of inactivation	-85 to -80mV (3)	-70 to -65mV (15)
t for max. peak I	5.32 ± 0.18ms (3)	0.80 ± 0.07ms (15)
Recovery from inactivation	Up to 250ms (3)	Within 3ms (7)
Action of 10mM CoCl₂	Block	None
Action of 10nM TTX	None	Block

3.2 Modification of the whole-cell current by the pyrethroid insecticide Deltamethrin.

3.2.1 Sodium Currents.

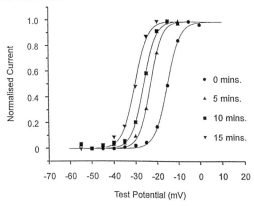

Figure 6 *1μM deltamethrin caused a time dependent hyperpolarising shift in activation voltage of the sodium current recorded in M. domestica neurons. Currents were elicited using step depolarisations from a holding potential of -100mV to potentials ranging between -70 and +60mV at 0.5Hz. After application of deltamethrin, the experiment was repeated in triplicate at 5 minute intervals for 15 minutes. Data were normalised relative to the maximum current and the curves were fitted with a modified Boltzmann function.*

The effects of deltamethrin on voltage-activated sodium currents were examined in isolated housefly neurons. Neurons were allowed to equilibrate for 10 minutes after entering the whole-cell configuration and current-voltage relationships were recorded in triplicate immediately prior to applying deltamethrin. Following the bath application of deltamethrin at a concentration of 1μM (n=5) current properties were measured at 5 minute intervals. Voltage protocols were performed in triplicate, averaged and plotted against the corresponding test potential at each time interval

Deltamethrin resulted in a rapid hyperpolarising shift in the voltage-dependence of activation (figure 6). After 15 minutes half-maximal currents (mean ± SEM) were found to be significantly shifted (P<0.01, 1-way ANOVA) from a potential of -15.12 ± 3.01mV to -31.08 ± 3.69mV.

3.2.2 Calcium currents Application of 1μM deltamethrin to isolated cells from *M. domestica* caused a significant (P<0.01, 1-way ANOVA) hyperpolarising shift in the mid-point of the LVA-calcium current activation curve (figure 7a). This change was observed in all (n = 3) of the cells tested. Rundown prevented longer experimental time-courses. However even after 30 mins of application to cells exhibiting HVA-calcium currents no effect of 1μM deltamethrin was evident on the activation properties of the current (figure 7b).

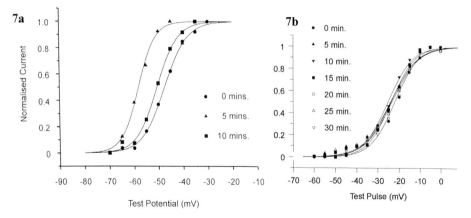

Figure 7. *Calcium currents were evoked using 30ms depolarising test pulses from a holding potential of -100mV to potentials from -70mV to +60mV in 5mV increments at a frequency of 0.5Hz. Voltage-protocols were performed in triplicate at each time interval and the mean current was normalised relative to the maximum current.* **Figure 7a** *1μM deltamethrin caused a time dependent hyperpolarising shift in activation voltage of the LVA-calcium current.* **Figure 7b** *1μM deltamethrin caused no change in the activation properties of HVA current.*

Two main conclusions may be reached from this study: i. that housefly neurons have at least two types of voltage activated calcium currents, in accordance with the two types of calcium current previously reported in cockroach DUM cells[16] ii. that the LVA channel type appears to be sensitive to pyrethroids and may be worthy of further study as a potential insecticide target.

4 ACTIONS OF DELTAMETHRIN ON INTRACELLULAR CALCIUM LEVELS
IN ISOLATED HOUSEFLY NEURONS

The implication of the experiments described above is that pyrethroid insecticides might mediate some of their toxicity via a calcium-mediated mechanism. It could be argued that modification of Ca^{++} entry into cells would provide a particularly potent toxic pathway due to the potential for Ca^{++} dependent release of Ca^{++} from intracellular stores and perturbation of the numerous cellular processes involving Ca^{++}[17]. To establish whether pyrethroids are capable of modulating $[Ca^{++}]_i$ we have used ratiometric fluorescence imaging with the calcium sensitive dye FURA-2. This dye fluoresces under UV illumination, however the intensity of fluorescence varies as the dye binds Ca^{++}, the intensity at 340nm increasing whilst that at 380nm diminishes. The ratio of the fluorescence at these two wavelengths therefore gives a measure of $[Ca^{++}]_i$ which is independent of the cell volume or loading efficiency. Fluorescence imaging has been used to monitor changes in $[Ca^{++}]_i$ in response to activation of insect ligand gated ion channels[18,19].

4.1 Method

Insect neurons were dissociated as described above except that the final resuspension and plating was carried out in housefly normal saline onto the surface of clean glass 22mm square coverslips. After cells had adhered to the coverslip they were incubated for up to 36 hours in Schneider's medium. The medium was replaced with medium containing $2\mu M$ FURA-2AM in Schneider's medium and incubated for 30 mins. The coverslip was then transferred to a perfusion chamber on the stage of a Zeiss Epifluorescence microscope. Neurons were visualised and selected for ratiometric imaging. Fluorescence was imaged at 340 and 380 nm and pairs of images (averages of 8 exposures) were collected at 2 second intervals and their ratios were analysed using "Ionvision" software (Improvision). Drugs were applied via the perfusion system and the cells were depolarised by raising the extracellular potassium concentration in the bathing saline to 80mM. Where indicated sodium channels were blocked with $1\mu M$ tetrodotoxin.

4.2 Fluctuations in $[Ca^{++}]_i$ induced by Deltamethrin

Deltamethrin (100nM) affected neuronal $[Ca^{++}]_i$ in two ways: i. Initiation of spontaneous oscillations in $[Ca^{++}]_i$ (figure 8, figure 9) which can be blocked by the calcium channel blocker verapamil. ii. Potentiation of the amplitude of depolarisation induced increases in $[Ca^{++}]_i$ (figure 8). These actions of deltamethrin are unaltered in the presence of tetrodotoxin, implying that the mechanism does not involve the action of voltage gated sodium channels. Furthermore verapamil appears to inhibit the deltamethrin induced spontaneous oscillations pointing to the likely involvement of calcium channels in the actions of deltamethrin.

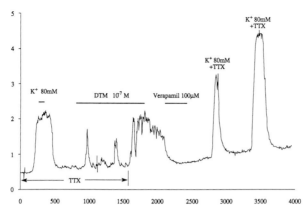

Figure 8 *Ratiometric analysis of FURA-2 fluorescence in isolated housefly neurons. Changes in intracellular calcium concentration $[Ca^{++}]_i$ are expressed as 340/380 ratiometric units (vertical axis) against time (horizontal axis). Depolarisation of the cells by elevating $[K^+]_o$ resulted in an increase in $[Ca^{++}]_i$. Addition of deltamethrin resulted in an increase in spontaneous oscillations of $[Ca^{++}]_i$ which can be blocked by verapamil. Subsequent K^+ depolarisations resulted in a potentiation of the induced elevation of $[Ca^{++}]_i$*

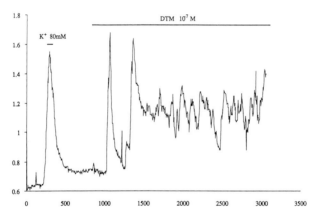

Figure 9 *Ratiometric analysis of FURA-2 fluorescence in isolated housefly neurons. Changes in intracellular calcium concentration $[Ca^{++}]_i$ are shown in 340/380 ratiometric units (vertical axis) against time (horizontal axis). Cells with spontaneous oscillations of $[Ca^{++}]_i$ often respond to deltamethrin by increrasing the frequency and amplitude of these oscillations.*

It is evident from these results that pyrethroids can modulate $[Ca^{++}]_i$ independently of their actions on sodium channels. These data could be interpreted in terms of a modification of VGCC seen above, however given the lipophilicity of pyrethroids it is also possible that they directly modulate intracellular calcium handling, as recently reported for a number of other pharmacological agents in insect neurons[20]. Further work using both electrophysiology and fluorescence imaging in combination with selective pharmacological agents would enable these processes to be dissected. The use of housefly neurons for these studies also provides the opportunity to exmine the actions of pyrethroids in resistant strains.

In conclusion, excitable cells in insects express several types of channels with different properties which are capable of gating Ca^{++}. The variability of calcium channels, their pharmacological diversity and the crucial role of these ions in cell signalling should make them an attractive target for the discovery and development of insecticides.

References

1. R. Anwyl, *J.Physiol. (Lond.)*, 1977, **273**, 367.

2. K. Kits and P.N.R. Usherwood, *J.Exp. Biol.,*1988, **138** ,499.

3. I. R. Duce, P.L. Donaldson and P.N.R. Usherwood, *Brain Res.,* 1983, **263** , 77.

4. T. Piek, *Comp. Biochem. Physiol .,* 1971, **72C,** 311.

5. R.B. Clark, P.L. Donaldson, K.A.F. Gration, J.J. Lambert, T. Piek, R.. Ramsey W. Spanjer and P.N.R. Usherwood, *Brain Res.,* 1982, **241,** 105.

6. H. Washio *J.Gen. Physiol.,* 1972, **59,** 121.

7. S. Hagiwara and L. Byerly, *Ann. Rev. Neurosci.,* 1981, **4,** 69.

8. F.M. Ashcroft, *J. Exp. Biol.,* 1981, **93,** 257.

9. H-T. Leung and L. Byerly, *J. Neurosci.,* 1991, **11,** 3047.

10. J.M. Skeer, R.I. Norman and D.B. Sattelle, *Biol Rev.,* 1996, **71,** 137.

11. J.M. Skeer N. Pruitt and D.B. Sattelle, *Insect Biochemistry,* 1992, **22,** 539.

12. M.de Waard, C.A. Gurnett and K.P. Campbell, "Ion Channels Vol 4 editor T. Narahashi", Plenum Press, New York, 1996.

13. M. Grabner, A. Bachmann, F. Rosenthal, J. Striessnig, F. Scheffauer, W.J. Koch, A. Schwartz and H. Glossmann, *FEBS. Letts.,* 1994, **339,** 189.

14. W. Zheng, G.Feng, D.Ren, D.F. Eberi, F.Hannan, M.Dubald and L.M. Hall, *J. Neurosci.,* 1995, **15,** 1132

15. T. Narahashi, *Trends in Pharmacol.Sci. ,*1992, **13,** 236

16 D. Wicher and H. Penzlin, *J. Neurophysiol.,* 1997, **77,** 186.

17. P.B. Simpson, R.A.J. Challiss and S.R. Nahorski, *Trends in Neurosci.,*1995, **18,** 299.

18 J.A. David and R.M. Pitman, *J.Exp. Biol.,* 1996, **199,** 1921.

19 F. Grolleau, B. Lapied, S.D. Buckingham, W.T. Mason and D.B. Sattelle, *Neurosci. Letts.,* 1996, **220,** 142

20. M. Heine and D. Wicher, *Neuroreport,* 1998, **9,** 3309.

Acknowledgements

The work presented here was supported by SERC, and BBSRC CASE studentships to SPMW and AJT and a Nuffield Student Bursary to JW. We should also like to thank Dr M.E. Adams (University of California Riverside) for training in the production of isolated housefly neurons.

Elucidation of the Bioactive Site and Potential Applications of Sodium Channel Modifiers from Scorpion Venom

Michael Gurevitz[1*], Oren Froy[1], Noam Zilberberg[1], Boaz Shaanan[2], Michael E. Adams[3], Jacob Anglister[4], Marcel Pelhate[5], Nor Chejanovsky[6] and Dalia Gordon[7]

[1] DEPARTMENT OF PLANT SCIENCES, FACULTY OF LIFE SCIENCES, TEL-AVIV UNIVERSITY, RAMAT-AVIV 69978, TEL-AVIV, ISRAEL
[2] DEPARTMENT OF BIOLOGICAL CHEMISTRY, INSTITUTE OF LIFE SCIENCES, HEBREW UNIVERSITY OF JERUSALEM, JERUSALEM 91904, ISRAEL
[3] DEPARTMENT OF ENTOMOLOGY, UNIVERSITY OF CALIFORNIA RIVERSIDE, CA 92521, USA
[4] DEPARTMENT OF STRUCTURAL BIOLOGY, THE WEIZMANN INSTITUTE OF SCIENCE, REHOVAT 76100, ISRAEL
[5] LABORATOIRE DE NEUROPHYSIOLOGIE, FACULTE DE MEDICINE, UNIVERSITE D'ANGERS, F-49045, FRANCE
[6] INSTITUTE OF PLANT PROTECTION, THE VOLCANI CENTER, ARO, BET-DAGAN 50250, ISRAEL
[6] DEPARTMENT D'INGENIERIE ET D'ETUDES DES PROTEINS, CEA, SACLAY F-91191, GIF-SUR-YVETTE, CEDEX, FRANCE
*Author for correspondence

Ongoing overuse of neurotoxic chemical insecticides, such as organophosphates, carbamates, and pyrethroids poses unacceptable risks to the environment and to human health resulting from non-target toxicity and insect resistance build up. Evidently, there is an urgent need for safer alternatives, which target insects more specifically and able to displace the hazardous chemicals or reduce their utilization. Such alternatives exist in venomous arthropods and are used for prey of insects or defence. The anti-insect selective polypeptide toxins found in scorpions are biodegradable and non-toxic to warm-blooded animals. Hence, characterization of their bioactive domains and mobilization into insect pest targets are of major interest due to the applicative potential.[1-5]

Sodium channel modifiers from scorpion venom
Scorpion venoms contain basic neurotoxic polypeptides of 60-70 amino acid residues constrained by four disulfide bonds. They share a similar 3-D core but display a wide array of pharmacological effects and sequences.[6-11] The α and β classes of sodium channel toxins are active, at various ratios, against both insects and mammals, whereas excitatory[12-13] and depressant[14-16] toxins, considered as two distinct groups among the β class, show absolute selectivity to insect sodium channels. Their phylogenetic

preference is of particular interest in the study of insect sodium channels and may be exploited as potential insecticides. The functional variations among the toxins and their distinct receptor binding sites provides a wide array of interacting polypeptides that are useful tools for the study of channel gating. Our study is focused on representative scorpion toxins belonging to three major pharmacological groups:

Alpha neurotoxins show variability in their apparent toxicity to mammals and insects, in their primary structures (Fig. 1), and in their binding features to neuronal membrane preparations.[17-20] This is the most studied group among scorpion neurotoxins and is useful in functional mapping of the sodium channel structure.[1,2,17,18,21] The mode of action of α-toxins is characterized by their ability to slow down the inactivation phase of the sodium current of the action potential.[22,23] Although most alpha toxins exhibit toxicity towards mammals, some representatives show anti-insect preference. LqhαIT[24,25] for example, binds to a single class of high affinity sites on insect neural membranes {Kd=0.2-0.5 nM and 0.03-0.04 nM in locust and cockroach, respectively}[17,26], and competes weakly with other α-toxins for binding to rat brain synaptosomes. AaHII, the most potent anti-mammalian scorpion α-neurotoxin, competes for 125I-LqhαIT binding site on insect sodium channels, suggesting that the two scorpion α-toxins bind to homologous, non-identical receptor-sites on insect and mammalian sodium channels.[17] LqhαIT is toxic to mice at relatively high concentrations as opposed to other scorpion α-neurotoxins such as AaHII,[17,20] and yet appears to recognize an α-toxin binding-site on both insect and mammalian sodium channels.

Excitatory neurotoxins are characterized by 1) induction of contracture upon injection only in insects.[27] Insect specificity is also manifested in toxin-receptor binding assays[12] indicating exclusive binding to receptors in insect nervous tissues;[28] 2) generation of excitatory paralysis of insects by inducing repetitive activity in motor nerves via a shift in voltage-dependent activation and reduction in inactivation;[14,29] 3) effect on insect neural preparations upon binding to a single class of high affinity (Kd=1-3 nM) and low capacity (1.2-2.0 pmole/mg protein) sites;[28] 4) a typical shift in the position of one disulphide bridge[30] compared to the strictly conserved positions of the four disulphide bonds in scorpion toxins belonging to other pharmacological groups. Three highly homologous excitatory toxins have been described thus far: AaHIT from *Androctonus australis* Hector,[31] LqqIT1 from *Leiurus quinquestriatus quinquestriatus*,[32] and LqhIT1 from *Leiurus quinquestriatus hebraeus*.[33]

Depressant neurotoxins are characterized by 1) induction of a short transient phase of contracture followed by a prolonged flaccid paralysis specific to insects;[15,34] 2) induction of transient repetitive firing in insect motoneurons (*Musca domestica*, *Heliothis virescens*), followed by a decreased amplitude of excitatory junctional potentials.[16,35] These toxins have no effect on mammalian sensory neurons up to mM concentrations; 3) recognition of two non-interacting binding sites on locust neural membranes: a high affinity (Kd=0.9±0.6 nM) low capacity (Bmax=0.1±0.07 pmole/mg) binding site as well as a low affinity (Kd=185±13 nM) high capacity (Bmax=10±0.6 pmole/mg) binding site.[36,37] Their high affinity binding site on sodium channels of locust neural membranes is in close proximity to the binding site of the excitatory toxin, AaHIT, and they are capable of displacing one another in competition experiments.[37,38] Four highly homologous depressant neurotoxins (LqhIT2 from

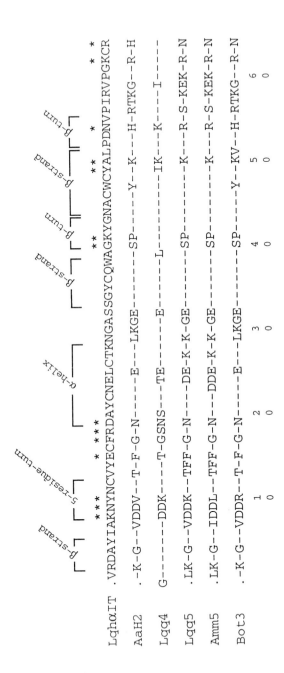

Fig. 1. Alignment of the amino acid sequences of several alpha scorpion neurotoxins. Residues homologous to those in LqhαIT are designated by dashes. Dots indicate gaps in the aligned sequences. Modified sites are designated by asterisks (modifications at positions 49, 50 and 54 were described previously[20] and secondary structure motifs[56] are indicated. AaHII, *Androctonus australis* Hector toxin 2; Lqq4 and Lqq5, *Leiurus quinquestriatus quinquestriatus* toxin 4 and toxin 5; Amm5, *Androctonus mauretanicus mauretanicus* toxin 5; Bot3, *Buthus occitanus tunetanus* toxin 3.[18]

Leiurus quinquestriatus hebraeus, LqqIT2 from *Leiurus quinquestriatus quinquestriatus*, BjIT2 from *Buthotus judaicus*, BeIT2 from *Buthus eupeus*), which induce a slow, progressive, flaccid paralysis in blowfly larvae, have been reported [for review see.[9,16]

Joint action of scorpion toxins with chemical insecticides

Although the multiple receptor-sites for chemical or scorpion toxins on sodium channels are topologically distinct, they display strong allosteric interactions.[1,3,19,39,40] For example: 1) the pyrethroids deltamethrin and cypermethrin and the insecticide DDT, each of which has been shown to increase the binding affinity of batrachotoxin, acting on sodium channel site 2;[41] 2) positive cooperativity has been shown among a synthetic pyrethroid, RU395668, a sea anemone toxin II acting at receptor site 3, and brevetoxin-2, acting at receptor site 5, which together enhance ~100 fold binding of batrachotoxin to synaptosomes;[42] 3) binding of the alpha mammalian toxin AaHII or the alpha anti-insect toxin LqhαIT to receptor site 3 on rat brain or locust channels, respectively, is cooperatively enhanced by the plant alkaloid veratridine, which binds to receptor site [21,26] Conversely, brevetoxin, which binds to receptor site 5, strongly inhibits the binding of AaHII and Lqq5 (two alpha mammalian toxins) to rat brain synaptosomes[3,39,40] but increases 2-fold the binding of LqhαIT to locust sodium channels.[39] In spite of the high affinity binding of LqhαIT on both cockroach and locust sodium channels, the allosteric enhancement by veratridine and brevetoxin has been observed only on locust sodium channels.[17,39] The observation that brevetoxin is able to decrease significantly the binding of α-toxins to rat brain sodium channels but to increase the binding of LqhαIT to a homologous receptor site on locust sodium channels, suggests that a combinatorial use of ligands may provide selective effects toward mammals and insects as well as among different insect species. Gaining anti-insect selectivity and increased efficacy is a major objective in insect pest control.

Genetic polymorphism and common anchestry of scorpion neurotoxins

Genomic clones representing the major classes of Buthidae scorpion toxins, namely, 'long' toxins affecting sodium channels (alpha, depressant, and excitatory) and 'short' toxins affecting potassium and chloride channels were isolated from a single scorpion segment and analysed.[33] In addition, a large number of cDNA clones has been isolated from cDNA libraries constructed from telson-derived poly(A)+ RNA of *Leiurus quinquestriatus hebraeus*,[43,33] *Androctonus australis* Hector,[31] and *Buthotus judaicus*.[44] Comparative analysis of nucleotide sequences clearly indicated a multiple number of distinct genes encoding each toxin and a very similar gene organization suggesting a common progenitor.[33] In light of the negligible changes in scorpion morphology over millions of years, the vast diversity of neurotoxin genes and their products may explain their evolutionary success of survival.

Production of recombinant scorpion neurotoxins

In order to elucidate the active sites and structural elements conferring anti-insect specificity of scorpion neurotoxins, a reliable expression system enabling genetic modification and biological assays is required.

Expression in Escherichia coli: Several representatives from the alpha, depressant, and excitatory groups of toxins have been produced using the pET-11 expression vector.[20,45,46] The recombinant toxins, LqhαIT,20 LqhIT2,45 and Bj-xtrIT,46 accumulating in an unsoluble, non-active form within inclusion bodies, were solubilized concomitant to denaturation by guanidinium hydrochloride and reduction by β-mercapto ethanol or dithiothreitol. Optimal conditions for in-vitro renaturation to gain a fully active dominant fold, were then exercised with each toxin analysing salt concentration, temperature, pH, and reducing agent concentrations. These experiments demonstrated that the reduction-oxidation state of a given scorpion neurotoxic polypeptide prior to, and perhaps throughout, folding was critical and had to be determined empirically. Furthermore, subtle differences in sequence and structure have been shown to play an important role in folding capacity.

The final folded recombinant LqhαIT, LqhIT2, and Bj-xtrIT were purified by C18-RP-HPLC and their physiological, biochemical, and structural characteristics analysed (see examples in Figures 2 and 3). In all cases, the recombinant toxins exhibited chemical and biological properties indistinguishable from those of the authentic native toxins despite an additional methionine residue constructed at their N-termini. Obviously, further analysis of structure-activity relationship of these toxins was dependent on their capability to withstand genetic alterations and still fold properly.

Expression in insect cells: It has been shown that a toxin gene incorporated into baculoviral entomopathogens increased their insecticidal efficacy.[47-52] In order to study the potential of this approach, three toxin cDNAs coding for LqhαIT, LqhIT2, and LqhIT1 have been constructed downstream of various promoters of the baculovirus *Autographa californica Multiple Nucleopolyhedrosis Virus* (AcMNPV). The recombinant viruses were used to infect either *Spodoptera frugiperda* insect cell line (Sf9) or *Spodoptera littoralis* and *Helicoverpa armigera* larvae.[51,52] Expression of the three toxins has been achieved and could be monitored by the toxic effects or immunochemically. These experiments revealed a significant increase in the insecticidal efficacy reducing the ET50, effective paralysis time 50%, of *Helicoverpa armigera* first instar larvae from ~90 hours, for the wild-type, to 59 hours for the virus producing the depressant toxin and 66 hours for the virus producing the excitatory toxin.[52] Interestingly, expression driven by an early viral promoter (p35) did not yield immuno-detectable recombinant toxin, but a clear paralytic effect could be monitored (ET50=73 hours). This observation suggests that baculovirus mediated production of a toxin in close proximity to its target site may overcome pharmacokinetic barriers encountered by the toxin when injected. It is noteworthy that 'feeding arrest' of the infected larvae was more prominent compared to lethality, a result of great promise when minimization of damage to crops is sought.

The bioactive surface of the alpha toxin LqhαIT

Despite the reported structures,[7,53-56] chemical modifications, and immunochemical studies[57-60] of various scorpion α-toxins, their active sites and domains conferring phylogenetic preference have never been described. We utilised the bacterial expression system to produce milligram amounts of active, purified toxin whose three-dimensional structure was determined by 2D-^{1}H-NMR.[56] This system was used for a genetic dissection followed by functional (Fig. 2) and structural (Fig. 3) analyses of

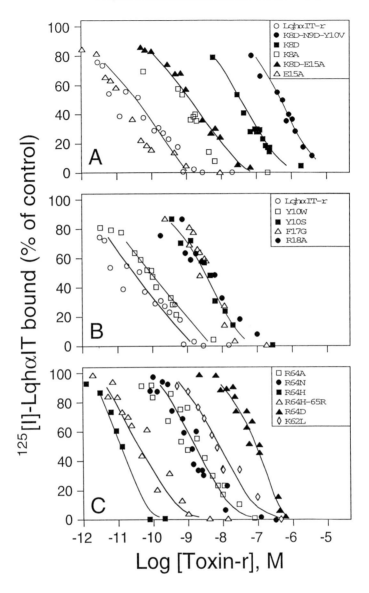

Fig. 2. Competitive inhibition of the binding of unmodified ^{125}I-labeled LqhαIT by various recombinant LqhαIT toxins. The unmodified toxin is compared to: mutants modified in turn structures (A); mutants modified at residues presumably interacting with the receptor-site (B); mutants modified at the C-terminal region (C). Cockroach neuronal membranes (25 mg membrane protein) were incubated for 60 min at 22°C in the presence of 0.03 nM of ^{125}I-labeled LqhαIT and increasing concentrations of unmodified or mutant toxins. Non-specific binding of ^{125}I-labeled LqhαIT, determined in the presence of 1 mM LqhαIT (corresponding to 15-25% of total binding), was subtracted. The binding was determined as described[17] and analysed by the LIGAND computer program.

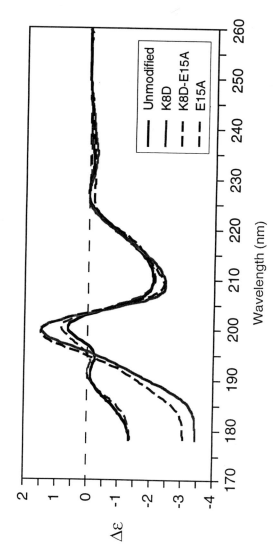

Fig. 3. Circular Dichroism spectra of unmodified and mutant LqhαIT toxins. The unmodified toxin is compared to: mutants modified at the five-residue turn and a suppressor mutant (A); mutants with minor structural changes (B); mutants modified at the 40-43 β-turn and at the C-terminal region (C). Spectra of some mutants that resembled that of the unmodified toxin, i.e., Y10W, D19N, D19H, R18A-D19N, R64N and R64HR, were omitted.

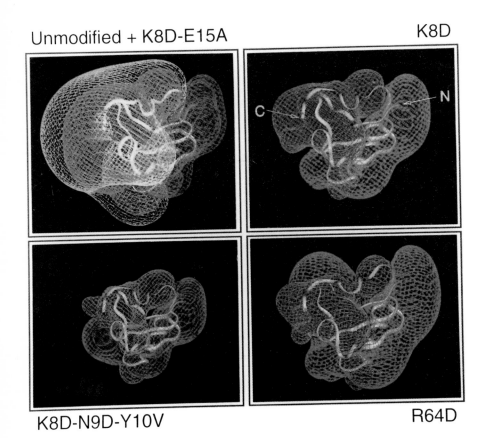

Fig. 4. The electrostatic potentials of LqhαIT and modificants. The positive (+1 Kcal/mol) surface of the unmodified toxin is shown as a white net (top left) and those of the mutants by blue nets. The negative (-1 Kcal/mol) surfaces are indicated by the red nets or by the purple net in the double mutant K8D-E15A. The structures and electrostatic potentials of the unmodified and K8D-E15A double mutant are superimposed. N and C stand for the N-terminus and C-terminus, respectively. The orange ribbons, oriented similarly in all variants, indicate the carbon backbones.

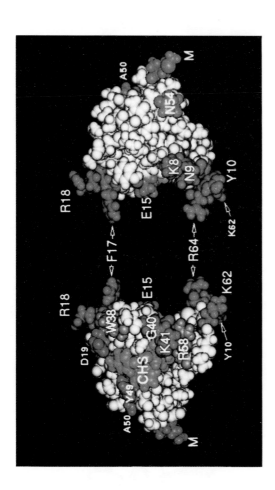

Fig. 5. The putative toxic-surface of LqhαIT. The model was constructed according to the solution structure of the toxin.[56] Genetically modified residues affecting the toxic surface are designated in red. Residues whose counterparts in similar toxins were affected by chemical modifications are colored in orange. Residues, whose substitution had no effect, are indicated in green. The "conserved hydrophobic surface", located on a different side of the molecule, appears in blue.

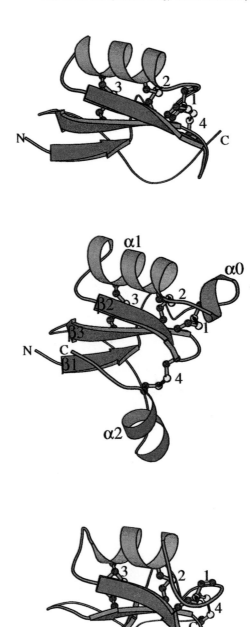

Fig. 6. Overall structures of toxins from various pharmacological groups. The alpha class is represented by AaHII (top); The excitatory group is represented by Bj-xtrIT (middle); CsE-v3 stands for the beta class (bottom). Similar structural elements are marked by the same colour. The disulfide bridges are indicated. Figure prepared using the program MOLSCRIPT.[10]

LqhαIT. Selection of sites for modification was based on comparison between two homologous α-toxins, AaHII and LqhαIT (Fig. 1), displaying two extremes in their phylogenetic preferences but a very similar three-dimensional configuration.[56] AaHII, the strongest anti-mammalian scorpion α-neurotoxin,[2,3] and LqhαIT, the most insecticidal toxin among the alpha group,[2,3,20,24] compete very poorly with each other for their binding sites on insect or mammalian sodium channels. This pharmacological difference can be attributed to non-homologous residues or structural motifs located on their surfaces. Site-directed modifications were introduced to LqhαIT in order to elucidate the molecular surface involved in recognition of the receptor-site on the sodium channel. All toxin variants were HPLC-purified using the toxicity assay on blowfly larvae as a quick and direct measure for activity. Binding assays to a cockroach neuronal membrane preparation were used as a measure for direct activity at the receptor site (Fig. 2), and possible structural alterations were assessed by circular dichroism spectroscopy (Fig. 3). This approach together with the determined structure in solution[56] highlighted both aromatic (Y10 and F17) and positively charged (K8, R18, K62 and R64) residues that (a) may interact directly with putative recognition points at the receptor-site on the sodium channel (Fig. 5);[61] (b) are important for the spatial arrangement of the toxin polypeptide, and (c) contribute to the formation of an electrostatic potential involved in biorecognition of the receptor site (Fig. 4). The latter was supported by a suppressor mutation (E15A) that restored a detrimental effect caused by a K8D substitution.[61] The feasibility of producing anti-insect scorpion neurotoxins with augmented toxicity was demonstrated by the substitution of the C-terminal arginine with histidine. Mutations at Y49, N50, A54 indicated that the anti-insect/anti-mammalian toxicity ratio could be manipulated.[20]

The putative bioactive surface of the excitatory toxin Bj-xtrIT
Scorpion excitatory neurotoxins show total specificity against arthropods and serve as invaluable probes of insect sodium channels. Despite their significance and potential for application, the clarification of their active site and three-dimensional structure was hampered by difficulties associated with their functional expression. Recently, we isolated and characterised an atypically long excitatory toxin, Bj-xtrIT, whose bioactive features resembled those of classical excitatory toxins, despite only 49% sequence identity. Using the bacterial expression system, we found Bj-xtrIT very useful for production and modification. The structure of Bj-xtrIT has been determined at 2.1Å resolution by X-ray crystallography10 highlighting a unique structural module composed of the carboxy-terminal region, whereas the main scaffold of the toxin was found very similar to those of other pharmacologically distinct toxins (Fig. 6). Genetic alterations have been introduced to the carboxy-terminal tail indicating its importance for activity.[46] On the basis of the bioactive role of the toxin tail and a structural comparison of Bj-xtrIT with a model of a classical excitatory toxin, AaHIT, a conserved surface surrounding and including the carboxy-terminus, is suggested to form the toxic site.

Scorpion toxins as future potential biopesticides
Elucidation of bioactive sites of scorpion insecticidal toxins may facilitate the design of selective insecticides or nonpeptide, small agonists and assist in generating a large

collection of insect killers, whose alternate use may minimize resistance build-up among insect pests. Therefore, the study of depressant and excitatory toxins is of practical value. The efficient expression system established for the depressant, LqhIT245 and the excitatory, Bj-xtrIT,[46] toxins is very useful for mutagenesis and structural studies. A collection of depressant toxin sequences has been established and used for comparative analysis and mutagenesis. This study has revealed specific regions playing a role in bioactivity.[62] However, the three-dimensional structure of depressant toxins has not been determined thus far, which is a barrier for determination of the molecular surface involved in receptor site recognition. The determined X-ray structure and putative toxic surface of Bj-xtrIT enables site-specific modifications and generation of variants.

In light of the synergistic effects obtained between certain scorpion toxins and pyrethroids[63] or other sodium channel modulators [veratridine and brevetoxin[17,26,39]; a substantial reduction in use of hazardous chemical insecticides seems possible upon concomitant sensitisation of the channels by scorpion toxins mobilised to these targets by baculoviral vectors.

Acknowledgements

These studies were supported by Grants IS-2486-94C (MG and MEA) and IS-2530-95C (NC) from BARD, The United States-Israel Binational Agricultural Research & Development Fund; Grant 891-0112-95 from the Israeli Ministry of Agriculture (MG); and Grant 466/97 from The Israel Academy of Sciences and Humanities (MG).

References

1. W. D. Catterall, *Annu. Rev. Biochem.*, 1986, **55**, 953-985.

2. W. D. Catterall, *Pharmacol. Rev.*, 1992, **72**(4) Suppl. S15-S48.

3. D. Gordon, In: *Toxins and Signal Transduction*, 'Cellular And Mollecular Mechanisms of Toxin Action', (P. Lazarovici, and Y. Gutman, Eds.), Amsterdam, Harwood Press, 1997. p. 119.

4. M. Gurevitz and N. Zilberberg, *J. Toxicol. Toxin Rev.*, 1994, **13**(1), p. 65.

5. M. Gurevitz, N. Zilberberg, O. Froy, D. Urbach, E. Zlotkin, B. D. Hammock, R. Herrmann, H. Moskowitz and N. Chejanovsky, 'Modern Agriculture and the Environment', (D. Rosen and E. Tel-Or, Eds.), Lancaster, UK, Kluwer Academic Publ., 1996, p. 81.

6. J. C. Fontecilla-Camps, R. J. Almassy, F. L. Suddath and C. E. Bugg, *Toxicon*, 1982, **20**, 1.

7. J. C. Fontecilla-Camps, C. Habersetzer-Rochat and H. Rochat, *Proc. Natl. Acad. Sci. USA*, 1988, **85**, 7443.

8. J. C. Fontecilla-Camps, *J. Mol. Evol.*, 1989, **29**, 63.

9. M-F. Martin-Eauclaire and F. Couraud, 'Handbook of Neurotoxicology', (L. W. Chang and R. S. Dyer, Eds.), New York, Marcel Dekker Press, 1995, p. 683.

10. D. Oren, O. Froy, E. Amit, N. Kleinberger-Doron, M. Gurevitz and B. Shaanan, *Structure*, 1998, accepted.

11. O. Froy, T. Sagiv, M. Poreh, D. Urbach, N. Zilberberg and M. Gurevitz, 1998, Submitted.

12. E. Zlotkin, Z. Teitelbaum, H. Rochat and F. Miranda, *Insect. Biochem.*, 1979, **9**, 347.

13. E. Zlotkin, *Insect. Biochem.*, 1983, **13**, 219.

14. D. Lester, P. Lazarovici, M. Pelhate and E. Zlotkin, *Biochim. Biophys. Acta*, 1982, **701**, 370.

15. E. Zlotkin, M. Eitan, V. P. Bindokas, M. E. Adams, M. Moyer, W. Burkhardt and E. Fowler, *Biochemistry*, 1991, **30**, 4814.

16. E. Zlotkin, M. Gurevitz, E. Fowler, M. Moyer and M. E. Adams, *Arch. Insect Biochem. Physiol.*, 1993, **22**, 55.

17. D. Gordon, M-F. Martin-Eauclaire, S. Cestele, C. Kopeyan, E. Carlier, R. Benkhalifa, M. Pelhate and H. Rochat, *J. Biol. Chem.*, 1996, **271**, 8034.

18. M. J. Dufton and H. Rochat, *J. Mol. Evol.*, 1984, **20**, 120.

19. G. Strichartz, T. Rando and G. K. Wang, *Annu. Rev. Neurosci.*, 1987, **10**, 237.

20. N. Zilberberg, D. Gordon, M. Pelhate, M. E. Adams, T. Norris, E. Zlotkin and M. Gurevitz, *Biochemistry*, 1996, **35**, 10215.

21. W. A. Catterall, *Annu. Rev. Pharmacol. Toxicol.*, 1980, **20**, 15.

22. E. Koppenhofer and H. Schmidt, *Pflgers Arch.*, 1968, **303**, 133.

23. E. Koppenhofer and H. Schmidt, *Pflgers Arch.*, 1968, **303**, 150.

24. M. Eitan, E. Fowler, R. Herrmann, A. Duval, M. Pelhate and E. Zlotkin, *Biochemistry*, 1990, **29**, 5941.

25. M. Gurevitz, D. Urbach, E. Zlotkin and N. Zilberberg, *Toxicon*, 1991, **29**, 1270.

26. D. Gordon and E. Zlotkin, *FEBS Lett.*, 1993, **315**, 125.

27. E. Zlotkin, H. Rochat, C. Kupeyan, F. Miranda and S. Lissitzky, *Biochimie*, 1971, **53**, 1073.

28. D. Gordon, E. Jover, F. Couraud and E. Zlotkin, *Biochim. Biophys. Acta*, 1984, **778**, 349.

29. M. Pelhate and E. Zlotkin, *J. Physiol. (London)*, 1982, **319**, 30.

30. H. Darbon, E. Zlotkin, C. Kopeyan, J. Van Rietschoten and H. Rochat, *Int. J. Pept. Prot. Res.*, 1982, **20**, 320.

31. P. E. Bougis, H. Rochat and L. A. Smith, *J. Biol. Chem.*, 1989, **264**, 19259.

32. C. Kopeyan, P. Mansuelle, F. Sampieri, T. Brando, E. M. Bahraoui, H. Rochat and C. Granier, *FEBS Lett.*, 1990, **261**, 423.

33. O. Froy, T. Sagiv, M. Poreh, D. Urbach, N. Zilberberg and M. Gurevitz, 1998, Submitted.

34. R. Benkhalifa, M. Stankiewicz, B. Lapied, M. Turkov, N. Zilberberg, M. Gurevitz and M. Pelhate, *Life Sci.*, 1997, **61**, 819-830.

35. D. Lee, E. Zlotkin, M. Gurevitz and M. E. Adams, 1998, Submitted.

36. E. Zlotkin, D. Kadouri, D. Gordon, M. Pelhate, M-F. Martin and H. Rochat, *Arch. Biochem. Biophys.*, 1985, **240**, 877.

37. D. Gordon, H. Moskowitz, M. Eitan, C. Warner, W. A. Catterall and E. Zlotkin, *Biochemistry*, 1992, **31**, 7622-7628.

38. H. Moskowitz, R. Herrmann, E. Zlotkin and D. Gordon, *Insect Biochem. Molec. Biol.*, 1994, **24**, 13.

39. S. Cestele, R. Benkhalifa, M. Pelhate, H. Rochat and D. Gordon, *J. Biol. Chem.*, 1995, **270**, 15153.

40. S. Cestele, F. Sampieri, H. Rochat and D. Gordon, *J. Biol. Chem.*, 1996, **271**, 18329.

41. G. B. Brown, J. E. Gaupp and R. W. Olsen, *Mol. Pharmacol.*, 1988, **34**, 54-59.

42. A. Lombet, C. Mourre and M. Ladzunski, *Brain Res.*, 1988, **459**, 44.

43. N. Zilberberg, E. Zlotkin and M. Gurevitz, *Insect Biochem. Molec. Biol.*, 1992, **22**, 199.

44. N. Zilberberg, E. Zlotkin and M. Gurevitz, *Toxicon*, 1991, **29**, 1155.

45. M. Turkov, S. Rashi, N. Zilberberg, D. Gordon, R. Benkhalifa, M. Stankiewicz, M. Pelhate and M. Gurevitz, *Prot. Express. Purific.*, 1997, **10**, 123.

46. O. Froy, N. Zilberberg, M. Turkov, D. Gordon, M. Stankiewicz, M. Pelhate, E. Loret, D. E. Oren, B. Shaanan and M. Gurevitz, 1998, Submitted.

47. S. Maeda, S. L. Volrath, T. N. Hanzlik, S. A. Harper, K. Majuma, D. W. Maddox, B. D. Hammock and E. Fowler, *Virology*, 1991, **164**, 777.

48. L. M. D. Stewart, M. Hirst, M. L. Ferber, A. T. Merryweather, P. J. Cayley and R. D. Possee, *Nature*, 1991, **352**, 85.

49. M. D. Tomalski and L. K. Miller, *Nature*, 1991, **352**, 82.

50. B. F. McCutchen, P. V. Choudary, R. Crenshaw, D. Maddox, S. G. Kamita, N. Palekar, S. Volrath, E. Fowler, B. D. S. Hammock and S. Maeda, *Bio/Technology*, 1991, **9**, 848.

51. N. Chejanovsky, N. Zilberberg, H. Rivkin, E. Zlotkin and M. Gurevitz, *FEBS Lett.*, 1995, **376**, 181-184.

52. E. Gershburg, D. Stockholm, O. Froy, S. Rashi, M. Gurevitz and N. Chejanovsky, *FEBS Lett.*, 1998, **422**, 132.

53. V. S. Pashkov, V. N. Maiorov, V. F. Bystrov, A. N. Hoang, T. M. Volkova and E. V. Grishin, *Biophys. Chem.*, 1988, **31**, 121-131.

54. D. Housset, C. Habersetzer-Rochat, J. P. Astier and J. C. Fontecilla-Camps, *J. Mol. Biol.*, 1994, **238**, 88.

55. C. Landon, B. Cornet, J. M. Bonmatin, C. Kopeyan, H. Rochat, F. Vovelle and M. Ptak, *Eur. J. Biochem.*, 1996, **236**, 395.

56. V. Tugarinov, I. Kustanovich, N. Zilberberg, M. Gurevitz and J. Anglister, *Biochemistry*, 1997, **36**, 2414.

57. F. Sampieri and C. Habersetzer-Rochat, *Biochim. Biophys. Acta*, 1978, **535**, 100.

58. H. Darbon, E. Jover, F. Couraud and H. Rochat, *Int. J. Pept. Prot. Res.*, 1983, **22**, 179.

59. M. El Ayeb, E. M. Bahraoui, C. Granier and H. Rochat, *Biochemistry*, 1986, **25**, 6671.

60. M. El Ayeb, H. Darbon, E. M. Bahraoui, O. Vargas and H. Rochat, *Eur. J. Biochem.*, 1986, **155**, 289.

61. N. Zilberberg, O. Froy, D. Gordon, E. Loret, D. Arad and M. Gurevitz, *J. Biol. Chem.*, 1997, **272**, 14810.

62. D. Strugatsky, N. Zilberberg, M. Turkov, E. Loret, D. Gordon, M. Stankiewicz, M. Pelhate and M. Gurevitz, Submitted.

63. D. Lee, M. Gurevitz and M. E. Adams, 1998, Submitted.

Agonist-specific Coupling of G-Protein Coupled Receptors to Multiple Second Messenger Systems

P.D. Evans, V. Reale, J.E. Rudling and K. Kennedy

THE BABRAHAM INSTITUTE, LABORATORY OF MOLECULAR SIGNALLING, DEPARTMENT OF ZOOLOGY, UNIVERSITY OF CAMBRIDGE, DOWNING STREET, CAMBRIDGE CB2 3EJ, UK

1 INTRODUCTION

The phenomenon of "agonist-specific coupling" [1,2] (also called "agonist trafficking" [3]) challenges our currently established concepts of receptor pharmacology, since it appears that many G-protein coupled receptors may exhibit different pharmacological profiles depending upon which second messenger systems are used to assess them. It is proposed that the binding of different agonists to these receptors can result in different conformational changes in the structure of the receptor which favour its interactions with different G-proteins. This can be seen as a development of both the extended ternary complex[4] and the multistate allosteric[5] models for receptor conformation. In the former model the number of conformational states of the receptor is defined, whereas in the latter it is proposed that there can be an infinite number of states which the receptor can oscillate between, only some of which are capable of activating G-proteins. In agonist-specific coupling the receptor would adopt different conformations either as a result of the induced fit between an agonist and the receptor, or as a result of the agonist stabilizing a particular conformation spontaneously adopted by the receptor. These different agonist promoted conformations would then couple the receptor preferentially to specific second messenger pathways.

The most compelling evidence in support of this phenomenon comes from studies where structurally related agonists for a given receptor show a reversed potency for different second messenger pathways. Thus, a cloned *Drosophila* octopamine/tyramine receptor has been shown to be differentially activated by the biogenic amine, octopamine, and its immediate metabolic precursor, tyramine, which are both naturally occurring biogenic amines within the insect nervous system.[1] Equally, a cloned vertebrate pituitary adenylyl cyclase activating peptide (PACAP) type 1 receptor shows a reversed second messenger potency for its two endogenous ligands PACAP-27 and PACAP-38.[6] Evidence has also been presented for a similar phenomenon mediated by synthetic agonists for a range of other G-protein coupled receptors from vertebrates, including the α_{2A}-adrenergic,[7] muscarinic,[8] prostaglandin E,[9] 5-HT$_{1C}$[10] and 5-HT$_{2A}$[11] receptors and also a cloned *Drosophila* D1-like receptor.[12] In the latter cases where the phenomenon has only been demonstrated in response to synthetic agonists, it is more difficult currently to speculate about the functional significance of the observed effects. However, it may indicate that there are other endogenous agonists yet to be discovered for these receptors, in addition to their well known classical endogenous activators.

2 INVERTEBRATE G-PROTEIN COUPLED RECEPTORS

2.1 The *Drosophila* Octopamine/Tyramine Receptor

A biogenic amine activated G-protein coupled receptor has been cloned from the *Drosophila* central nervous system and shown to be activated by both octopamine[13] and its naturally occurring immediate metabolic precursor, tyramine.[14]   In binding studies with the α_2-adrenergic antagonist, [³H]-yohimbine, which binds to this receptor, membrane preparations made from a range of vertebrate clonal cell lines expressing this receptor showed a higher affinity for tyramine than for octopamine.[1,14]   This suggested the possibility that this receptor was actually a receptor for tyramine rather than octopamine, since evidence has been presented to suggest that a separate tyraminergic modulatory system (see refs 15,16) may exist in insects alongside the more well established octopaminergic system.[17,18]   However, when studies were carried out on the ability of this receptor to couple to different second messenger systems when expressed in Chinese Hamster Ovary (CHO) cells, it was found that the receptor could be coupled both to an inhibition of adenylyl cyclase activity and to the generation of an intracellular Ca^{2+} signal due to the release of Ca^{2+} from intracellular stores, by separate G-protein coupled pathways.[1,19]   The coupling of the receptor to the inhibition of adenylyl cyclase activity was found to be pertussis toxin-sensitive, whereas its coupling to the generation of the intracellular calcium signal was pertussis toxin-insensitive.[1]   When the relative abilities of tyramine and octopamine to activate these two second messenger systems were compared, tyramine was almost two orders of magnitude more potent than octopamine at inhibiting adenylyl cyclase activity, in line with the results obtained in the binding studies with [³H]-yohimbine (Fig. 1).   However, surprisingly, octopamine was equipotent with tyramine at generating Ca^{2+} signals when the peak Ca^{2+} response was measured (Fig. 1) and was almost an order of magnitude more potent than tyramine when kinetic parameters of the response, such as time to peak for the signal and lag time to a response were considered.[1]   Thus, the two endogenously occurring biogenic amines, octopamine and tyramine, which differ structurally by only the presence of a single hydroxyl group on the β-carbon of the side chain of octopamine, can differentially couple this receptor to different second messenger systems when it is expressed in CHO cells.

The above observations have several important implications in terms of insect neurobiology.   It is not clear whether this particular *Drosophila* receptor is primarily an octopamine or a tyramine receptor.   The possibility exists that it could be a multifunctional receptor depending upon its location in the insect nervous system and on whether it is exposed locally to neuronally released octopamine or tyramine.   It might then function as an octopamine receptor in some locations and as a tyramine receptor in others.   Alternatively, it could be involved in a novel form of modulation whereby its responses to octopamine could be modified depending upon how much of its precursor molecule tyramine is co-released with it from octopaminergic neurones.

2.2 Cellular specificity

It is also possible that the ability of the *Drosophila* octopamine/tyramine receptor to be coupled differentially to different second messenger systems by different agonists could be influenced by cell specific factors, such as their local G-protein environments. Indeed, an extension of this idea could be the possibility that agents that alter the expression levels of specific G-proteins in neurones might switch the second messenger

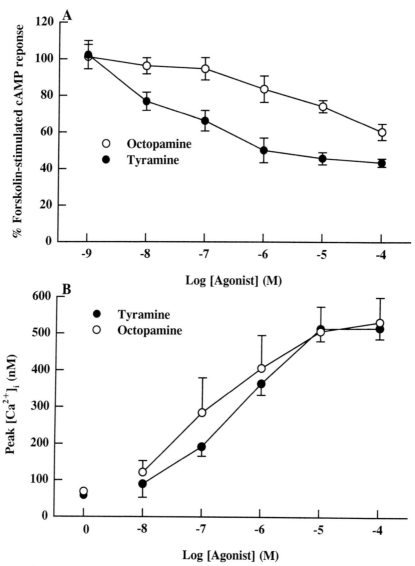

Figure 1 *(A) The effects of (±)-para-octopamine and para-tyramine on cyclic AMP production in Chinese Hamster Ovary cells stably expressing the cloned Drosophila octopamine/tyramine receptor. Both amines cause a dose-dependent inhibition of cyclic AMP production. Data represent mean ± S.E. , n≥3. (B) Dose response plots for the effects of (±)-para-octopamine and para-tyramine on peak intracellular Ca^{2+} levels in Chinese Hamster Ovary cells stably expressing the cloned Drosophila octopamine/tyramine receptor. Data represent mean ± S.E. of values obtained from at least 25 individual cells. (Modified from Ref 1).*

coupling responses of a single cell. To begin to explore these possibilities we have started to express the cloned *Drosophila* octopamine/tyramine receptor in a range of other cellular environments, including *Xenopus* oocytes.[16]

When *Xenopus* oocytes expressing the *Drosophila* octopamine/tyramine receptor are exposed to either octopamine or tyramine, they respond with the generation of oscillatory currents superimposed upon a maintained inward current. These currents are due to the receptor mediated release of Ca^{2+} from intracellular stores which activates the endogenous inward Ca^{2+}-dependent chloride current of the oocyte. Octopamine and tyramine are equipotent at generating these responses, having the same thresholds for activation of between 10^{-8} and 10^{-9} M, and the same maximal responses at 10^{-4} M. However, if we examine the ability of the biogenic amines to alter oocyte cyclic AMP levels, we find that neither octopamine nor tyramine are capable of changing cyclic AMP levels in the oocytes expressing this receptor. This contrasts with oocyte experiments in which a vertebrate β-adrenergic receptor is expressed and where the β-adrenergic agonist isoproterenol induces a substantial increase in oocyte cyclic AMP levels. However, if the *Drosophila* octopamine/tyramine receptor is coexpressed with the vertebrate β-adrenergic receptor in the same oocytes, neither tyramine nor octopamine can reduce the isoproterenol-mediated increases in oocyte cyclic AMP levels. In fact, both biogenic amines actually potentiate the isoproterenol-induced elevations in cyclic AMP levels by a Ca^{2+}-dependent effect that can be blocked by the Ca^{2+} buffering agent BAPTA.[16]

Thus, it appears that the *Drosophila* octopamine/tyramine receptor when expressed in *Xenopus* oocytes, is not capable of expressing the phenomenon of agonist-specific coupling. It seems likely that this is due to the specific inability of the receptor to couple to a G-protein pathway capable of inhibiting adenylyl cyclase activity in the oocyte rather than to the absence of the signalling components for this pathway in the oocyte. This idea is supported by the observation that other receptors, such as vertebrate pituitary somatostatin receptors[20] and δ-opioid receptors,[21] can reduce β-adrenergic-stimulated cyclic AMP levels when expressed in *Xenopus* oocytes via an interaction with G_i-like G-proteins. However, current thinking in the field of cellular specificity of second messenger responses indicates that the presence or absence of other cellular components, such as specific scaffolding proteins necessary for the formation of "transducisome" complexes[22] could also underlie such a cellular specificity of signalling responses. A wide range of scaffolding proteins, such as the 14-3-3 proteins, the PDZ domain proteins and those found in the caveolar complex, are currently being proposed to function as binding sites for specific receptors, G-proteins and effector molecules to produce functional signalling complexes.[22-24] It will be of much interest to see if the lack of one or more scaffolding proteins could underlie the absence of agonist-specific coupling by the cloned *Drosophila* octopamine/tyramine receptor when expressed in *Xenopus* oocytes.

2.2 The *Drosophila* Dopamine D1-like Receptor

In terms of the cellular specificity of the phenomenon of agonist-specific coupling it is interesting to note that a recently cloned *Drosophila* D1-like dopamine receptor (DopR99B) does show this phenomenon, at least for synthetic agonists, when expressed in *Xenopus* oocytes.[12,25] This receptor is unusual in that it groups structurally with the *Drosophila* octopamine/tyramine receptor in dendrograms and also lies very close to it on the right arm of *Drosophila* chromosome 3. This contrasts with a previously cloned *Drosophila* D1-like dopamine receptor[26,27] which groups structurally with vertebrate D1-

like dopamine receptors and has a different chromosome location.

When expressed in *Xenopus* oocytes, activation of the DopR99B receptor leads to a time-dependent and dose-dependent increase in cyclic AMP levels. However, it also leads to the generation of large inward currents due to the activation of the endogenous oocyte Ca^{2+}-dependent chloride current due to a receptor-mediated Ca^{2+} release from intracellular stores. These two second messenger pathways are again activated by separate G-protein coupled pathways. The buffering of internal oocyte Ca^{2+} levels with BAPTA leads to an almost complete inhibition of the inward current response to dopamine, whilst the cyclic AMP responses are unaltered. Conversely, pretreatment of the oocytes with pertussis toxin, which selectively blocks signalling through G_i or G_o mediated pathways, abolishes the dopamine-mediated cyclic AMP responses but not the receptor-mediated Ca^{2+} release effects. This suggests that the elevation of cyclic AMP levels in oocytes expressing the DopR99B receptor is unusual in that it appears to be mediated by pertussis sensitive G-proteins. However, this response is also blocked selectively and dose-dependently by the injection of a fragment of β-adrenergic receptor kinase which binds $\beta\gamma$-subunits of G-proteins.[28] This suggests that the observations can be explained by $\beta\gamma$-subunits, released from pertussis toxin sensitive G-proteins, activating particular isoforms of adenylyl cyclase in the oocytes. Previous studies in other cell types have shown a $G_{\beta\gamma}$-subunit-mediated stimulation of the type II and type IV forms of adenylyl cyclase activity.[29]

In pharmacological terms, both second messenger effects mediated by this receptor show a similar profile for activation by endogenously occurring catecholamines with a rank order of potency of dopamine > noradrenaline > adrenaline > tyramine. Both responses also showed a similar potency ratio for a range of synthetic agonists. Surprisingly, however, there were differences in the rank order of potency for a range of synthetic agonists on the activation of the two second messenger pathways (see Table 1). Compounds such as the D1-like dopamine agonists, Chloro-APB and Bromo-APB, were very effective agonists of the inward current responses, but produced no cyclic AMP responses. Conversely, a D2-like dopamine agonist, ($\pm$)-PPHT, produced increases in cyclic AMP levels whilst having no effects on inward currents.

Thus, the *Drosophila*, D1-like dopamine receptor, DopR99B, like a range of vertebrate G-protein coupled receptors, also shows agonist-specific coupling for a range of synthetic agonists. The physiological significance of these observations is unclear at the present time but they suggest the possibility that other endogenous agonists, besides dopamine, may exist for this receptor.

3 VERTEBRATE G-PROTEIN COUPLED RECEPTORS

It is clear that the phenomenon of agonist-specific coupling is not confined to invertebrate G-protein coupled receptors since, as mentioned above, it has been observed for the endogenously occurring forms of the neuropeptide PACAP on its Type 1 receptor and for a range of such vertebrate receptors with synthetic agonists. Of particular interest from a pesticide neurotoxicological point of view, is the fact that a cloned human α_{2A}-adrenergic receptor that has previously been shown to exhibit this phenomenon for synthetic agonists,[7] may also show this effect when the actions of noradrenaline are compared with those of some of its naturally occurring structural homologues, such as *meta*-octopamine.[30] Octopamine occurs naturally in the sympathetic nervous system of vertebrates at concentrations in the range of 0.1 to 0.01 times those of noradrenaline and

Table 1 *Effects of agonists on inward currents and cAMP responses initiated in Xenopus oocytes expressing the Drosophila DopR99B receptor*

Agonists (10 μM)	% of inward current response to 1 μM Dopamine (n)		% of cAMP response to 10μM Dopamine (n)	Receptor Type Specificity
($\pm$)-6-Chloro-APB	89.4$\pm$3.8%	(6)	1.9$\pm$1.2% (10)	D1-like
R(+)-6-Bromo-APB	73.3$\pm$9.1%	(6)	3.7$\pm$2.9% (10)	D1-like
($\pm$)-6-Chloro-PB	19.6$\pm$7.7%	(5)	13.0$\pm$7.6% (10)	D1-like
Quinelorane	11.3$\pm$3.0%	(8)	3.2$\pm$2.1% (10)	D2-like
($\pm$)-Bromo-criptine	7.5$\pm$2.6%	(5)	4.3$\pm$1.6% (10)	D2-like
Quinpirole	4.1$\pm$2.3%	(6)	2.0$\pm$0.8% (10)	D2/D3
R(+)-SKF-38393	1.8$\pm$1.2%	(6)	5.3$\pm$1.5% (10)	D1-like
($\pm$) Isoproterenol	1.3$\pm$0.9%	(6)	3.5$\pm$1.5% (10)	β-adrenergic
PD-128,907	0	(6)	1.3$\pm$0.9% (10)	D3
($\pm$)-PPHT	0	(4)	16.1$\pm$6.5% (10)	D2-like

The size of the inward current response to a 2 min pulse of agonist is expressed as a percentage $\pm$ SE of the response to a 2 min control dopamine pulse given to the same oocyte. The mean response to a 2 min control pulse of 1 μM dopamine was 331.4 $\pm$ 15.6 nA (n=73).

The size of the cAMP response to a 30 min exposure to 10 μM agonist in the presence of 100 μM IBMX after a 30min preincubation in the presence of 100 μM IBMX alone is expressed as a percentage $\pm$ SE of the response to a control dopamine exposure. The mean response to a 30 min control exposure to 10 μM dopamine was an increase of 2.57 $\pm$ 0.42 pmoles cAMP/oocyte.

All measurements were made 5 d after injection of oocytes with DopR99B cRNA

(Data reproduced from Ref 12)

it is co-released with noradrenaline upon sympathetic nerve stimulation.[31,32] In the majority of cases that have been examined, the sympathetically released octopamine has only been shown to be a weak agonist of α-adrenergic receptors and has been assumed to have the same spectrum of actions as noradrenaline.[33] However, recent evidence suggests that there may be differences in the second messenger pathways activated by a cloned human α_{2A}-adrenergic receptor expressed in CHO cells when activated by *meta*-octopamine or (-)-noradrenaline.[30] These two agonists differ structurally by only the presence of an extra hydroxyl group at the *para*-position on the catecholamine ring of noradrenaline. Thus, noradrenaline can couple the receptor in a dose-dependent fashion to both an inhibition and to a stimulation of adenylyl cyclase activity. The coupling to the stimulation of adenylyl cyclase activity can be clearly seen after the inhibition of the inhibitory G-protein coupled pathway by pretreatment of the cells expressing this receptor with pertussis toxin. Conversely, *meta*-octopamine specifically couples the receptor only to an inhibition of adenylyl cyclase activity (Fig. 2).[30]

We have also compared the effect of substitution of the Ser[200] and Ser[204] residues of the cloned human α_{2A}-adrenergic receptor with alanine, on the abilities of (-)-noradrenaline and (±)-*meta*-and (±)-*para*-octopamine to couple the receptor expressed in CHO cells to G-protein linked second messenger pathways mediating either an increase or a decrease in cyclic AMP levels. The results are consistent with a role for Ser[204] of the human α_{2A}-adrenergic receptor in receptor activation through an interaction with the *para*-hydroxyl of the catecholamine ring of adrenergic ligands. They also emphasise the importance of both the Ser[200] and Ser[204] residues of the receptor in exerting an inhibitory influence on the ability of (±)-*para*-octopamine and (±)-*meta*-octopamine respectively, to induce a receptor-agonist conformation capable of inhibiting forskolin-stimulation of cyclic AMP levels, irrespective of whether Ser[200] is directly involved in the binding of the *meta*-hydroxyl on the catecholamine ring of adrenergic ligands. Such site-directed mutagenesis studies also indicate the importance of Ser[204] in TMV of the human α_{2A}-adrenergic receptor in the prevention of *meta*-octopamine from generating a receptor-agonist conformation that can increase cyclic AMP levels. This emphasises the importance of this receptor residue in the agonist-specific coupling of the receptor to different second messenger pathways.[34]

Activation of the human α_{2A}-adrenergic receptor by octopamine is likely to be particularly important under conditions such as hepatic and renal encephalopathy, where the circulating levels of octopamine are substantially increased[35,36] and approach the concentrations at which (-)-*meta*-octopamine has been shown to be effective at inhibiting cyclic AMP production.[30] Such levels are also in excess of the threshold concentrations for the effectiveness of octopamine stereoisomers on α-adrenergic receptors in a number of whole tissue preparations.[32] Thus, it is possible to predict that interactions between circulating catecholamines and octopamines, both at the receptor-agonist binding and intracellular transduction levels, may determine the final cellular response to human α_{2A}-adrenergic receptor activation *in vivo*. In addition, the ability of octopamine to couple the receptor selectively to the inhibition of cyclic AMP production, suggests a possible modulatory role for these compounds through the activation of α-adrenergic receptors. This mode of action may explain why specific octopamine receptors have not been identified to date, despite the presence and capacity for neurosecretion of octopamine, in vertebrate nervous systems.

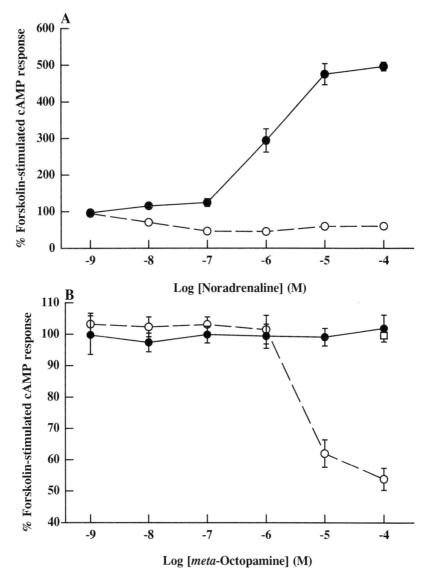

Figure 2 *The effects of (-)-noradrenaline (**A**) and (±)-meta-octopamine (**B**) on cyclic AMP production in Chinese Hamster Ovary cells stably expressing the cloned human α_{2A}-adrenergic receptor. (**A**) In the absence of pertussis toxin (PTX) pretreatment (open symbols), (-)-noradrenaline caused inhibition of cyclic AMP production, while pretreatment with PTX (filled symbols) revealed a dramatic stimulation of cyclic AMP production. (**B**) (±)-meta-octopamine caused a dose-dependent inhibition of cyclic AMP production in the absence of PTX pretreatment (open symbols); pretreatment with PTX (filled symbols) abolished inhibition of cyclic AMP production, but failed to reveal stimulation of cyclic AMP production. The α_2-adrenergic antagonist, rauwolscine (□), abolished octopamine-sensitive inhibition of cyclic AMP production in the absence of PTX pretreatment. Data represent mean±S.E., n=4 (**A**), n≥6 (**B**). (Modified from Ref 29).*

4 CONCLUSIONS

In general terms the phenomenon of agonist-specific coupling of G-protein coupled receptors to different second messenger systems means that a single receptor could have different pharmacological profiles depending upon which second messenger is used to assay it. In addition, in different parts of the nervous system the same receptor could have different pharmacological profiles depending on the G-protein environment of the cell or on the availability of specific scaffolding proteins required for the establishment of different transducisome signalling complexes specific for linking receptor activation to particular second messenger pathways.

In practical terms, the phenomenon could lead to the development of highly specific drugs that could couple receptors specifically to beneficial second messenger pathways and not to those that generate unwanted side effects. Equally, it is conceivable that highly potent novel insect control agents could be developed that again specifically couple target receptors to the activation of second messenger pathways that maximally disrupt insect central nervous system function and thus lead to a maximal crop protective effect. Finally, the demonstration of agonist-specific coupling of human α_{2A}-adrenergic receptors to specific second messenger pathways by *meta*-octopamine has obvious implications for the neurotoxicology of any novel insect control agents designed to exert their actions via the activation of insect octopaminergic receptors.

An understanding of the precise molecular mechanisms underlying the phenomenon of "agonist-specific coupling" of various G-protein coupled receptors to different second messenger systems will undoubtedly require structural studies based on the crystallization of specific receptors in the presence and absence of various agonists. Such studies will, hopefully, allow us to understand how different agonist-receptor conformations bias the coupling abilities of the receptors to different G-proteins. However, even such studies based on molecular snapshots will not allow us to distinguish between a specific agonist-induced conformation of a receptor and an agonist stabilization of a particular conformation spontaneously adopted by the receptor.

5 REFERENCES

1. S. Robb, T. R. Cheek, F. L. Hannan, L.M. Hall, J. M. Midgley and P. D. Evans, *EMBO J.*, 1994, **13**, 1325.
2. P. D. Evans, S. Robb, T. R. Cheek, V. Reale, F. L. Hannan, L. S. Swales, L. M. Hall and J. M. Midgley, *Prog. Brain Res.*, 1995, **106**, 159.
3. T. Kenakin, *Trends Pharmacol. Sci.*, **16**, 232.
4. P. Samama and R. J. Lefkowitz, 1997, "α_{2A}-adrenergic receptors: Structure, Function and Therapeutic Implications", Eds. S. M. Lanier and L. E. Limbird, Harwood Academic Publishers, Amsterdam, 1997, p.77.
5. U. Gether, S. Lin and B. K. Kobilka, 1997, "α_{2A}-adrenergic receptors: Structure, Function and Therapeutic Implications", Eds. S. M. Lanier and L. E. Limbird, Harwood Academic Publishers, Amsterdam, 1997, p.31.
6. D. Spengler, C. Waeber, C. Pantaloni, F. Holsboer, J. Bockaert and P. H. Seeburg, 1993, *Nature*, **365**, 170.
7. M. G. Eason, M. T. Jacinto and S. B. Liggett, 1994, *Mol. Pharmacol.*, **45**, 696.
8. D. Gurwitz, H. Haring, E. Heldman, C. M. Fraser, D. Manor and A. Fisher, 1994, *Eur. J. Pharmacol.*, **267**, 21.

9. M. Negishi, A. Irie, Y. Sugimoto, T. Namba and A. Ichikawa, 1995, *J. Biol. Chem.*, **270**, 16122.

10. K. A. Berg, S. Maayani and W. P. Clarke, 1995, *Soc. Neurosci. Abstr.*, **21**, 1365.

11. K. A. Berg, E. D. Loh, J. D. Cropper, S. Maayani and W. P. Clarke, 1996, *Soc. Neurosci. Abstr.*, **22**, 1777.

12. V. Reale, F. Hannan, L. M. Hall and P. D. Evans, 1997, *J. Neurosci.*, **17**, 6545.

13. S. Arakawa, J. D. Gocayne, W. R. McCombie, D. A. Urquhart, L. M. Hall, C. M. Fraser and J. C. Venter, 1990, *Neuron*, **4**, 343.

14. F. Saudou, N. Amlaiky, J. -L. Plassat, E. Borrelli and R. Hen, 1990, *EMBO J.*, **9**, 3611.

15. T. Roeder, 1994, *Comp. Biochem. Physiol.*, **107C**, 1.

16. V. Reale, F. Hannan, J. M. Midgley and P. D. Evans, 1997, *Brain Res.*, **769**, 309.

17. P. D. Evans, "Comprehensive Insect Physiology, Biochemistry and Pharmacology", Eds. G. A. Kerkut and L. I. Gilbert, Pergamon Press, Oxford, 1985, Vol. 11, p.499.

18. P. D. Evans, "Comparative Molecular Neurobiology", Ed. Y. Pichon, Birkhäuser Verlag, Basel, 1993, p.286.

19. S. Robb, T. R. Cheek, J. C. Venter, J. M. Midgley and P. D. Evans, 1991, *Pest. Sci.*, **32**, 369.

20. M. M. White and T. Reisine, 1990, *Proc. Natl. Acad. Sci. USA*, **87**, 133.

21. M. Tamir and L. Kushner, 1993, *Biochem. Res. Commun.*, **193**, 1224.

22. S. Tsunoda, J. Sierralta, Y. Sun, R. Bodner, E. Suzuki, A. Becker, M. Socolich and C. S. Zuker, 1997, *Nature*, **388**, 243.

23. J. M. Anderson, 1996, *Current Biology*, **6**, 382.

24. W. F. C. de Weerd and L. M. F. Leeb-Lundberg, 1997, *J. Biol. Chem.*, **272**, 17858.

25. G. Feng, F. Hannan, V. Reale, Y. Y. Hon, C. T. Kousky, P. D. Evans and L. M. Hall, 1996, *J. Neurosci.*, **16**, 3925.

26. F. Gotzes, S. Balfanz and A. Baumann, 1994, *Receptors and Channels*, **2**, 131.

27. K. S. Sugamori, L. L. Demchyshyn, F. McConkey, M. A. Forte and H. B. Niznik, 1995, *FEBS Lett.*, **362**, 131.

28. W. J. Koch, B. E. Hawes, J. Inglese, L. M. Luttrell and R. J. Lefkowitz, 1994, *J. Biol. Chem.*, **269**, 6193.

29. D. M. F. Cooper, N. Mons and J. W. Karpen, 1995, *Nature*, **374**, 421.

30. C. N. Airriess, J. E. Rudling, J. M. Midgley and P. D. Evans, 1997, *Brit. J. Pharmacol.*, **122**, 191.

31. K. E. Ibrahim, M. W. Couch, C. M. Williams, M. J. Fregly and J. M. Midgley, 1985, *J. Neurochem.*, **44**, 1862.

32. C. M. Williams, M. W. Couch, C. M. Thonoor and J. M. Midgley, 1987, *J. Pharm. Pharmacol.*, **39**, 153.

33. C. M. Brown, J. C. McGrath, J. M. Midgley, A. G. B. Muir, J. W. O'Brien, C. M. Thonoor, C. M. Williams and V. G. Wilson, 1988, *Brit. J. Pharmacol.*, **93**, 417.

34. J. E. Rudling, C. N. Airriess and P. D. Evans, 1997, *Soc. Neurosci. Abstr.*, **23**, 2323.

35. D. W. Kinniburgh and N. D. Boyd, 1979, *Clin. Biochem.*, **12**, 27.

36. H. Hörtnagl, H. Lochs, G. Kleinberger, J. M. Hackl, A. F. Hammerle, H. Binder and F. Wewalka, 1981, *Klin. Wochenschr.*, **59**, 1159.

Physiological and Pharmacological Studies Using *Ascaris suum* and *Ascaridia galli* Muscle Preparations

R.J. Walker, N. Trim, J. Brooman, D.J.A. Brownlee, C.J. Franks, Z.A. Bascal and L. Holden-Dye

SCHOOL OF BIOLOGICAL SCIENCES, UNIVERSITY OF SOUTHAMPTON, BASSETT CRESCENT EAST, SOUTHAMPTON SO16 7PX, UK

Over the past ten to twelve years there has been increasing interest in the search for new anthelmintics which is linked to an increase in resistance to existing compounds. To assist in the development of novel target sites, the basic physiology and pharmacology of the nervous and muscle systems have been analysed. In our studies we have mainly used *Ascaris suum* as the test species but in some experiments we have also used *Ascaridia galli* for comparison. For the experiments using somatic body wall muscle, both tension recordings using muscle strips and intracellular recordings from muscle cells have been made.

1.1 Acetylcholine and GABA

The classical transmitters at the somatic body wall muscle system are acetylcholine (ACh) and gamma-aminobutyric acid (GABA) which act as excitatory and inhibitory transmitters respectively. The pharmacological profiles of these receptors have been investigated and summarised. (1) Briefly the ACh receptor of *A. suum* resembles the mammalian neuronal nicotinic receptor where ganglionic agonists are most potent while some muscarinic agonists induce weak hyperpolarization. The most potent antagonists are benzoquinonium, a neuromuscular blocker, and mecamylamine, a ganglion blocker. Histrionicotoxin, neosurugatoxin and N-methyl-lycaconitine, are other potent antagonists with IC-50 values in the range 0.17 - 0.65 μM. Interestingly two other neuronal or ganglionic blockers, hexamethonium and dihydro-β-erythroidine, were either inactive or possessed a very low potency.

The GABA *A. suum* receptor is activated by agonists which are active at the mammalian GABA-A receptor, for example, (S)-(+)-dihydromuscimol and ZAPA ((Z)-3-[(aminoiminomethyl)-thio]-2-propenoic acid hydrochloride) are more potent than GABA while muscimol is slightly less potent. There is a good correlation between the potency of agonists at the *Ascaris* GABA receptor and their affinity for binding at the mammalian GABA-A receptor. In terms of antagonist profile, the *Ascaris* GABA receptor and the mammalian GABA-A receptor, are very different. For example, bicuculline is inactive while picrotoxin has a very low potency at the *Ascaris* GABA receptor. However a series of azole derivatives, for example, SN606078, 2-(2,6-dichloro-4-trifluoromethylphenyl)-4-(4,5-dicyano-1H-imidazol-2-yl)-2H-1,2,3-triazole, did show clear antagonism at the *Ascaris* GABA receptor in the low μM range, with IC-50 values of 5.5μM. (2) This compound may act as an open channel blocker of the GABA-gated chloride channel in *A.suum*.

Another compound which blocks the *Ascaris* GABA receptor is the anthelmintic ivermectin but the IC-50 for this block is relatively high, ie, 8.86 μM, and so it is unlikely that ivermectin exerts its anthelmintic effect at this site.

GABA also has an inhibitory effect on pharyngeal pumping in *A. suum*. (3) GABA exerts this effect in the range 1 - 1000 μM, with an IC-50 of 23 μM, and the duration of this inhibition is concentration-dependent. Glutamate has a similar inhibitory effect but is less potent with an IC-50 value of 491 μM. Interestingly following the perfusion of low concentration of ivermectin (1 pM), which have no direct effect, the threshold for inhibition for both GABA and glutamate are enhanced at least ten fold. High concentrations of ivermectin (1μM) have a direct inhibitory action on pharyngeal pumping. High concentrations of picrotoxin (500 - 1000 μM) reduce the response to both GABA and glutamate. The observation that pM ivermectin can enhance the inhibitory effect of both GABA and glutamate on pharyngeal pumping suggests that this anthelmintic may exert its primary effect at this site. Cessation of pharyngeal pumping would mean that *A. suum* can no longer feed.

1.2 5-Hydroxytryptamine (5-HT)

In addition to ACh and GABA there is good evidence that 5-HT plays a key physiological role in *A. suum*. 5-HT can modulate the excitatory action of ACh on body wall muscle. (5) For example, 5-HT (1000 μM) can reduce the tension increase induced by the response to 30 μM ACh. This action of 5-HT can be reversed following washing. Little is known regarding the mechanism of action of 5-HT on ACh excitation though 5-HT does increase basal cAMP levels in somatic muscle of *A. suum* and this effect is concentration-dependent in the range 100 - 1000 μM. Interestingly dopamine (10 μM) also increases basal levels of cAMP in this tissue.

5-HT has a direct excitatory action on the pharyngeal muscle of *A. suum*. An isolated muscle preparation has been developed to investigate the physiology and pharmacology of this muscle. (6) The threshold for this 5-HT effect is 10 μM with a maximal stimulatory effect at around 1000 μM. Tryptamine, 8-OH DPAT, sumatriptan and 5-carboxyamido-tryptamine all failed to stimulate pharyngeal pumping, though the 5-HT$_2$ antagonist, ketanserin, did block the action of 5-HT. Interestingly 5-HT had no effect on basal levels of cAMP in this muscle. 5-HT has been identified in neurones in the enteric nervous system which innervates the pharyngeal muscle (7,8) and so is very likely to play a major role in the normal physiology of pharyngeal pumping.

1.3 Nitric Oxide (NO)

As with other invertebrate phyla, there is evidence, using NADPH diaphorase stain as a marker, that NO may play a physiological role in many tissues. Positive staining for NADPH diaphorase has been demonstrated in the nerve cord and somatic muscle of *A. suum*. (9) Neurones that stain for NADPH diaphorase also show positive immunoreactivity for RFamides. (10) Biochemical studies provide further evidence in that *A. suum* nerve cord can synthesise citrulline from arginine when co-factors including NADPH, calcium, calmodulin, H$_4$B, flavin adenine dinucleotide (FAD) and flavin mononucleotide (FMN) are present. When NO donors are applied to *A. suum* body wall muscle strips, there is surprisingly an increase in basal tone with a decrease in amplitude of ACh-induced muscle contractions. However further studies are required before a role for NO in nematodes can be established.

1.4 Neuroactive Peptides

Immunocytochemical studies using antibodies raised against mammalian neuropeptides first suggested that similar peptides may be present in *A. suum*. These studies have suggested the presence of a number of mammalian peptide families in nematodes but to date only one family has been identified and members sequenced, the RFamide family. (11, 12) This family was first identified in a mollusc but is likely to occur in most if not all phyla, including chordates. (13) To date at least 18 RFamides have ben identified in *A. suum* with three additional RFamides in *Panagrellus redivivus*. 18 genes have been identified in *Caenorhabditis elegans* which are responsible for a number of additional RFamides. (14) This represents a formidable number of peptides, all presumably with a physiological role in nematodes. It is as yet unclear the extent to which individual RFamides occur in all nematode species or are restricted to a group or even to a single species. Far more work is required on a range of nematodes before a pattern can emerge though it would appear that AF-2 probably occurs widely through the phylum. (15) A list of the peptides identified in *A. suum* and *P. redivivus* is given in Table 1.

1.5 Effect of AF-1 and AF-2 on body wall muscle

Both AF-1 and AF-2 are excitatory on *A. suum* body wall muscle, increasing muscle tone in both cases, though the latter also has an inhibitory component. (16) The inhibitory, relaxing, phase is brief and precedes the excitatory effect but is not always observed. The excitatory actions of AF-2 have been studied in detail, using the body wall muscle of *A. suum*, where it enhances the frequency and amplitude of spontaneous contractions. These actions can be long lasting, for example, in excess of an hour. The threshold for this response is around 10 nM. AF-2, 100 nM, also potentiates ACh-induced contractions and excitatory junction potentials (ejps) recorded in the muscle. In the presence of 100 nM, AF-2, the threshold at which ejps are elicited is greatly reduced. With intracellular recording, AF-2 did not potentiate muscle cell depolarizations produced by ACh but did induce spontaneous muscle cell action potentials in quiescent cells. Overall the evidence suggests that AF-2 possesses both pre- and postsynaptic actions on this nerve muscle preparation. AF-2 also increases phasic activity in body wall muscles of *A. galli*.

1.6 Effects of AF-3 and AF-4 on body wall muscle

The actions of AF-3 and AF-4 have been examined on the body wall muscle of both *A. suum* and *A. galli*. (17) Both peptides contract *A. suum* muscle with EC-50 values of 24 nM and 37 nM, respectively, for AF-3 and AF-4. These peptides are considerably more potent than ACh which has an EC-50 value of 13 μM. Intracellular recording from muscle cells demonstrated that AF-3 and AF-4 both depolarize the muscle cells with EC-50 values of 681 nM and 901 nM respectively. Mecamylamine was found to block the ACh excitation without any effect on the peptide responses, suggesting the peptides act on a separate receptor to ACh. The ionic mechanisms associated with the ACh depolarization and the depolarization due to the peptides were different, providing further evidence that these peptides do not activate the body wall nicotinic ACh receptor. AF-3 and AF-4 also

Table 1 *Sequences of RFamide peptides which have been identified in A. suum (AF) and P. redivivus (PF) and their actions on A. suum body wall muscle. Note that AF-8 and PF-3 are the same sequence.*

Peptide	Sequence	Action on muscle
AF-1	KNEFIRFamide	excitation
AF-2	KHEYLRFamide	biphasic
AF-3	AVPGVLRFamide	excitation
AF-4	GDVPGVLRFamide	excitation
AF-5	SGKPTFIRFamide	biphasic
AF-6	FIRFamide	inhibition
AF-7	AGPRFIRFamide	no effect
AF-8	KSAYMRFamide	excitation
AF-9	GLGPRPLRFamide	excitation
AF-10	GFGDEMSMPGVLRFamide	excitation
AF-11	SDIGISEPNFLRFamide	inhibition
AF-12	FGDEMSMPGVLRFamide	not tested
AF-13	SDMPGVLRFamide	excitation
AF-14	SMPGVLRFamide	excitation
AF-15	AQTFVRFamide	
AF-16	ILMRFamide	no effect
AF-17	FDRDFMRFamide	excitation
AF-18		
AF-19	AEGLSSPLIRFamide	inhibition
AF-20	GMPGVLRFamide	excitation
PF-1	SDPNFLRFamide	inhibition
PF-2	SADPNFLRFamide	inhibition
PF-3	KSAYMRFamide	excitation
PF-4	KPNFIRFamide	inhibition

contract body wall muscle strips from *A. galli*, with EC-50 values of 721 nM and 371 nM respectively. The EC-50 value for ACh-induced contraction on *A. galli* muscle was 13 μM, the same value as for *A. suum* muscle. Intracellular recordings from *A. galli* muscle again showed that all three compounds depolarised these muscle cells, with EC-50 values of 14 μM, 5 μM and 10 μM respectively for ACh, AF-3 and AF-4. This suggests that both AF-3 and AF-4 may have a functional role in the control of body wall muscle in a range of nematodes.

1.7 Role of cAMP in the actions of AF-3

The possible role of adenylate cyclase in the excitatory action of AF-3 on *A. suum* body wall muscle has been investigated. (18) This peptide has a potent and long lasting excitatory effect on the muscle, suggesting the possible involvement of a second messenger system. The effect of AF-3 was examined on the basal level of cAMP in body wall muscle. AF-3, 1 μM, decreased basal levels of cAMP from 1721 pmol mg^{-1} protein to 1148 pmol mg^{-1} protein. Lower concentrations of peptide, for example, 100 nM, also reduced cAMP levels but not significantly. Forskolin, 10 μM, raised cAMP levels to 3242 pmol mg^{-1} protein and this increase could be reduced by AF-3. AF-3, 1 μM, failed to alter basal levels of cAMP in *A. galli* though this concentration of peptide did reduce forskolin-induced potentiation of cAMP levels in this species. The effect of 3-isobutyl-1-methylxanthine (IBMX), a phosphodiesterase inhibitor and forskolin on AF-3 muscle tension responses were also investigated. Control responses to AF-3 showed that the second contraction was always lower than the first, being around 75% of the first response. IBMX, 500 μM, had no effect on resting tension but this concentration did significantly inhibit 1 μM AF-3 contractions, compared with controls. Forskolin, 10 μM, had a similar inhibitory action to IBMX on the AF-3 contractions. AF-3 enhanced ACh-induced contractions of *A. suum* body wall muscle and this enhancement was reduced by IBMX, 500 μM. In some experiments this enhancement effect of AF-3 on ACh contractions was not evident until the peptide had been removed. Similarly AF-3, 1 μM, potentiated the action of ACh on *A. galli* muscle but again before this potentiation can be seen the peptide has to be removed. These results provide good evidence for at least certain of the actions of AF-3 being associated with a decrease in the activation of adenylate cyclase.

1.8 Effect of PF-1 and PF-2 on neuromuscular transmission

Although PF-1 and PF-2 have been isolated from *P. redivivus*, they both have potent actions on *A. suum* body wall muscle and so it is likely that either these peptides or peptides with similar structures are present in *A. suum*. PF-1 relaxes body wall muscle with a threshold of 1 nM. (19) In the presence of PF-1 the ACh contraction is reduced but returns to normal following washing. PF-1, 1 μM, also reduced ACh-induced contractions of *A. galli* body wall muscle. At a concentration of 1 μM PF-1 can relax the muscle for over three hours. This relaxation is not associated with an increase in chloride conductance and so PF-1 does not act through the release of GABA. Preliminary experiments suggest that PF-1 relaxation may be associated with an increase in potassium conductance. For example, in the presence of tetraethylammonium, 5 mM, and 4-aminopyridine, 250 μM, the hyperpolarization induced by 1 μM PF-1 was reversibly blocked. Intracellular recordings have also been made from body wall muscle where PF-1 hyperpolarizes the membrane potential and reduces ejps recorded (figure 1) following

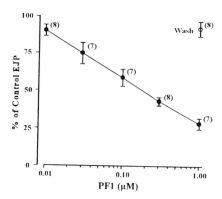

Figure 1 *Concentration-dependent effect of PF-1 on amplitude of ejps recorded from A. suum body wall muscle cell. Mean amplitude of ejps determined before each application of PF-1. Reversal (o) shown following wash for 15 minutes.*

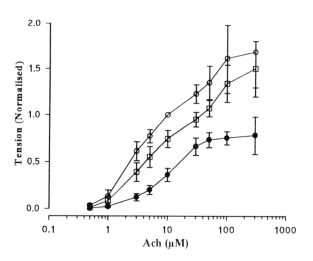

Figure 2 *Effect of SEPNFLRFamide on ACh contractions of A. galli body wall muscle strip. Increases in isometric tension by ACh (o) were reduced in the presence of SEPNFLRFamide (1μM;•). The antagonism by the peptide was reversed partially following wash (□). n=6 ± SEM; data normalised to control ACh 10μM.*

stimulation of the nerve cord just anterior to the retrovesicular ganglion. (20) This effect on ejps was concentration-dependent in the range 10nM to $1\,\mu$M PF-1. The EC-50 for PF-1 inhibitory effect on ejps was 311 nM. The action of PF-2 was similar to PF-1. PF-1 had no effect on ACh-induced depolarization, suggesting the action on ejps was presynaptic. These experiments suggest that inhibitory RFamides can modulate the action of excitatory motoneurones and so help to regulate locomotion in *A. suum*.

A structure-activity study was undertaken to try and determine the importance of the different N-terminal amino acids in the ability of PF-1 to reduce ACh-induced contractions of *A. galli* body wall muscle. The potency of the peptide sequences tested was as follows where PF-1 was the most potent: SDPNFLRFamide > SADPNFLRFamide > SEPNFLRFamide > SDVNFLRFamide > SDRNFLRFamide > SDENFLRFamide > PNFLRFamide. (4) Figure 2 is an example showing the effect of SEPNFLRFamide on ACh-induced contractions of *A. galli* muscle. Since the six amino acid sequence, that is PNFLRFamide, is the least active, it is clear that the first two N-terminal amino acids, serine and aspartate, are of key importance in activating this peptide receptor. The replacement of an aspartate by a glutamate also reduces potency as does replacement of the proline by either a valine, arginine or glutamate. This is not surprising as the presence of the proline has a large influence on the shape of the peptide and so its ability to interact with its receptor. However PNFLRFamide still contains the proline but in the absence of additional N-terminal amino acids it either cannot combine with the receptor or if it can then it is unable to activate it.

1.9 Effects of PF-4 on body wall muscle

PF-4 is one of the peptides identified from *P. redivivus* which relaxes *A. suum* body wall muscle, Table 1. (21, 22) Unlike PF-1 and PF-2, PF-4 rapidly relaxes the muscle with a threshold of around 10 nM and an EC-50 value of 98 nM which is considerably lower than that of GABA which has an EC-50 of 59 μM. While the rapid hyperpolarization induced by PF-4 is similar to that of GABA, the peptide hyperpolarization is followed by a depolarization to a steady plateau which slowly return to the resting membrane potential. The maximum hyperpolarization and conductance increase to PF-4 is greater than that of GABA. Interestingly the increase in input conductance to PF-4 and to a supramaximal concentration of GABA were additive, suggesting a different mechanism. The membrane potential reversal potential for the fast PF-4 response was measured in different concentrations of external chloride and found to have a slope of 29.6 mV for a ten fold change in chloride concentration, a value which is very close to the slope predicted for a chloride-dependent event. This value was similar to the reversal potential for GABA which is a pure chloride event. The late PF-4 response is unlikely to be due to chloride since in the presence of a hyperpolarization due to a supramaximal concentration of GABA, the muscle still depolarized when a supramaximal concentration of PF-4 was added. For example, the membrane potential in the presence of 1 mM GABA was 61.8 mV while in the presence of this concentration of GABA plus 10 μM PF-4, the membrane potential was 47.5 mV. In addition ivermectin blocked the response to GABA but had no effect on the hyperpolarization due to PF-4. These data suggest that GABA and PF-4 act through separate receptor systems even though their initial fast hyperpolarizations are chloride events. Since PF-4 has such a potent action on *A. suum* muscle it is likely that, as with PF-1 and PF-2, *A. suum* either contains this peptide or a closely related one which activates the same receptor.

From this work it can be suggested that the pharynx system is a potential target site for new anthelmintics. The neuropeptide system is a second site for the development of anthelmintics which could act as agonists, antagonists or modulate the second messenger system.

Acknowledgements

We are grateful to the BBSRC, Hoechst Roussel Vet and the Wellcome Trust for financial support.

References

1. R. J. Walker, L. M. Colquhoun, H. R. Parri, R. G. Williams and L. Holden-Dye, Neurotox '91 (ed. I.R. Duce), Elsevier Science Applied, London, 1992, pp. 105-121.

2. Z. A. Bascal, L. Holden-Dye, R. J. Willis, S. W. G. Smith and R. J. Walker, *Parasitol.*, 1996, **112**, 253-259.

3. D. J. A. Brownlee, L. Holden-Dye and R. J. Walker, *Parasitol.*, 1997, **115**, 553-561.

4. C. J. Franks, PhD Thesis, University of Southampton, 1996.

5. J. E. Brooman, PhD Thesis, University of Southampton, 1997.

6. D. J. A. Brownlee, L. Holden-Dye, I. Fairweather and R. J. Walker, *Parasitol.*, 1995, **111**, 379-384.

7. D. J. A. Brownlee, I. Fairweather, C. F. Johnston and C. Shaw, *Parasitol.*, 1994, **108**, 89-103.

8. D. J. A. Brownlee, I. Fairweather, L. Holden-Dye and R. J. Walker, *Parasitol. Today*, 1996, **12**, 343-351.

9. Z. A. Bascal, A. Montgomery, L. Holden-Dye, R. G. Williams and R. J. Walker, *Parasitol.*, 1995, **110**, 625-637.

10. Z. A. Bascal, A. Montgomery, L. Holden-Dye, R. G. Williams, M. C. Thorndyke and R. J. Walker, *Parasitol.*, 1996, **112**, 125-134.

11. A. O. W. Stretton, C. Cowden, P. Sithigorngul and R. E. Davis, *Parasitol.*, 1991, **102**, S107-S116.

12. C. Cowden and A. O. W. Stretton, *Peptides*, 1995, **16**, 491-500.

13. R. J. Walker, *Comp. Biochem. Physiol.*, 1992, **102C**, 213-222.

14. D. J. A. Brownlee, L. Holden-Dye and R. J. Walker, *Advances in Parasitol.*, 1998, in press.

15. C. Keating, L. Holden-Dye, M. C. Thorndyke, R. G. Williams and R. J. Walker, *Parasitol.*, 1995, **111**, 315-321.

16. F.-Y. Pang, J. Mason, L. Holden-Dye, C. J. Franks, R. G. Williams and R. J. Walker, *Parasitol.*, 1995, **110**, 353-362.

17. N. Trim, L. Holden-Dye, R. Ruddell, and R. J. Walker, *Parasitol.*, 1997, **115**, 213-222.

18. N. Trim, J. E. Brooman, L. Holden-Dye and R. J. Walker, *Mol. Biochem. Parasitol.*, 1998, in press.

19. C. J. Franks, L. Holden-Dye, R. G. Williams, F.-Y. Pang and R. J. Walker, *Parasitol.*, 1994, **108**, 229-236.

20. L. Holden-Dye, C. J. Franks, R. G. Williams and R. J. Walker, *Parasitol.*, 1995, **110**, 449-455.

21. A. G. Maule, C. Shaw, J. W. Bowman, D. W. Halton, D. P. Thompson, T. G. Geary and L. Thim, *Biochem. Biophys. Res. Commun.*, 1994, **200**, 973-980.

22. L. Holden-Dye, D. J. A. Brownlee and R. J. Walker, *Br. J. Pharmacol.*, 1997, **120**, 379-386.

Effects of Hexachlorocyclohexanes on Human GABA$_A$ Receptors

K.A. Wafford[1], P.D. Maskell[2], L.S. Aspinwall[2], D.J. Beadle[2] and I. Bermudez[2]

[1] MERCK SHARP & DOHME RESEARCH LABORATORIES, NEUROSCIENCE RESEARCH CENTRE, TERLINGS PARK, EASTWICK ROAD, HARLOW, ESSEX CM20 2QR, UK
[2] SCHOOL OF BIOLOGICAL AND MOLECULAR SCIENCES, OXFORD BROOKES UNIVERSITY, GIPSY LANE CAMPUS, OXFORD OX3 0BP, UK

1 INTRODUCTION

The GABA$_A$ receptor is a transmembrane protein complex that forms an ion channel that is selectively permeable to chloride ions. Cloning of the GABA$_A$ receptor subunit cDNAs has revealed considerable heterogeneity, with at least six α-, four β-, three γ-, one δ and one ε subunits, providing a molecular basis for multiple GABA$_A$ receptor subtypes which distribute throughout the brain[1].

The Cl$^-$ channel is directly gated by γ-aminobutyric acid (GABA). The GABA$_A$ receptor also contains several allosteric sites important for the modulatory action of various classes of drugs such as benzodiazepines, β-carbolines, the convulsants picrotoxin and t-butylbicyclophosphorothionate (TBPS), barbiturates, neurosteroids, propofol and alcohols[2]. Organochlorine insecticides such as γ-hexachlorocyclohexane (γ -HCH or lindane) are also known to bind the GABA$_A$ receptor inducing convulsions of the Grand Mal type[3,4] and inhibiting GABA-induced chloride fluxes in a wide range of mammalian brain preparations[5,6,7] and in *Xenopus* oocytes expressing rat[8] and human[9] GABA$_A$ receptors. Studies showing that γ-HCH displaces ^{35}S-TBPS from its binding site in rat brain membrane homogenates[10,11], together with the convulsant effects of γ-HCH, suggest that this insecticide exert its actions by binding the convulsant or picrotoxin site of the GABA$_A$ receptor.

Other HCH isomers have been reported to have only weak (β-HCH) or act as CNS depressants (α- and δ-HCH)[12]. The site of action of these isomers in the mammalian CNS has not been determined as yet, although studies showing them to potentiate GABA-activated chloride channels in *Xenopus* oocytes[8] and in primary cultures of cortical[7] and dorsal root ganglion neurones[13], show that they too may interact with the GABA$_A$ receptor. Recently, we have studied the effects of HCH isomers in recombinant human GABA$_A$ receptors in detail and our findings prompted us to propose the γ-HCH as a partial inverse agonist of the picrotoxin site and that δ-HCH binds the barbiturate locus or a site closely linked to it.

1.1 The effect of γ-HCH

γ-HCH suppresses GABA-induced currents in dorsal root ganglion neurones[13], insect neurones[14,15], and oocytes expressing mammalian GABA$_A$[8] or *Drosophila*[16,17] receptors. γ-HCH also inhibits GABA currents in oocytes expressing human α1β2γ2S, α1β3γ2S and α6β3γ2S GABA$_A$ receptors with an EC$_{50}$ of about 1 µM (Table 1), which is in agreement with values reported for other mammalian preparations[8,13]. γ-HCH is a partial inhibitor of GABA$_A$ receptors, suppressing EC$_{50}$ GABA responses by a maximum of 34% (Table 1). Partial inhibition of GABA-induced currents by γ-HCH has also been observed in *Xenopus* oocytes expressing rat or bovine GABA$_A$ receptors[8]. However, full γ-HCH induced inhibition has been reported for dorsal root ganglion neurones[13] and *Xenopus* oocytes expressing a *Drosophila* GABA receptor subunit[16]. Efficacy, therefore, may be influenced by receptor subunits, although we have not found a significant effect of α1, α6, β2 or β3 subunits (Table 1).

1.1.1 The Site of Action of γ-HCH.   γ-HCH inhibits [^{35}S]TBPS binding in neuronal membranes[10,11] and GABA-mediated ^{36}Cl$^-$ fluxes in neurones[5,7]. In addition, γ-HCH relieves picrotoxin inhibition in *Xenopus* oocytes expressing α1β3γ2S in a competitive manner[9]. These results are consistent with the idea that γ-HCH binds the picrotoxin locus[9].

The binding site of picrotoxin has not been identified, as yet. However, it is likely to be in the M2 region of the Cl$^-$ channel, since site-directed mutagenesis studies of the putative M2 domain of ρ receptors[18], β glycine receptor subunits[19] and a *Drosophila* GABA subunit[17] cause significant changes in picrotoxin affinity and efficacy. It is significant that mutations of the picrotoxin site (alanine 302) in a *Drosophila* GABA subunit decreases the potency of both picrotoxin and γ-HCH inhibition[16,17], which further support the proposal that these two compounds ligand the same locus in the GABA$_A$ receptors.

1.1.2 The Mechanism of Action of γ-HCH.   The mechanism underlying the inhibition of the GABA$_A$ receptor by picrotoxin has not been determined with precision, as yet. A number of studies suggest that picrotoxin is a non-competitive inhibitor, as judged by the effect of picrotoxin on GABA concentration-effect curves[20,21] and ^{3}H-muscimol binding[22]. More recently, biophysical studies of picrotoxin action have suggested a complex mechanism that may involve allosteric blockade of the chloride channel[13,23]. Since we have shown that γ-HCH binds the picrotoxin locus to inhibit the GABA$_A$ receptor in a similar fashion to picrotoxin, it is reasonable to assume that γ-HCH also interacts allosterically with the GABA$_A$ receptor. By analogy to the pharmacological concepts used for other allosteric sites of the GABA$_A$ receptor and the non-competitive inhibitors fluorinated methyl-butyrolactones[24], we define picrotoxin as a full inverse agonist of the picrotoxin (convulsant) modulatory site. In contrast, γ-HCH is a partial inverse agonist of the picrotoxin site, since it both partially blocks GABA responses mediated by GABA$_A$ receptors[8,9] and relieves picrotoxin-induced inhibition of human GABA$_A$ receptors[9].

1.2 The Effect of Depressant HCH Isomers on GABA$_A$ Receptors

There is strong experimental evidence that the α and δ HCH isomers depress the CNS by positive allosteric modulation of GABA$_A$ receptors. Thus, for example, δ-HCH potentiates GABA responses in *Xenopus* oocytes expressing rat and bovine GABA$_A$[8], 1992), *Drosophila* GABA[25] receptors, dorsal root ganglion[13] and cortical[7]

Table 1. The effect of γ-HCH on recombinant human GABA$_A$ receptors

Receptor Type	EC$_{50}$ (μM)	Maximal Inhibition of GABA responses (%)
$\alpha1\beta2\gamma2S$	0.87 ± 0.1	45 ± 4
$\alpha1\beta3\gamma2S$	1 ± 0.3	34 ± 4
$\alpha6\beta2\gamma2S$	1.3 ± 0.2	30 ± 2

neurones. We also observed α- and δ-HCH-dependent potentiation of human $\alpha1\beta3\gamma2S$, $\alpha1\beta2\gamma2S$ and $\alpha6\beta3\gamma2S$ GABA$_A$ receptors. Interestingly, δ-HCH produces a parallel shift of GABA concentration-response curves on $\alpha1\beta2\gamma2S$ receptors with a significant increase in the efficacy of GABA. Increases in maximal GABA responses are also caused by barbiturates[26,27] and propofol[28], but not by flunitrazepam[26].

δ-HCH potentiation is not influenced by α-subunit composition, which is in contrast to other positive allosteric modulators of the GABA$_A$ receptor such as barbiturates[27] and benzodiazepines[29]. Also the potentiation by δ-HCH is unaffected by the benzodiazepine antagonist Ro15-1788[8], suggesting the mechanism to be unrelated to that of benzodiazepines. β subunits do not appear to influence δ-HCH-dependent potentiation, we have found no significant difference in the potentiation of GABA EC$_{20}$ responses in $\alpha1\beta2\gamma2S$ or $\alpha1\beta3\gamma2S$ receptors (Table 2). The lack of effect of the β subunit on δ-HCH-dependent potentiation of the GABA$_A$ receptor is consistent with the proposal that binding site of δ-HCH is closely related to the barbiturate site; the latter site appears to be unaffected by the subtype of β subunit[27].

1.2.1 The Binding Site of δ-HCH in the GABA$_A$ Receptor. Do the δ- and γ-HCH isomers bind the same locus in the GABA$_A$ receptor? Several lines of evidence argue against the idea of an identical binding locus for the δ and γ isomers. Firstly, a A302S mutant of a *Drosophila* GABA subunit receptor shows reduced susceptibility to inhibition by picrotoxin and γ-HCH without changes in its affinity towards the positive allosteric modulator δ-HCH[17]. Secondly, ρ receptors are endowed with a picrotoxin binding locus but lack a site for positive allosteric modulation by the δ isomer[8,18]. We have observed inhibition of δ-HCH-dependent effects by the γ-HCH, as well as the inhibition of picrotoxin antagonism by the δ isomer[9], which suggest that the two sites may be close together or overlapping. Indeed, our observation that the inhibition of δ-HCH potentiation by γ-HCH is of a non-competitive nature (inhibition cannot be overcome at high concentrations, and the δ-HCH EC$_{50}$ is not affected) clearly indicates two separate binding sites linked together by an allosteric relationship. However, it is also possible that the δ-HCH activity at the picrotoxin site is masked by its potentiating effect, and only when pentobarbital is used as an agonist is the inhibition observed.

Our pharmacological studies of δ-HCH action indicate a close relationship between the δ-HCH locus and those of barbiturate and propofol, as judged by the lack of effect of δ-HCH on barbiturate potentiation and the slight inhibition of propofol potentiation[9]. Although neither the barbiturate or propofol allosteric sites have been defined with precision, they appear to be separate loci[28], with the α and β subunit probably contributing to the barbiturate site[27,30] and propofol sites[31]. It is possible to

Table 2. The effects of δ-HCH on EC_{20} GABA responses by recombinant $GABA_A$ receptors.

Receptor	EC_{50} (μM)	Maximum % increase in GABA EC_{20}
$\alpha 1\beta 2\gamma 2S$	17 ± 1	260 ± 53
$\alpha 1\beta 3\gamma 2S$	15 ± 4	216 ± 31
$\alpha 6\beta 3\gamma 2S$	14 ± 3	342 ± 52

envisage a locus by studying its subunit dependence. Our studies have so far found that the effects of the HCH are not significantly affected by changes in the α or β subunits so far studied. It is unlikely that the δ-HCH site is linked to other sites such as the benzodiazepine site asflumazenil, an antagonist of the benzodiazepine site, has no effect on δ-HCH-mediated potentiation of GABA responses[9].

1.2.2. Direct Activation of Human GABA_A Receptor by δ-HCH. At concentrations higher than 1 μM, δ-HCH activates $GABA_A$ receptors in the absence of GABA. This effect is similar to the direct activation of $GABA_A$ receptors by barbiturates[25,27] and propofol[25,32]. It is not clear at present whether the direct effects of barbiturates and propofol are mediated by sites different from those mediating their positive allosteric effects. It is clear, however, that direct activation of $GABA_A$ receptors by barbiturates[27,33] and propofol[32] is not mediated through the GABA binding site[34], which suggests that the site for direct activation by the δ isomer is a separate locus from the agonist site. Recent evidence suggest that homomeric β-subunits form receptors which can be gated by barbiturates and propofol[35,36], but only weakly by GABA, which suggests a role for the β-subunit in this activation. In the case of δ-HCH, $\beta 2$ or $\beta 3$ containing $\alpha 1\beta x\gamma 2S$ $GABA_A$ receptors do not respond differentially to activating concentrations of δ-HCH.

1.3 The Effects of β-HCH on $GABA_A$ Receptors

We have found the β isomer to be essentially inactive on either GABA responses or [^{35}S]TBPS binding, confirming previous suggestions that this isomer is essentially a non-GABAergic HCH isomer[8,13]. However, a depressant action for the β isomer has been well substantiated[37,38] and Pomés *et al.*[7] demonstrated a biphasic action (positive modulation at concentrations lower than 1 μM and inhibition at higher concentrations) of β-HCH on GABA-dependent $^{36}Cl^-$ uptake into primary cultures of rat neocortical neurones. It is unlikely that these differences stem from subunit composition, as judged from our studies on the δ and γ isomers. It is however feasible that the intracellular pathway profile of the cells studied play a role in the differential effect of the β-HCH, since it is known that HCHs interact with intracellular targets such as ryanodine-sensitive calcium channels[39], which in turn may lead to changes (e.g. receptor phosphorylation) in the function of $GABA_A$ receptors.

1.4 Conclusions

HCH isomers act differentially at $GABA_A$ receptors. γ-HCH is a partial inhibitor of the receptor, binding the picrotoxin site, where it behaves as a partial inverse agonist. In contrast, δ-HCH is a positive allosteric modulator of the receptor. δ-HCH binds a site that is closely related to the barbiturate site, as judged by the lack of effect of δ-HCH on barbiturate potentiation and identical effect of γ-HCH on barbiturate and δ-HCH potentiation. The δ-HCH binding locus is unlikely to be identical to the barbiturate site as the subunit dependence of the two sites differs.

References

1.　R. M. McKernan and P. J. Whiting, TINS.,1996, **19**, 139.
2.　P. J. Whiting, R. M. McKernan and K. A. Wafford, Int. Rev. Neurobiol., 1995, **38**, 95.
3.　J. M. Tussel, C. Suñol, E. Gelpi, E. Rodríguez-Farré, Arch. Toxicol., 1987, **60**, 432.
4　J. Portig and C. Schnorr, Toxicology, 1988, **52**, 309.
5.　I. M. Abalis, M. E. Eldefrawi and T. M. Eldefrawi, J. Toxicon. Environ. Health, 1986, **18**, 13.
6.　J. R. Bloomquist, P. M. Addams and D. M. Sunderland, Neurotoxicol., 1986, **7**, 11.
7.　A. Pomés, E. Rodriguez-Farré, C. Suñol, J. Pharmacol. Exp. Therp., 1994, **27**, 1616.
8.　R. M. Woodward, L. Polenzani, L. and R. Miledi, Mol. Pharmacol., 1992, **41**,1107.
9.　L. S. Aspinwall, I. Bermudez, L. A. King and K. A. Wafford, J. Pharmacol. Exp. Ther., 1997, **282**, 1557.
10.　L. J. Lawrence and J. E. Casida, Life Sci., 1984, **35**, 171.
11.　J. C. Llorens, C. Suñol, J. M., Tussell, and E. Rodríguez-Farré, Toxicol. Teratol., 1990, **12**, 607.
12.　B. McNamara S. and Krup, J. Pharmacol. Exp. Ther., 1948, **92**, 140.
13.　K. Nagata and T. Narahashi, Brain Res., 1995, **704**, 85.
14.　K. A.Wafford, S. C. R. Lummis, and D. B. Sattelle, Pestic. Sci., 1988, **24**, 338.
15.　I. Bermudez, C. Hawkins, A. M. Taylor and D. J. Beadle, Receptor Res., 1991, **11**, 221.
16.　H-G. Zhang, R. H. ffrench-Constant and M. B. Jackson, J. Physiol., 1994, **479**, 65.
17.　D. Belleli, A. G. Hope, H. Callachan, C. Hill-Venning, and J. J. Lambert, Br. J. Pharmacol., 1995, **116**, 442P.
18.　T-L Wang, A. S. Hackam, W. B. Guggino and G. R. Cutting, Proc. Natl. Acad. Sci. USA., 1995, **92**, 11751.
19.　I. Pribilla, T. Tagaki, D. Langosch, J. Bormann, J. and H. Betz, EMBO J., 1992, **11**, 4305.
20.　A. Constanti and A. Nigri, Br. J. Pharmacol., 1976, **57**, 347.
21.　J. P. Gallagher, H. Higashi and S. Nishi, J. Physiol., 1978, **275**, 263.
22.　U. Quast and O. Brenner, J. Neurochem., 1983, **41**, 418.

23. C. F. Newland and S. G. Cull-Candy, J. Physiol., 1992, **447**, 191.

24. K-W Yoon, D. J Canney, D. F. Covey and S. M. Rothman, J. Pharmacol. Exp. Thr., 1990, **255**, 248.

25. D. Belleli, H. Callachan, C. Hill-Venning, J. A. Peters, and J. J. Lambert, Br. J. Pharmacol., 1996, **118**, 563.

26. A. L. Horne, P. C. Harkness, K. L. Hadingham, P. Whiting and J. A. Kemp, Br. J. Pharmacol., 1993, **108**, 711.

27. S. A. Thompson, P. J. Whiting and K. A. Wafford, Br. J. Pharmacol., 1996, **117**, 521.

28. A. Concas, G, Santoro, G., M. Serra, E. Sanna, and G. Biggio, Brain. Res., 1991, **542**, 225.

29. K. A. Wafford, P. J. Whiting, P. J. and J. A. Kemp, Mol. Pharmacol., 1993, **43**, 240.

30. J. Amin, J. and D. S. Weiss, Nature, 1993, **366**, 565.

31. E. Sanna, M. P. Mascia, R. L., Klein, P. J. Whiting, G. Biggio and R. A. Harris, J. Pharmacol. Exp. Therp., 1995, **274**, 353.

32. B. A. Orser, L-Y-Wang, P. S. Pennefather and J. F. MacDonald, J. Neurosci., 1994, **14**, 7747.

33. D. A. Mathers and J. L. Barker, Science, 1980, **209**, 507.

34. S. Ueno, J. Bracamontes, C. Zorumski, D. S Weiss and J. H. J. Steinbach, J. Neurosci., 1997, **17**, 625.

35. B. J. Krishek, S. J. Moss and T. G. Smart, Mol. Pharmacol., 1996, **49**, 494.

36. E. Sanna, F. Garau and R. A. Harris, Mol. Pharmacol., 1995, **47**, 213.

37. H. W. Volland, J. Portig and K. Stein, K, Toxicol. Appl. Pharmacol., 1981, **57**, 425.

38. L. G. Stark, T. E. Albertson and R. M. Joy, Neurobehav. Toxicol. Teratol., 1986, **81**, 487.

39. I. N. Pessah, F. Ch. Mohr, M. Schiedt and R. M. Joy, J. Pharmacol. Exp. Ther., 1992, **262**, 661.

Modulation of Insect Ligand-gated Ion Channels

R.M. Pitman, S.J.B. Butt and J.A. David

SCHOOL OF BIOMEDICAL SCIENCES, UNIVERSITY OF ST. ANDREWS, ST. ANDREWS, FIFE KY16 8LB, UK

1 INTRODUCTION.

Acetylcholine is probably the major fast excitatory neurotransmitter in insects, since it is released by most sensory nerve fibres and a number of interneurones[1]. Much of the early work on cholinergic transmission focussed upon the actions of ACh mediated by receptors that share many similarities with vertebrate nicotinic receptors; ACh and nicotinic agonists activate a ligand-gated ion channel that has a cation selectivity similar to that of nicotinic receptors at vertebrate neuromuscular junctions[2, 3]. Activation of these receptors by neurally released transmitter or applied ACh generates rapid membrane depolarization and excitation. In the insect nervous system, gamma-aminobutyric acid (GABA) appears to play a role complementary to that of ACh operating through nicotinic receptors. Inhibitory motoneurones and many inhibitory interneurones release GABA that acts rapidly via ligand-gated chloride channels with characteristics in common with vertebrate $GABA_A$ and $GABA_C$ receptors[4].

Although a considerable volume of information is available on the role of nicotinic and GABA ligand-gated ion channels in the insect nervous system, the role of other types of receptor is far less extensive. For example, while it had been well known that insects are sensitive to muscarine (the active ingredient of fly agaric mushroom, extracts of which traditionally have been used to kill flies) and that muscarinic binding sites are present in the insect CNS[5], the role of muscarinic receptors has been something of a puzzle, since muscarinic agonists have a comparatively weak effect upon the membrane potential of most insect neurones. Recently, however, it has become clear that muscarinic receptors do exert a number of actions upon insect neurones, but that these are relatively subtle compared to the effects of nicotinic receptor activation[6]. For example, muscarinic receptors can modulate transmitter release from cholinergic synaptic terminals[7-10], modulate transmembrane ion currents[11, 12] and alter neuronal excitability[13, 14]. We have recently found that muscarinic receptors can also exert a powerful modulatory action both upon nicotinic cholinoceptors and GABA receptors[15].

The biogenic amines serotonin, dopamine and octopamine are widespread in the insect nervous system[16-19]. Despite this, attempts to establish their physiological function in insects has only achieved relatively limited success. This possibly could be because their effects, like those mediated by muscarinic receptors, are less immediate and dramatic than those produced by activation of ligand-gated ion channels. Thus, although dopamine and serotonin do activate characteristic membrane currents in central neurones, these appear to be less ubiquitous and more complex than responses mediated by ligand-gated ion channels[20, 21]. As yet the physiological roles of these currents are unclear. Amines, however, have been shown to produce effects that can be directly related to neural function. Octopamine, for example, has been shown to modulate the excitable properties of central neurones[22] and, when injected into specific neuropilar regions, this amine can elicit specific locomotor patterns[23]. Biogenic amines also have been shown to alter the amplitude of cholinergic excitatory postsynaptic potentials (EPSPs) recorded from identified cockroach interneurones; dopamine and octopamine cause an amplitude increase, while serotonin decreases the amplitude of evoked EPSPs[24]. In light of these effects of amines upon cholinergic transmission we have performed experiments to study the intracellular mechanisms by which this modulation occurs and to compare it with modulation mediated by muscarinic receptors.

2 MATERIALS AND METHODS

Experiments were performed on the metathoracic 'fast' coxal depressor motoneurone, D_f [25], of adult male cockroaches (*Periplaneta americana*). The thoracic ganglia and the first three abdominal ganglia were isolated and the third thoracic desheathed on its ventral surface for electrophysiological recording[26]. Experiments were performed in circulating oxygenated saline containing: NaCl 214.0 mM; KCl 3.1 mM; $CaCl_2$ 9.0 mM; and TES buffer 10 mM (pH 7.2). Intracellular recordings from D_f somata were made with borosilicate glass microelectrodes (Clark Electromedical, Pangbourne, U.K.) filled with 2M potassium acetate (resistance 12-20 MΩ).

ACh and GABA were locally pressure-applied to the soma of the neurone from a glass microelectrode filled with a 100 mM solution of the agonist (by applying 0.5-1 Bar pulses of 10-200 ms duration). Other drugs were added to a side compartment of the chamber (total volume 2ml), where the oxygenation system mixed and diluted these agents before they reached the preparation. Their concentrations, therefore, are expressed as final values attained after dilution in the experimental chamber.

A CED 1401 computer interface (Cambridge Electronic Design) and associated software were used for generating voltage command pulses, recording digitized data and for off-line analysis. Data were also recorded on tape using a VCR coupled to a Medical Systems pulse code modulator.

To monitor changes in intracellular Ca^{2+} levels, cells were pre-loaded with fluo-3 at the beginning of each experiment by a 45 s period in which pressure pulses were applied (20 ms, 0.5 Bar, 2 Hz) through microelectrodes containing 10 mM fluo-3 pentaammonium salt. An extruded quartz rod (tip diameter, 2 mm) was used to direct light (excitation wavelength 490 nm) at the cell soma. Fluorescence emitted by fluo-3 was collected by manipulating an optical fibre (0.25 mm diameter) to within 1 mm of the cell. The collected light was filtered (transmitted light >510 nm) and amplified using a photomultiplier tube (Thorn EMI). The photomultiplier output was then amplified and recorded digitally on computer using the CED1401 interface and associated software.

In experiments to establish the effects of rapid, brief increases in $[Ca^{2+}]_i$ upon responses mediated by nicotinic ACh receptors and GABA receptors, neurones were pre-loaded with the photo labile Ca^{2+} chelator nitr-5 by pressure-injection (20 ms, 0.5 Bar pulses at 2 Hz for 30 s) from a microelectrode containing 58 mM nitr-5 (tetrapotassium salt, Calbiochem) in 30 mM $CaCl_2$. Ca^{2+} was photolytically released from nitr-5 with 50 ms UV light pulses applied to the neurone through an extruded quartz rod (tip diameter, 2 mm). A solenoid-operated shutter (Cairn Research Ltd) was used to deliver pulses of UV light from a continuous UV light source.

3 RESULTS

3.1 Modulation of nicotinic ACh responses and GABA responses by muscarinic agonists.

When ACh is locally applied to the soma of the 'fast' coxal depressor motoneurone (D_f), it produces a membrane depolarization that is associated with in increase in cation conductance (Figure 1). This is produced by activation of ligand-gated ion channels with characteristics broadly similar to vertebrate nicotinic receptors[2].

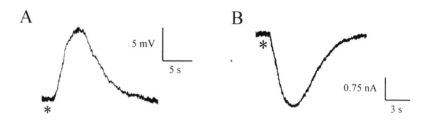

Figure 1 *(A) Voltage response of motoneurone D_f to local pressure application of ACh (1.5 Bar, 100 ms pressure pulses). (B) Response of the neurone to ACh recorded under voltage-clamp conditions. Holding potential = -80 mV. Asterisks indicate point at which ACh was applied.*

Although bath application of muscarinic agonists like McN-A-343 (McN) have little effect upon the membrane potential of motoneurone D_f, they can cause dramatic reduction in the amplitude of depolarizations (or inward currents) produced by activating nicotinic receptors (Figure 2A). This effect cannot be attributed to a direct action of the agonists upon nAChRs, since the muscarinic antagonist pirenzepine (10^{-5} M) has no significant effect upon nicotinic responses, but blocks the modulatory action of muscarinic agonists[15]. Furthermore, depression of nicotinic responses is not merely a consequence of an increase in the membrane conductance of the neurone, since this modulation could be observed under voltage clamp conditions, when the amplitude of nicotinic currents is independent of any influence muscarinic agonists might have upon membrane conductance.

Besides modulating nicotinic currents, muscarinic agonists also modulate GABA responses. For reasons as yet unclear, however, GABA currents in some preparations are enhanced by muscarinic agonists, while in others, they are depressed. The same variability in modulation of GABA responses is seen when ACh is bath applied to preparations pre-treated with α-bungarotoxin (to block its nicotinic actions) (Fig. 2B). The modulatory action of muscarinic agonists upon GABA responses, like that on nicotinic currents, appears to involve a muscarinic receptor, since it is blocked by pirenzepine.

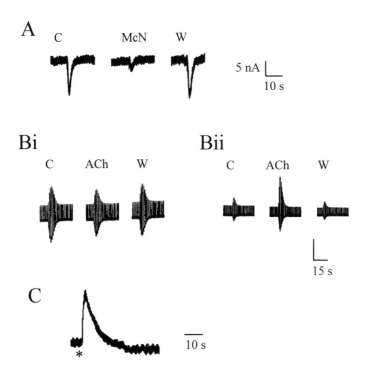

Figure 2 *(A) Modulatory effect of bath application of the muscarinic agonist McN (10^{-4} M) on nicotinic ACh currents evoked by pressure-application of ACh (30 ms pulses at 1 per minute). Each trace shows a response to a single application of ACh. C = control nicotinic current, McN = nicotinic current in the presence of McN and W = nicotinic current after washing McN from the preparation. Voltage-clamp holding potential = -80 mV.*
(B) Modulation of GABA-induced currents by activation of muscarinic receptors. GABA was pressure-applied at 1 minute interval. Each panel shows the response to a single application. To monitor any change in GABA reversal potential, the membrane was voltage-clamped at a holding potential of -110 mV and stepped to -70 mV at 1.5 s intervals. Muscarinic receptors were activated by bath application of 10^{-4} M ACh (after the preparation had been pre-incubated with α-bungarotoxin). C = control GABA current, ACh = GABA current in the presence of ACh and W = GABA current after washing ACh from the preparation. (Bi) ACh depressed GABA-induced currents in this neurone. (Bii) GABA currents were enhanced by ACh in this neurone. Vertical calibration: Bi 20 nA, Bii, 10 nA. (C) Transient elevation in $[Ca^{2+}]_i$ induced by application of the muscarinic agonist McN (10^{-4} M applied at asterisk) determined by measuring fluorescence intensity (increase shown upward) of a cell pre-loaded with fluo-3. The cell was voltage-clamped at -80 mV.

Application of the muscarinic agonist McN causes a transient rise in intracellular calcium concentration ($[Ca^{2+}]_i$) as indicated by the change in fluorescence signal emitted by neurones pre-loaded with the calcium-sensitive dye fluo-3 (Figure 2C). The duration of the modulatory effect of McN upon both ACh and GABA currents, however, outlasts this increase in $[Ca^{2+}]_i$ by an order of magnitude. To establish whether a rise in $[Ca^{2+}]_i$ is an essential step in the mAChR-mediated modulation of nicotinic and GABA currents motoneurone D_f was pre-loaded with the photolabile Ca^{2+} chelator nitr-5. $[Ca^{2+}]$ in the neuronal cytosol was rapidly elevated by flash photolysis (using 50 ms light pulses) of nitr-5. Photolytically released Ca^{2+}, like muscarinic agonists, always decreased nicotinic currents. Calcium released in this way also mimicked the McN-mediated modulation of GABA currents in individual neurones (i.e. McN and elevation in $[Ca^{2+}]_i$ each augmented GABA currents in some neurones and each depressed them in others). One possible trigger for muscarinic receptor-evoked rise in $[Ca^{2+}]_i$ could be an increase in inositol 1,4,5-trisphosphate (InsP$_3$) production. This hypothesis is supported by two lines of evidence. Firstly, McN has been shown to increase IP$_3$ production in the cockroach CNS[27]. Secondly, pretreatment with 10 mM lithium (that produces a prolonged elevation of InsP$_3$ in the insect CNS by inhibiting its degradation[28-31] caused the modulatory effect of McN on both nicotinic and GABA responses to become irreversible. This result would be expected if InsP$_3$ degradation were blocked.

3.2 Modulation of nicotinic responses by biogenic amines.

The biogenic amines dopamine, octopamine and serotonin have little effect upon the input resistance or membrane potential of motoneurone D_f when applied at relatively low concentrations. However, they are all able to cause a depression in the amplitude of nicotinic ACh responses that superficially resembles that produced by muscarinic receptor activation (Figure 3).

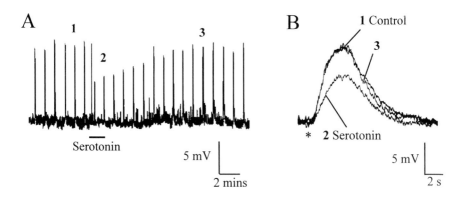

Figure 3 *(A)   Modulatory effect of serotonin on ACh responses recorded from motoneurone D_f. Each vertical deflection is the membrane potential change produced by a single pressure pulse of ACh.   Horizontal bar indicates duration of serotonin administration.   Numbers indicate responses that are shown on an expanded scale in panel (B).   (B) Selected ACh responses from panel (A) shown on an expanded time-scale. Asterisks indicate point at which ACh was applied.*

In the case of serotonin, the threshold for its modulatory action is below 10^{-6} M. The modulation produced by amines, however, appears to be brought about by completely different intracellular mechanisms from that mediated by muscarinic agonists. Dopamine, when bath applied to the neurone, causes a large transient fall in $[Ca^{2+}]_i$[32]. Therefore the modulatory action of dopamine cannot be triggered by a rise in $[Ca^{2+}]_i$. It appears that all three amines produce their modulatory effects either via the same receptor or the same second messenger pathway, since serotonin produces a depression of nicotinic responses which is not further enhanced by co-administration with dopamine or octopamine. Since all three amines do appear to share similar mechanisms and because serotonin is the most potent of the three, most work has centred upon this amine. Evidence that the serotonin-induced modulation of nocotinic responses involves a G-protein was obtained by intra-cellular injection of GDP-β-S. This non-hydrolysable analogue of GDP competitively binds to the GTP-binding site of G-proteins and renders them inactive. Injection of this compound reversibly reduced the modulatory effect of serotonin on nicotinic responses. It appears that the action of serotonin is mediated by cyclic nucleotides, since membrane soluble analogues of cyclic AMP and cyclic GMP both mimic the effects of serotonin and occlude its effects. Recently two findings have suggested that the serotonin-mediated modulation of nicotinic responses involves phosphorylation. Firstly, application of the protein kinase A (PKA) inhibitor 8-bromoadenosine-5',5'-cyclic monophosphorothioate, Rp isomer (Rp-8-Br-cAMPS) depresses the effects of serotonin. Secondly, the protein phosphatase inhibitor cantharidin enhances and prolongs the down-regulation of nicotinic responses by serotonin, presumably because it blocks a dephosphorylation reaction.

4. DISCUSSION

Our observations demonstrate that insect nicotinic cholinergic receptors and GABA receptors may both be modulated by activation of muscarinic receptors via a mechanism that apparently involves an increase in the turnover of membrane phospholipids and a rise in $[Ca^{2+}]_i$. Serotonin, dopamine and octopamine, like muscarinic agonists, also produce a modulatory suppression of nicotinic ACh responses, but appear to do so by quite separate intracellular signalling pathways. Amine-mediated modulation probably involves either cyclic AMP or cyclic GMP or both nucleotides activating protein kinases that directly or indirectly alter nicotinic receptor function by a process of phosphorylation. This would be consistent with previous observations that serotonin, dopamine and octopamine can all elevate cyclic nucleotide synthesis in cockroach nerve cords[33]. Figure 4 diagrammatically summarizes the mechanisms by which we propose that muscarinic agonists and biogenic amine exert their modulator effects on nicotinic ACh receptors.

Modulation of GABA receptors appears to be less straightforward than that of nico-tinic ACh receptors in two respects. Firstly, in the uniquely identifiable coxal depressor motoneurone, D_f, muscarinic agonists produce up-regulation of GABA responses in some preparations and down-regulation in others. The only obvious explanation for this is that the direction of modulation depends on the past history of the neurone. The second complexity in GABA modulation is that although amines have little or no modulatory effect upon GABA responses in motoneurone D_f, dopamine markedly enhances GABA responses recorded from the first basalar motoneurone of the locust *Schistocerca gregaria*[34]. The most likely reason for this difference between the two preparations is that the subunit composition of GABA receptors differs between insect species or even between individual neurones.

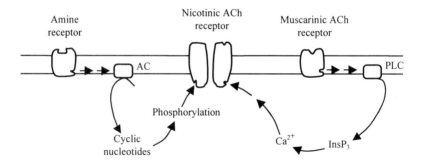

Figure 4 *Diagram summarizing the proposed routes through which muscarinic ACh receptors and amine receptors modulate nicotinic ACh receptor function. AC = adenylyl cyclase, PLC = phospholipase C, InsP₃ = inositol trisphosphate*

Our observations suggest that insect nicotinic ACh receptors may have multiple sites at which they can be modulated via different second messenger pathways. However, we do not at present have sufficient evidence to implicate cyclic nucleotides in modulation of insect GABA receptors. This situation with insect nicotinic ACh receptors appears to be similar to that found in vertebrate ligand-gated ion channels. Vertebrate nicotinic receptor subunits possess a number of consensus sequences some of which may be phosphorylated by PKA[35], protein kinase C (PKC) [36] and protein tyrosine kinase[37]. Phosphorylation of such sites can increase the rate of receptor desensitization[38]. Vertebrate GABA_A receptors, similarly possess both sites for PKA and for PKC-mediated phosphorylation[39, 40]. The effects of receptor phosphorylation vary between preparations, presumably depending upon the subunit composition of the particular GABA receptors involved; for example phosphorylation by PKA can enhance, depress or have no influence upon GABA responses recorded from different neurone types[39].

Although our experiments have been limited to a pharmacological approach, there is no *a priori* reason to suppose cholinergic and GABAergic synaptic transmission should not be modulated in a similar manner to that described here. This could provide a mechanism by which ACh (acting upon muscarinic receptors) or amines and could reduce the efficacy of transmission across a given cholinergic synapse.   Under circumstances in which muscarinic receptor produce an enhancement of GABA responses, the two processes could act synergistically to make it reduce the probability that postsynaptic neurones will be activated. The work presented here indicates that neurotransmitters and neuromodulators acting through G-protein-linked receptors have the potential to exert a profound modulatory influence upon fast transmission mediated by ligand-gated ion channels. Such processes could have a major influence on neural function.

References

1.   R.M. Pitman 'Comprehensive Insect Physiology, Biochemistry and Pharmacology,
     Insect Pharmacology', Ed G.A. Kerkut and L.I. Gilbert, Pergamon, Oxford, 1985,
     Vol. 11, Chapter 2, p. 5.
2.   J.A. David, and D.B. Sattelle, *J. exp. Biol.*, 1990, **151**, 21.

3. E.D. Gundelfinger, *Trends Neurosci.*, 1992, **15**, 206.
4. F. Shotkoski, H.G. Zhang, M.B. Jackson and R.H. ffrench-Constant, *FEBS Letters,* 1996, **380**, 257.
5. F. Hannan and L. Hall, 'Comparative Molecular Neurobiology', Ed. Y. Pichon, Birkhäuser, Basel, 1993, pp. 98-145
6. B.A. Trimmer, *Trends Neurosci.,* 1995, **18**, 104.
7. B. Hue, B. Lapied and C.O. Malécot, *J. exp. Biol.*, 1989, **142**, 447.
8. H Le Corronc, B. Lapied and B. Hue, *J. Insect Physiol.* 1991, **37,**647.
9. B. Leitch and R.M. Pitman, *J. Neurobiol.*, 1995, **28**, 455.
10. D. Parker and P.L. Newland, *J. Neurophysiol.,* 1995, **73**, 586.
11. J.A. David, and R.M. Pitman, *Brain Res.*, 1995, **669**, 153.
12. J.A. David, and R.M. Pitman, *J. Neurophysiol.* 1995,**74**, 2043.
13. H. Le Corronc and B. Hue, *J. exp. Biol.,* 1993 **181**,257.
14. B.A. Trimmer, and J.C. Weeks, *J. Neurophysiol.*,1993. **69**, 1821.
15. J.A. David and R.M. Pitman, *Proc. R. Soc.* Lond. **B**, 1996, **263**, 469.
16. G.R. Dymond and P.D. Evans, *Insect Biochem.,* 1979, **9**, 535.
17. J.R. BAKER, and R.M. Pitman, *Comp. Biochem. Physiol.*, 1989, **92C** 237.
18. C.A. Bishop and M. O'Shea, *J. Neurobiol.* 1983, **14**, 251.
19. P.D. Evans, *Adv. Insect. Physiol.*, 1980, **15**, 317.
20. J.P.L. Davis and R.M. Pitman, *J. exp. Biol.*, 1991, **155**, 203.
21. I. Bermudez, D.J. Beadle and J.A. Benson, *J. exp. Biol.,* 1992, **165**, 43.
22. J.M. Ramirez and K.G. Pearson, *Brain Res.,* 1991, **549**, 332.
23. S. Sombati and G. Hoyle, *J. Neurobiol.,* 1984, **15**, 481.
24. J.L. Casagrand and R.E. Ritzmann, *J. Neurobiol.,* 1992, **23**, 644.
25. K.G. Pearson and J.F. Iles, *J. exp. Biol.,* 1970, **52**, 139.
26. R.M. Pitman, *J. Physiol., Lond.*, 1975, **247**, 511.
27. J.A. David and R.M. Pitman, *J. Physiol., Lond.*, 1994, **480**, 97P.
28. A.H. Drummond and C.A. Raeburn, *Biochem. J.*, 1984, **224**, 129.
29. B.A. Trimmer and M.J. Berridge, *Insect Biochem.*, 1985, **15**, 811.
30. B.A. Brami U. Lei and G. Hauser, *Biochim. biophys. Res. Commun.*, 1991, **174**, 606.
31. K. Muraki Y. Imaizumi and M. Watanabe, *Pflügers Arch.*, 1992, **420**, 461.
32. R.M. Pitman, J.A. David, L.S. Prothero and S.J.B. Butt, *J. Physiol., Lond.*, 1997, **504**, 4S
33. J.A. Nathanson and P. Greengard, *Science, N.Y.,* 1973, **180**,308.
34. L.S. Prothero, J.C. McLelland, J.A. David, and R.M. Pitman, *Soc. Neurosci. Abstr.*, 1995, **21**, 1374.
35. R.L. Huganir and P. Greengard, *Proc. Natn Acad. Sci. U.S.A. –Biol. Sci.*, 1983, **80**, 1130.
36. A. Safran, R. Sagi-Eisenberg, D. Neumann and S. Fuchs, *J. Biol. Chem.*, 1987, **262**, 10506.
37. J.F. Hopfield, D.W. Tank, P. Greengard and R.L. Huganir, *Nature, Lond.*, 1988, **336**, 677.
38. I.B. Levitan, *A. Rev. Physiol.*, 1994, **56**, 193.
39. L.A. Raymond, C.D. Blackstone and R.L. Huganir, *Trends Neurosci.*, 1993, **16**, 147.
40. M.D. Browning, M. Bureau, E.M. Dudek and R.W. Olsen, *Proc. Natn. Acad. Sci. U.S.A.*, 1990, **87**, 1315.

Molecular Biology

Use and Risk Assessment of Genetically Modified Baculoviruses

J.S. Cory

ECOLOGY AND BIOCONTROL GROUP, NERC INSTITUTE OF VIROLOGY AND
ENVIRONMENTAL MICROBIOLOGY, MANSFIELD ROAD, OXFORD OX1 3SR, UK

1 INTRODUCTION

The failure to reduce the quantity of field and stored-product crops lost to insects, despite the continuing development of chemical insecticides, is a testimony to our need for novel and more effective control agents. One avenue of research which holds great potential is the expansion of the use of microbial insecticides. Microbial insecticides includes organisms which cause disease such as viruses, bacteria, protozoa and fungi and also other micro-parasites such as nematodes. Whilst there is undoubtedly still considerable scope for the expansion of the use of these organisms in their natural form, the most interesting and promising recent developments have been in the construction of genetically modified microbial pesticides. The use of naturally occurring microbial insecticides is likely to be most beneficial on crops with relatively high damage thresholds where the natural ecology of the pest:pathogen interaction can be manipulated. However, the development of faster-acting genetically modified insecticides raises the possibility that they can compete more directly with the synthetic chemical insecticides in high value crops where a faster knockdown is required, thereby expanding microbial insecticide use into a new market. At the forefront of this research is the development of genetically modified baculoviruses (GMBVs). Baculoviruses are invertebrate specific viruses which have a narrow host range compared to other forms of insect control. Most baculoviruses have been isolated from insects, particularly the Lepidoptera (butterflies and moths) and they have a long history of use in their unmodified form.

2 LABORATORY STUDIES

The first aim of the genetic modification of baculoviruses has been to increase their speed of action. Like all pathogens, they need time to multiply and during this period unacceptable crop damage can occur. Several routes to genetic improvement have been taken involving gene deletion as well as gene addition. Baculoviruses, like all organisms, strive to maximize their reproductive success. This does not necessarily mean (in fact it is unlikely) that the characteristics they develop are going to be those which are optimal for insect pest control. For example, there is usually a trade-off between virus productivity and the time taken for the insect to die, so under certain circumstances it may pay the virus to keep the insect alive as long as possible to maximise yield. And this has indeed been found to be the case with baculoviruses. Baculoviruses possess at least one gene which prolongs caterpillar development, thereby increasing yield, the ecdysteroid UDP-glucosyltransferase gene, otherwise known as the *egt* gene. If this gene is deleted, both virus yield and time-to-death are reduced[1]. Deletion of this gene has therefore been proposed as one route for the improvement of insect baculoviruses and is now commonly used in conjunction with the addition of toxin genes (see Table 1).

Table 1. *Addition and deletion of genes to increase the speed of kill of baculoviruses*

Gene added deleted	Virus	Effect on speed of kill	Ref
Egt gene deletion	AcNPV	22% reduction	1
Diuretic hormone	BmNPV	20% reduction	2
Juvenile hormone esterase (JHE)	AcNPV	Only in 1st instars	3
JHE + *egt* minus	AcNPV	As for *egt* minus alone	4
Modified JHE	AcNPV	20-35% reduction	5
Eclosion hormone + *egt* minus	AcNPV	As for *egt* minus alone	6
Prothoracotropic hormone (PTTH)	AcNPV	No effect	7
Chitinase (polyhedrin minus)	AcNPV	20% reduction (injected)	8
Bacillus thuringiensis δ-endotoxin	AcNPV	No effect	9,10
Scorpion toxin (*Buthus*)	AcNPV	No paralytic activity	11
Scorpion toxin AaHIT (*Androctonus*)	AcNPV	25-30% reduction	12,13
	BmNPV	38% reduction	14
Scorpion toxin AaHIT (DA26)	AcNPV	40% reduction	15
Mite toxin Txp-1 (*Pyemotes*)	AcNPV	41% reduction	16
Mite toxin Txp-1 (synthetic prom)	AcNPV	55% reduction	17
Mite toxin Txp-1 (*egt* minus)	HzNPV	40% reduction	18
Spider toxins (*Tegenaria, Diguetia*)	AcNPV	10-33% reduction	19
Scorpion toxin LqhIT1 and 2	AcNPV	25-30% reduction	20

However, the main thrust of BV modification has been the incorporation of foreign genes. Several groups have investigated the expression of genes encoding hormones or enzymes which are derived from insects, with the intention of interrupting insect growth or metabolism. These are summarized in Table 1. On the whole these have been fairly unsuccessful although they may prove to be useful tools in the study of insect endocrinology and physiology. Far more successful has been the work using insect selective toxins. The first successful constructs involved two toxins, one from the North African Scorpion, *Androctonus australis*[12] and the other from the itch mite *Pyemotes tritici*[16]. The toxin from *A. australis*, AaHIT or AaIT, was chosen because there was already a considerable body of knowledge about its host range and mode of action[21,22]. It is a small neuropeptide which causes contractile paralysis in insects. The initial laboratory results with an AaHIT expressing baculovirus demonstrated that speed of action was reduced by approximately 25%[12]. Since then research has concentrated on optimizing the action of these toxins primarily by altering their temporal expression by using different promoters, both baculovirus-derived and from other sources[17]. AaHIT, although an excellent model system, is not as effective on Lepidoptera as it is on other insects. The search for more effective toxins has therefore continued with recent studies investigating baculovirus expression of depressant toxins from scorpion venom[20] and toxins derived from spiders[19] (Table 1). Results from these studies are hard to compare directly due the different viruses and promoters used and the range of methodologies, species and ages of host used to assess any changes. There must be a limit below which speed of action cannot be reduced as the virus needs a certain period during which it must multiply before an effect can be evident and it is likely that some of the recombinant baculoviruses that have been produced must be approaching this. These results look extremely promising, although their real test will come in how effective they are in the field.

3. FIELD TESTS

Whilst the search for novel toxin genes and the genetic modification of baculoviruses has continued apace, field trials and risk assessment/ecological studies have lagged behind. From the insecticide point of view, this is of concern as it is quite possible that differences in efficacy demonstrated in laboratory assays will not be found in the field. This is usually as a result of the variability inherent in the natural system or because of the effect of additional factors which come into play in the field, which will usually act to reduce pathogen-induced mortality. To date, field trials have been restricted to baculoviruses containing one toxin - AaHIT.

The first trials with any genetically modified virus were carried out by the NERC Institute of Virology and Environmental Microbiology in 1986[23]. These trails were followed by the first field test of GMBV with enhanced activity in 1993. This trial showed that a baculovirus (*Autographa californica* NPV, known as AcNPV) expressing AaHIT acted significantly more rapidly than the parent wild-type, resulting in a significant reduction in crop (cabbage) damage[24]. Interestingly, this trial also demonstrated a feature that could not be deduced from laboratory assays; that toxin-expression had a behavioural effect on the insects. In the field the paralysed insects fell off the plants before they died and were unable to climb back up again, thereby enhancing the efficacy of the virus.

Since this trial, two of the major companies involved in the development of genetically modified insecticides in the US, American Cyanamid and DuPont Agricultural Products, have carried out small-scale field tests on a range of crops and target species. Most of the data on the American Cyanamid trials have been published[15,25] but those from DuPont are not yet available. Most of the American Cyanamid work has focused on two constructs; an *egt* deletion mutant and a second recombinant with contains an *egt* deletion and expresses AaHIT. Field trials on the AcNPV *egt* deletion mutant alone in 1993 and 1994 did show a reduction in pest (cabbage looper) numbers in the field as compared to the wild type virus, however, the results were disappointing by comparison with laboratory and greenhouse tests[26]. The first American Cyanamid field trials incorporating the AaHIT toxin (plus *egt* deletion) took place in 1995 in Georgia and Texas on cotton, one of the key insecticide crop targets. Results showed reductions in crop damage which were greater than for the wild type virus or the *egt* deletion mutant. The studies also confirmed that high application rates of the AaHIT-producing virus had no adverse effect on other groups of non-target arthropods[25]. In 1996 the US EPA (Environmental Protection Agency) approved small-scale trials in 12 States on a range of pests on cotton, tobacco, lettuce and cabbage. In cotton and tobacco the AaHIT/*egt* minus construct consistently resulted in pest control equivalent to a chemical treatment at doses of 1.2×10^{12} polyhedra per hectare (relatively high)[25]. The situation in vegetables is more complex as crops can be attacked by a wide range of pests. Results in these crops, whilst showing some improvement compared to the untreated control, were inconclusive, partly due to the influence of species in the pest complex which are not highly susceptible to AcNPV[25].

4. RISK ASSESSMENT

GMBVs contain novel combinations of genes; we therefore need to know whether their wide-scale release into the environment will present any risks. Detailed studies on naturally occurring baculoviruses, which have been developed and registered for pest control over the last two decades, have provided us with a body of data on their safety to humans and other non-target organisms. The restricted host range of baculoviruses is well-established; some baculoviruses appear to infect only single species, whereas others, such as AcNPV, have a wider host range[27]. However, even those with a wider host range are restricted to species from within the order from which they were isolated, in this case the Lepidoptera (butterflies and moths). Laboratory host range testing has also shown that not all species within this range are equally susceptible and lie along a continuum from highly infectable to refractory[23]. So the prime risk from releasing GMBVs is whether they are going to affect these susceptible non-target organisms, causing environmental perturbation.

Various approaches have been adopted for risk assessment, however, the group at IVEM decided that as the issues raised by GMO release are essentially ecological, a quantitative ecological approach was the most appropriate. The 'new', genetically modified, organism can be viewed as a potential invader into target or non-target populations and ecological theory can be used as a basis for assessing whether this invader is likely to gain a foothold. The background to this approach is described in Cory *et al.*[27] and Cory and Hails[28]. As a starting point we can use simple mathematical models which describe the interaction between insect (host) and virus (pathogen) in terms of a few key parameters[29]. The key parameters in the simplest interaction are, virus productivity, transmission (which combines host susceptibility with the likelihood of acquiring an infective dose) and virus persistence. Using these parameters it is possible to describe two terms which define the invasion process: R_0, the basic reproductive rate of the pathogen and H_T, the host population density threshold required for virus invasion[27]. These three parameters will be discussed below.

4.1 Yield

Virus yield can be easily measured in the laboratory. These studies show that there is a clear trade-off with speed of kill: the more rapidly a virus kills, the less virus progeny (polyhedra) are produced. The earlier death of larvae killed by a toxin-producing baculovirus results in considerably reduced yield compared to those insects killed by the parent wild type virus[30]. The effect of this would be to lower the basic reproductive rate of the virus (R_0) and raise the host threshold necessary for virus invasion (H_T). However, as would be expected, laboratory testing has focused on insect pest species which are highly susceptible to the pathogen. For risk assessment, it is necessary to know whether it is possible to extrapolate from the behaviour in highly susceptible hosts to the less susceptible species, which are likely to make up the majority of the non-targets. Very little work has been done on the behaviour of natural or GM BVs in less susceptible hosts. We have carried out an initial study on the cabbage moth, *Mamestra brassicae*, a host of intermediate susceptibility to AcNPV. One unexpected finding from this study was that the toxin-producing virus does not kill faster than the wild type parent[31]. Further testing is needed to ascertain why the toxin is not effective (for example, it is known that AaHIT is not equally effective for all Lepidoptera[21]) and to find out whether this is an isolated case. However, it does illustrate that the response of less susceptible hosts cannot necessarily be predicted from highly susceptible ones.

4.2 Transmission

Transmission is a more difficult parameter to estimate and it can only be measured in the field. In a small-scale field trial we compared transmission of wild type AcNPV and AcNPV expressing AaHIT in a permissive (*Trichoplusia ni*) and a semi-permissive host (*M. brassicae*). As predicted from our first field trial in 1993[24], the transmission parameter for the AaHIT recombinant virus is significantly lower that of the wild type (for both species), primarily as a result of the insects falling off the plants and removing the virus from the vicinity of other susceptible insects. Interestingly, in the field, the semi-permissive host actually produced more virus than the more susceptible host, as a result of it taking longer to die and also being a slightly larger species. However, transmission to *M.brassicae* is significantly lower than to *T. ni* and, curiously, transmission from *M. brassicae* cadavers is lower than from *T. ni* cadavers for both species (Hails *et al*, in prep.).

4.3 Persistence

Baculovirus persistence can also only be studied in the field. It is already known that persistence of the virus varies with microhabitat, for example, virus in the soil tends to be more protected from UV degradation than virus on foliage. This means that any virus existing in these protected pockets could form a reservoir, which could play a role in virus-host dynamics if it is translocated from the reservoir to a site where it could initiate infection (for discussion see Hails *et al.*[32]). Because caterpillars infected with the toxin-producing viruses drop off the plant, the spatial distributions of the wild type and recombinant viruses produced in the epizootic are different. This could affect virus persistence: in the short term it means that secondary cycling of the virus to foliar feeding insects is reduced, however, in the longer term, it is possible that the recombinant virus in the soil persists for longer than the wild type and may have the potential to initiate new cycles of infection. These are the type of questions we are currently addressing in our field trials.

5 CONCLUSIONS

The first generation of recombinant baculovirus insecticides look extremely promising and it is to be hoped that wider testing in the field will lead to their acceptance as viable and environmentally acceptable control agents in agricultural crops. The interest in genetically modified baculoviruses has also had the added bonus that it has increased interest in baculovirus ecology. If we understand more about the behaviour of these pathogens in natural populations we should be able to deploy both natural and genetically modified baculoviruses more effectively in the field. All of studies so far infer that the addition of toxin genes (and any other modifications to the baculovirus genome) results in a less competitive virus which should die out in competition with the wild type. Therefore it would appear that we are essentially pursuing a safe strategy which should not result in environmental perturbation. However, we still need more information on the behaviour of baculoviruses in hosts which cover the whole range of susceptibility, as well as information on the ecology of these viruses in natural populations. This information will be particularly important as the genetic modification of baculoviruses moves into the second phase, the modification of host range, which will raise a wider range of issues than altering speed of kill.

Acknowledgements

The ideas behind much of this research are the result of a productive collaboration with Rosie Hails at IVEM. The data reported here could not have been produced without a team effort, in particular, I would like to thank Rosie Hails, Steve Sait, Pedro Hernández-Crespo, Bernadette Green and Tim Carty for their hard work, ideas and enthusiasm.

References

1. D. R. O'Reilly and L. K. Miller, *Bio Technology* 1991, **9**, 1086-1089.
2. S. Maeda, *Biochem. Biophys. Res. Comm.*, 1989, **3**, 1177-1183.
3. B. D. Hammock, B. C. Bonning, R. D. Possee, T. N. Hanzlik, T. N. and S. Maeda, *Nature*, 1990, **344**, 458-461.
4. R. Eldridge, D. R. O'Reilly, B. D. Hammock and L. K. Miller, *Appl. Environ. Micro.* 1992a, **58**, 1583-1591.
5. B. C. Bonning and B. D. Hammock, *Annu. Rev. Entomol.*, 1996, **41**, 191-210.
6. R. Eldridge, D. R. O'Reilly and L. K. Miller, *Biol. Control*, 1992b, **2**, 104-110.
7. D. R. O'Reilly, T. K. Kelly, E. P. Masler, B. S. Thyafaraja, R. M. Robson, R. C. Shaw and L. K. Miller, *Insect Biochem. Mol. Biol.*, 1995, **25**, 475-485.

8. K. Gopalakrishnan, S. Muthukrishnan and K. J. Kramer, *Insect Biochem. Mol. Biol.*, 1995, **25**, 255-265.
9. A. T. Merryweather, U. Weyer, M. P. G. Harris, M. Hirst, T. Booth and R. D. Possee, *J. Gen Virol.* 1990, **71**, 1535-1544.
10. B. M. Ribiero and N. E. Crook, *J. Invertebr. Pathol.*, 1993, **62**, 121-130.
11. L. F. Carbonell, M. R. Hodge, M. D. Tomalski and L. K. Miller, *Gene*, 1988, **73**, 409-418.
12. L. M. D. Stewart, M. Hirst, M. L. Ferber, A. T. Merryweather, P. J. Cayley and R. D. Possee, *Nature*, 1991, **352**, 85-88.
13. B. F. McCutchen, P. V. Choudary, R. Crenshaw, D. Maddox, S. G. Kamita, N. Palekar, S. Volrath, E. Fowler, B. D. Hammock and S. Maeda, *Bio technology*, 1991, **9**, 848-852.
14. S. Maeda, S. L. Volrath, T. N. Hanzlik, S. A. Harper, K. Majima, D. W. Maddox, B. D. Hammock and E. Fowler, *Virology*, 1991, **184**, 777-780.
15. B. C. Black, L. A. Brennan, P. M. Dierks and I. E. Gard, In: *The Baculoviruses*. Ed. L. K. Miller, pp. 341-387, Plenum Press, New York, 1997.
16. M. D. Tomalski and L. K. Miller, *Nature*, 1991, **352**, 82-85.
17. A. Lu, S. Seshagiri and L. K. Miller, *Biol. Control*, 1996, **7**, 320-332.
18. H. J. R. Popham, L. Yonghong and L. K. Miller, *Biol. Control*, 1997, **10**, 83-91.
19. P. R. Hughes, H. A. Wood, J. P. Breen, S. F. Simpson, A. J. Duggan and J. A. Dybas, *J. Invertebr. Pathol.* 1997, **69**, 112-118.
20. E. Gershburg, D. Stockholm, O. Froy, S. Rashi, M. Gurevitz and N. Chejanovsky, *FEBS Letters*, 1998, **422**, 132-136.
21. R. Herrman, L. Fishman and E. Zlotkin, *Insect Biochem.*, 1990, **20**, 625-637.
22. E. Zlotkin, D. Kadouri, E. Gordon, M. Pelhate, M. F. Martin and H. Rochat, *Arch. Biochem. Biophys.* 1985, **240**, 877-887.
23. D. H. L. Bishop, M. L. Hirst, R. D. Possee and J. S. Cory, In: *50 Years of Microbials*, Eds. G. K. Darby, P. A. Hunter, and A. D. Russell, pp. 249-277, Cambridge University Press, Cambridge, UK, 1995.
24. J. S. Cory, M. L. Hirst, T. Williams, R. S. Hails, D. Goulson, B. M. Green, T. M. Carty, R. D. Possee, P. J. Cayley and D. H. L. Bishop, *Nature*, 1994, **370**, 138-140.
25. I. E. Gard, In: *Microbial insecticides: novelty or necessity?*, pp. 101-114, BCPC Symposium no. 68, 1997.
26. M. F. Treacy, J. N. All and G. M. Ghidiu, *J. Econ. Entomol.*, 1997, **90**, 1207-1214.
27. J. S. Cory, R. S. Hails and S. M. Sait, In: *The Baculoviruses*, Ed. L. K. Miller, pp. 301-339, Plenum Press, 1997.
28. J. S. Cory and R. S. Hails, *Curr. Op. Biotech.*, 1997, **8**, 323-327.
29. R. M. Anderson and R. M. May, *Phil. Trans R. Soc. London. Biol. Sci.* 1981, **291**, 451-524.
30. Y. Kunimi, J. R. Fuxa and B. D. Hammock, *Ent. Exp. et appl.*, 1996, **81**, 251-257.
31. P. Hernández-Crespo, S. M. Sait, R. S. Hails and J. S. Cory, *Appl. Environ. Micro.*, in review.
32. R. S. Hails, J. S. Cory, C. A. Donnelly, M. L. Hirst, M. R. Speight, D. Goulson and T. Williams, *Am. Nat.* in review.

Functional Assays for Cloned Insect Sodium and Calcium Channels

Linda M. Hall, Christer Ericsson and Hongjian Xu

DEPARTMENT OF BIOCHEMICAL PHARMACOLOGY, STATE UNIVERSITY OF NEW YORK AT BUFFALO, BUFFALO, NY 14260, USA

1 ION CHANNELS AS TARGETS FOR INSECTICIDES

Voltage-sensitive ion channels, especially those such as sodium and calcium channels which are involved in excitable cell depolarization, are generally excellent targets for insecticides. Indeed, many plants have developed insect defense mechanisms by producing toxins which act on these channels. For example, chrysanthemums make pyrethrums, the natural product which was the basis for synthetic pyrethroids. The Monk's Hood plant produces aconitine. Both of these toxins act on insect sodium channels. Tetrandrine, a plant derived product used in Chinese herbal medicine, acts on insect calcium channels[1]. There are likely to be many, as yet undiscovered, natural products which will target insect sodium or calcium channels. To identify new lead compounds from synthetic organic chemistry, from plant extracts, or from venom of spiders, scorpions and other venomous creatures, it is important to have rapid screening assays for the function of these target channels. Functional assays will help to identify the mechanism of action of new pesticides at the target site and are useful to compare the relative sensitivity of mammalian and insect targets. To this end we are developing functional assays for cloned insect sodium and calcium channels.

The cloning of several ion channel subunits and neurotransmitter receptors from insects has opened the door for the development of direct functional assays. In addition, having the gene for a pesticide target in hand has facilitated the identification of mutations causing resistance. In this manuscript, we discuss two examples of how Drosophila genetics has played a key role in the development of functional assays for new insecticide testing. The first example, using insect sodium channels, illustrates how Drosophila genetics identified and allowed the positional cloning of a novel insect sodium channel component required for robust expression of the channel in an heterologous expression system. The second example focuses on insect calcium channels and illustrates how a genetic approach provides an unambiguous answer to the question of whether blocking a particular channel will kill the insect. In addition, a genetic approach has allowed us to address the question of whether there is functional redundancy between the two different genes that encode similar calcium channel $\alpha 1$ subunits.

Our genetic studies have generated information of importance in the logical choice of new target systems. Functional studies are providing information of importance concerning pharmacological differences between insect and mammalian ion channels. Functional analysis of resistant mutants versus wild type allows us to identify structurally unrelated compounds which nevertheless show cross resistance. Finally, information concerning subunit interactions generated in the course of our work may lead to the development of novel ways to inhibit ion channel function.

2 INSECT SODIUM CHANNELS

2.1 Genetic Identification of Sodium Channel Auxiliary Subunits: The TipE Protein

Biochemical purification and subsequent gene cloning studies of mammalian voltage sensitive sodium channels demonstrated that these channels are composed of a large α subunit and two smaller, auxiliary subunits designated $\beta 1$ and $\beta 2$ as illustrated in Figure 1A[2,3].

Sodium Channel Components

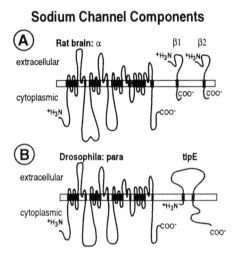

Figure 1 *Comparison of general structure of sodium channels from rat brain (A) versus Drosophila (B)*

Although some mammalian sodium channels, such as $\mu 1$ from skeletal muscle, express well in heterologous expression systems such as Xenopus oocytes, current levels are often low and channel kinetics are abnormally slow. Coexpression with the auxiliary β subunits increases current levels and restores normal channel kinetics.

The first insect sodium channel α subunit was cloned from Drosophila through positional cloning of the *para* gene[4]. However, it could not be functionally expressed in Xenopus oocytes. Several observations led us to postulate that there was a another factor required for sodium channel function both in Xenopus oocytes and in Drosophila. We postulated that factor was the product of the *tipE* (temperature induced paralysis locus E) gene. First, *tipE* gene mutants show a paralytic phenotype very similar to *para* mutations, that is rapid paralysis at the nonpermissive temperature followed by rapid recovery at the permissive temperature. Second, saxitoxin binding studies showed a reduction in number of membrane-associated sodium channels in *tipE* relative to wildtype[5]. Third, *tipE* mutants show synergistic effects on viability and nerve conduction when combined with various *para* mutant alleles[6]. To investigate the role of tipE in sodium channel function and regulation, we identified the cDNA for this gene by positional cloning involving: deletion mapping, chromosome walking, DNA sequencing of mutant and wild type genes, and finally by transformation rescue using the cloned candidate cDNA under the control of an inducible promoter[7,8].

The protein encoded by the *tipE* gene is unlike any other protein in the sequence databases, showing the power of a genetic approach to identify novel proteins. Hydropathy profiles combined with *in vitro* translation in the presence and absence of microsomes established the TipE protein as a heavily glycosylated, integral membrane protein with two transmembrane domains[8]. Figure 1B shows the transmembrane topology of the TipE protein is different from the mammalian auxiliary β subunits. For TipE both amino and carboxy termini are on the cytoplasmic side of the membrane and there is a large extracellular loop containing several sites for glycosylation.

2.2 Role of TipE in Sodium Channel Functional Assays

To determine the role of TipE in sodium channel function, the Xenopus oocyte expression system was used[8]. cRNA from *para* alone, *tipE* alone, or *para* plus *tipE* were injected into Xenopus oocytes and currents recorded after 2 to 6 days. As shown in Figure 2 (left panel), when *para* alone was injected, only very small currents of 200 to 300 nAmps were detected. No currents were seen when only tipE was injected (data not shown). However, when para cRNA was coinjected with tipE, peak currents of ~5 μAmps were detected. In the experiment in Figure 2, the peak current averaged 18-fold higher in the presence of TipE compared with in its absence. In general, peak current increased from 13 to 30-fold in the presence of TipE. These sodium currents were very sensitive to tetrodotoxin and were completely inhibited by 10 nM[8]. Although the sodium currents seen in the absence of TipE were small, they were proportional to the amount of *para* cRNA injected.

Using this Drosophila *para/tipE* expression system the comparative pharmacological specificity of insect sodium channels has been defined[9]. Insect channels differ from vertebrate channels in several ways. Although insect and some mammalian channels show similar affinity to toxin II from *Anemonia sulcata*, this toxin causes a 100-fold greater decrease in the rate of inactivation in the Drosophila channels than in mammalian channels. In comparison to rat brain II sodium channels, insect channels are >10-fold more sensitive to tetrodotoxin block and >100-fold more sensitive to the pyrethroid permethrin. This was the first direct demonstration that the selective toxicity of pyrethroid insecticides is due, in part, to increased target site affinity. Thus, this expression system can be used to address many long standing questions concerning toxin interactions with insect sodium channels.

Xenopus oocyte expression

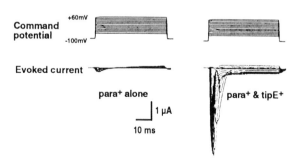

Figure 2 *Drosophila Para Sodium Current Stimulation by TipE Coexpression*

With the utility of the *para/tipE* expression system firmly established for the analysis of insect sodium channels, we are now interested in determining the mechanism of action of TipE. The absence of TipE results in very low sodium current expression in Xenopus oocytes[8] and in reduced numbers of membrane-associated channels in Drosophila homozygous for the *tipE* mutation[5]. How does tipE exert its effects? To address this question, we have made recombinant cDNA constructs carrying an epitope tagged para α subunit. This has allowed us to monitor α subunit incorporation into oocyte membranes in the presence and absence of TipE. Immunoprecipitation of epitope-tagged Para from solubilized membrane extracts of ^{35}S methionine labeled oocytes has shown that the total amount of Para protein synthesized and incorporated into membranes in the presence of TipE is only ~2-fold higher than in its absence (Ericsson and Hall, unpublished results). However, these same oocytes showed a 13-fold increase in sodium current levels. Thus, we conclude that in the presence of TipE more functional sodium channels are reaching the cell surface than in its absence. However, the increase in sodium currents cannot be due solely to increased rate of protein synthesis, increased incorporation of Para into membranes or decreased rate of Para protein degradation.

We propose two possible models shown in Figure 3 to explain TipE action. In Model I in the absence of TipE, the Para protein is synthesized and incorporated into membranes approximately normally. However, the protein does not move normally to the surface membrane. Instead, it accumulates in internal membranes where it does not function as an ion channel. Only a small number of the synthesized α subunits reach the surface. In this model TpE is acting like a chaperone to guide channels to the proper insertion site in the surface membrane. In Model II, the Para protein reaches the cell surface but does not function normally in the absence of TipE. Experiments are in progress to distinguish these two models using immunofluoresence with the epitope-tagged Para constructs to determine how expression in the presence of TipE affects trafficking to the cell surface.

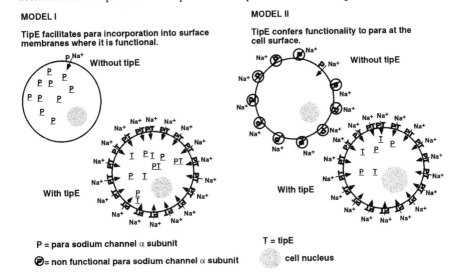

MODEL I

TipE facilitates para incorporation into surface membranes where it is functional.

MODEL II

TipE confers functionality to para at the cell surface.

P = para sodium channel α subunit

Ⓟ = non functional para sodium channel α subunit

T = tipE

cell nucleus

Figure 3 *Two Models for the Role of TipE in Sodium Channel Function.*

2.3 Requirement for the TipE Protein Across Insect Species

While the Drosophila sodium channel can be used effectively as a model system for insect sodium channels, assays using cloned sodium channels from insect pests will be required for testing species specific pesticides targeted against sodium channels. Recently, Smith and coworkers[10] have shown that the cloned housefly sodium channel can be expressed in Xenopus oocytes in the presence of Drosophila TipE. Do non-Dipteran insect sodium channels also require TipE for robust functional expression? In collaboration with the laboratories of Ke Dong (Michigan State University) and Alan Goldin (University of California-Irvine), we (Sinakevitch-Pean et al., poster presentation in this meeting) have tested the need for TipE in the functional expression of German cockroach Para sodium channels in Xenopus oocytes. The cockroach Para sodium channel protein shows an overall 78% sequence identity to the Drosophila Para[11]. We find that for the cockroach, just as for the Dipteran species, Drosophila TipE causes dramatic stimulation of sodium currents. Coexpressing cockroach Para sodium channel with TipE at cRNA concentrations that give peak currents of 2-3 μAmps, produces no detectable sodium currents when the cockroach Para is expressed alone This is the farthest cross species requirement for TipE that has been demonstrated to date. It is likely the TipE gene product or its homologue will be required for expression of all insect sodium channels including those of pests for which functional assays are a high priority.

The cockroach sodium channel α subunit/TipE expression system is also very useful for defining changes in channel properties and pharmacological specificity in cockroach channels with kdr[11,12] (Dong, 1997; Miyazaki et al., 1996) or *superkdr* mutations[13]. Briefly, Sinakevitch-Pean et al. (poster abstract from this meeting) have shown that there is little or no difference between wild-type cockroach sodium channels and those expressing *superkdr* mutations (L993F in domain II-S6 and M918T in the cytoplasmic IIS4-S5 loop) in terms of voltage-dependence of channel activation or voltage-dependence of channel inactivation. However, the wild-type channels are much more sensitive to the pyrethroid deltamethrin and to the site 2 neurotoxin aconitine. Thus, we have used this expression system to conclusively demonstrate that *superkdr* mutations in the sodium channel α subunit simultaneously cause resistance to both pyrethroids and site 2 neurotoxins. This system will provide an efficient way to determine whether existing mutations will cause cross-resistance to new candidate insecticides.

2.4 High Throughput Assay for Insect Sodium Channels

The assay of insect sodium channels using expression in Xenopus oocytes provides the fastest way to test new constructs and interesting resistant mutations. However, it is labor intensive since each cell to be recorded must be individually injected. For high throughput screening we are developing permanently transformed cell lines expressing FLAG epitope tagged Para alone, HA epitope tagged TipE alone and both in combination. To make these cell lines most suitable for use in high throughput screens, we are including a single point mutation in the ion selectivity filter of the α subunit to convert the selectivity from sodium to calcium as described for other sodium channels[14]. This will allow the use of well-characterized calcium-sensitive dyes in conjunction with robotic monitoring to rapidly test for compounds which interfere with channel function. Candidate compounds will then be tested on channels with the normal sodium selectivity filter to make certain that the change introduced for screening purposes does not affect interaction of the channel with candidate compounds of interest. In screening for new drugs acting on insect sodium channels, it will be extremely important to include in subsequent testing the various alternative *para* splice variants[15] to test for differences in sensitivity. Forms differing in sensitivity as a result of alternative splicing or RNA editing would provide a reservoir within the insect population for rapid development of resistance simply by shifting from one structural isoform to another.

3 CALCIUM CHANNELS

3.1 Calcium Channel Structure

Our initial knowledge of calcium channel subunit structure has come from purification and cloning of mammalian calcium channels from skeletal muscle and other tissues. (See reviews by Campbell et al.[16], 1988; Catterall, 1995[2].) As illustrated in Figure 4, the pore forming subunit, designated α1 in calcium channels has the same general architecture as the α subunit of sodium channels. (See Figure 1 for comparison.) The common features are that both sodium and calcium α/α1 subunits have 4 homologous repeats each with 6 transmembrane domains and a loop between transmembrane segments 5 and 6 which dips into the membrane to form part of the ion selective pore. In each case the S4 transmembrane segment has positively charged residues every third or fourth amino acid and is thought to be part of the voltage sensor which moves through the membrane in response to membrane depolarization. In addition to the pore forming α1 subunit, calcium channels have an α2-δ subunit encoded by a single gene and cleaved during posttranslational processing. The δ portion is membrane bound and is attached to the α2 subunit through disulfide bonds. In addition there is a totally cytoplasmic β subunit which interacts with the α1 subunit at the cytoplasmic loop between repeat domains I and II. Finally, mammalian skeletal muscle channels contain a membrane associated γ subunit which has not been found in neuronal N type[17] or P/Q type calcium channels[18]. For some calcium channels the auxiliary subunits (α2-δ, β, and γ) are needed to reconstitute channel properties in heterologous expression systems. Some subunits, like the cardiac α1 interact promiscuously with different auxiliary subunit structural isoforms. In other cases such as mammalian skeletal muscle, the α1 subunits are very selective and calcium channel currents can be measured only in the presence of specific auxiliary subunit isoforms[19].

What is known about insect calcium channel subunit structure? We have identified two different genes (Dmca1A and Dmca1D)[20] which encode Drosophila α1 subunits. These two insect α1 subunits resemble those from mammals. We have also cloned one gene encoding a β subunit (Ren, Chopra, and Hall, unpublished results). Each of these genes (two α1 and one β) undergo extensive alternative splicing and at least one of them may generate additional heterogeneity through RNA editing[20,21]. The Drosophila genome sequencing project suggests that there

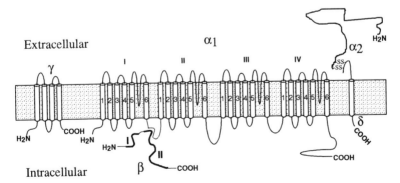

Figure 4 *Calcium Channel Structure as Determined for Mammalian Skeletal Muscle Dihydropyridine Receptors*

may be another $\alpha 1$ subunit gene in the region near to where Dmca1D maps. Our Xenopus oocyte expression studies strongly suggest that there is also an $\alpha 2$-δ subunit in the Drosophila genome since calcium channel currents from the cloned Dmca1D $\alpha 1$ and β subunits are dramatically stimulated by coexpression with mammalian $\alpha 2$-δ (M. Chopra and L.M. Hall, unpublished results). Taken together this work suggests that insect calcium channels have a subunit composition similar to mammals. That is, the functional channel consists of a complex of at least $\alpha 1$, $\alpha 2\delta$, and β subunits. The existence of a γ subunit in insects is undetermined at this time.

In Drosophila there are multiple genes encoding different forms of the same subunit type at least for the pore-forming $\alpha 1$ subunit and possibly for some of the others as well. We have identified two $\alpha 1$ subunits and have shown that they map to different chromosome locations. Preliminary evidence from the Drosophila genome project suggests the existence of a third $\alpha 1$ subunit gene. There may be still other calcium channel subunit genes to be discovered.

3.2 Are Calcium Channels Good Targets for New Insecticides?

Given the genetic heterogeneity of insect calcium channel components, a key question to be addressed is whether blockade of one subtype of insect calcium channel will lead to lethality? In light multiple genes encoding similar pore-forming subunits, the formal possibility exists that these subunits will be functionally redundant but pharmacologically distinct. Indeed, as shown in the dendrogram below, the two calcium channel $\alpha 1$ subunits sequenced to date, Dmca1A and Dmca1D, fall into two structurally different families distinct in their sensitivities to dihydropyridines. Those channels falling below the dotted line fall into the dihydropyridine-sensitive, L-type calcium channel category. Dmca1D is in this category. Indeed, Dmca1D is sensitive to blockade by dihydropyridine antagonists such as nifedipine (M.Chopra and L.M. Hall, unpublished results). Interestingly, the Dmca1D channel is insensitive to the dihydropyridine agonist Bay K8644 which is why in Figure 5 we categorize it as both sensitive (to antagonists) and insensitive (to agonists).

The pharmacological specificity of the other Drosophila $\alpha 1$ subunit Dmca1A has not yet been determined. However, as shown in Figure 5, it falls into the structural group that is generally insensitive to dihydropyridines. Thus, Dmca1A is likely to have a pharmacological profile distinct from Dmca1D. If these two channels were functionally redundant and pharmacologically distinct, a toxin which blocks one might not affect the

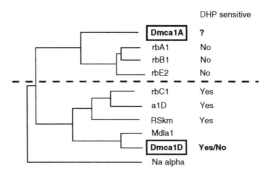

Figure 5 *Dendrogram Showing the Structural Relationship and Dihydropyridine Sensitivity of Calcium Channel $\alpha 1$ Subunits Cloned from Drosophila and Mammals*

other making killing of the insect more difficult since both channels would have to be inactivated to give killing. The most direct way to determine whether calcium channel genes such as Dmca1A and Dmca1D show functional redundancy is to determine the null mutant phenotype. In Drosophila this determination is often assisted by the existance of mutations in many genes. For example, the Dmca1D gene mapped to a region of the Drosophila genome which was saturated for mutations[22].

To determine whether any of the existing mutations affected the Dmca1D calcium channel α1 subunit, deletion mapping was performed as illustrated in Figure 6. Panel A illustrates the method for deletion mapping a recessive trait. If the mutant phenotype is expressed in a deletion heterozygote (upper panel in A), that mutation maps within the region of the deletion. If the wild-type phenotype is seen, the mutation maps outside the deleted region. A similar strategy of *in situ* hybridization to polytene chromosomes from deletion heterozygotes is used for mapping the cloned gene labeled with biotinylated nucleotides so that the hybridized probe can be readily detected. If the clone maps within the deletion, it will be seen hybridizing to the wild type chromosome only (the loop area) since the equivalent region is missing in the deleted chromosome (A, upper right panel arrow). If the cloned gene maps outside the deletion, it will be seen as a dark band hybridizing across both chromosomes (at arrow in lower right panel in A). Figure 6B summarizes the deletions tested (with the vertical bar indicating the extent of the deletion and the horizontal tics showing the ends each deletion). Also summarized are the mutant genes in that area which were tested.

The only gene which showed the same deletion mapping pattern as the cloned gene hybridization was *l(2)35Fa*, which has an embryonic lethal phenotype. Subsequent sequencing of DNA from this gene for several different mutant alleles identified point mutations in the Dmca1D α1 subunit[19,23]. This evidence in conjunction with transformation rescue of the mutant phenotype with a cosmid clone containing only this gene, provided convincing evidence that *l(2)35Fa* encodes the Dmca1D α1 subunit. This study also demonstrated that when this channel is not functioning, embryonic lethality results. Thus, there is no functional redundancy between

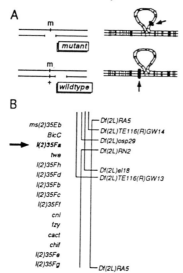

Figure 6 *Method for Deletion Mapping of Cloned Genes (Panel A) and Existing Mutations (Panel B) to Identify Candidate Genes Corresponding to Clones*

DmcalD and DmcalA. Similarly, null mutant alleles of DmcalA also result embryonic lethality[20] providing additional evidence for the lack of functional redundancy between these two different calcium channel α1 subunit genes. The fact that when either subunit activity is blocked the flies die as embryos make each of these calcium channel subunits excellent targets for the development of new classes of insecticides.

3.3 Insect Calcium Channel Functional Assays

Having established that both DmcalA and DmcalD calcium channels are good targets for insecticides, the next important step is to develop assays for testing agents which target these channels. Here we describe two assays. The first involves the Drosophila larval muscle preparation which allows immediate testing of compounds on two different calcium channel currents expressed in larval muscle. The second uses heterologous expression of cloned calcium channel subunits in Xenopus oocytes. As for sodium channel assays, future development of stably transformed cell lines will provide a rapid method for high throughput robotic testing of new compounds affecting these channels.

3.3.1 Larval Muscle Preparation. This preparation involves dissection of third instar larvae followed by two electrode voltage clamping of the large body wall muscles. These muscle cells express two distinct calcium channel currents[24] which can be separated pharmacologically or electrophysiologically as shown schematically in Figure 7. The A (Amiloride-sensitive) current is blocked by 1 mM amiloride or by a holding potential of - 30 mV allowing the D (Dihydropyridine sensitive) current to be studied in isolation. Alternatively, the D current is blocked with either 500 mM diltiazem or 10 µM nifedipine (a dihydropyridine antagonist) allowing study of the A current. Recent work from our laboratory using this preparation in conjunction with a missense mutation in the DmcalD gene has shown that the D current is produced by calcium channels containing the DmcalD α1 subunit[25]. Mutations in DmcalD are without effect on the A current suggesting that this current is due to channels with a non DmcalD α1 subunit. It remains to be determined what α1 subunit gene is involved in production of the A current. Although this open preparation allows testing of effects of compounds on two different calcium channel currents, it is labor-intensive and the preparation is relatively unstable. Therefore, the development of functional assays with the cloned Drosophila calcium channel subunit genes would provide a number of advantages.

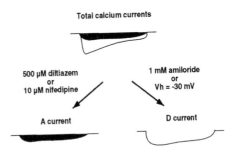

Total calcium currents

500 µM diltiazem
or
10 µM nifedipine

1 mM amiloride
or
Vh = -30 mV

A current   D current

Figure 7   *Separation of Calcium Channel Currents in Larval Muscle Using Pharmacological or Electrophysiological Methods*

3.3.2 Expression in Xenopus Oocytes. We have in hand clones encoding two different Drosophila calcium channel α1 subunits (including several splice variants of each)[20,21] plus numerous splice variants of one beta subunit (D. Ren and L.M. Hall, unpublished work). Initial work has focused on developing a Xenopus oocyte expression assay for the dihydropyridine-sensitive Dmca1D that is expressed in larval muscle[25], nervous system[21] and also affects Drosophila embryonic heart function[23]. As with the Drosophila sodium channel expression, initial attempts to express the Dmca1D calcium channel in Xenopus oocytes were problematic even when coexpression with the Drosophila β subunit and various combinations of mammalian subunits was attempted. Since there were no candidate mutants readily available that might encode the missing subunit, we took another strategy of making chimeras between the Drosophila Dmca1D α1 subunit and the readily expressed rabbit cardiac α1 subunit in order to define regions in the Drosophila α1 subunit causing expression problems. Using 16 chimeras, we narrowed the problem region to a small domain in one of the intracellular loops (Ren and Hall, unpublished observations). We were able to get robust expression from a chimeric α1 subunit containing 96% Drosophila sequence. Since the problem internal segment is not near any of the known calcium channel drug binding sites, we are currently using this chimera for initial characterization of this calcium channel pharmacology.

The interesting question remains as to why an internal segment must be mammalian in order to get expression in Xenopus oocytes. One possibility is that this segment must interact with an insect-specific component that has not yet been identified. Since this is a nonmembrane region, it is possible that a yeast two hybrid screen will be useful in the identification of this missing component. A second possibility is that we may have assembled incompatible splice variants in this region since it is a region where alternative splicing occurs.

3.4 Calcium Channel Pharmacology

Using the 96% Drosophila chimeric α1, one of the Drosophila β subunit splice variants, and mammalian α2δ subunit cDNAs, we have been able to get consistent robust expression of calcium channel currents in Xenopus oocytes. We find that these currents are insensitive to amiloride, but can be blocked with the dihydropyridine antagonist nifedipine and by diltiazem (M. Chopra and L.M. Hall, unpublished observations). This confirms our previous conclusion the Dmca1D is responsible for the dihydropyridine- and diltiazem-sensitive D current in larval muscle[19] and provides clear evidence that the Dmca1D channel current is insensitive to amiloride. Interestingly, the Drosophila channel is about 20-fold less sensitive to nifedipine than is the mammalian cardiac channel. In addition, the Drosophila channel is insensitive to the dihydropyridine agonist Bay K 8644. (M. Chopra and L.M. Hall, unpublished observations). These striking differences between the mammalian and insect L-type calcium channels suggests that at least some of the amino acid differences between the two should provide sites for the development insect-selective toxins. The two assays we describe for insect calcium channels should provide a means to evaluate various natural products and scorpion and spider toxins for their direct effects on insect calcium channels.

4 FUTURE DIRECTIONS IN SODIUM AND CALCIUM CHANNEL STUDIES

One of the recurring themes in our work has been observations of the importance of auxiliary subunit interaction in ion channel function. Mutations in the *tipE* gene reduce the number of functional sodium channels in neuronal membranes in the fly. Drosophila sodium currents expressed in the absence of TipE in Xenopus oocytes are dramatically lower than in its presence. Calcium channel expressed current levels are also dramatically affected by coexpression with auxiliary subunits. Thus, one novel way to inhibit channel function would be to develop reagents that interfere with subunit interactions. Coexpression with TipE has no effect on many mammalian sodium channels (skeletal muscle μ1 or rat brain II, for example) and mammalian sodium channel β subunits are without effect on the Drosophila Para sodium channel. The development of reagents which would interfere with TipE interaction with Para sodium channels offers the exciting potential for very specific effects on insect sodium channels. For such a program to be fruitful, a careful structure-function analysis of TipE is required.

The feasibility of disrupting subunit interactions can be tested first on the insect calcium channels because a substantial amount of work has gone into defining the regions of interaction between α1 and β subunits in mammalian channels[26,27]. Since the sites of interaction are well-defined on both the α1 and β subunits, we reasoned that it should be possible to block the interaction of β with α1 by producing excess amounts of the short interaction site (I-II loop) from α1. If this loop retains proper configuration, it may interact with free β subunits and acting as a dominant negative mutation would prevent normal interaction between β with α1. The idea for this is illustrated in Figure 8. We have produced a mini gene from the I-II loop of the Dmca1D α1 subunit that prevents Drosophila β subunit stimulation of the Drosophila calcium channel expression in Xenopus oocytes. It will be interesting to test this construct for effects *in vivo* using transformation rescue.

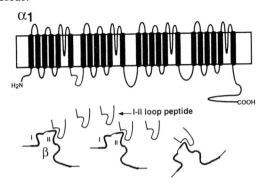

Figure 8 *Strategy for Development of Molecular Biological Reagents to Interfere with Insect Specific Ion Channel Subunit Interaction. The Drosophila Calcium Channel α1 Subunit I-II Loop Interferes with β Stimulation of Calcium Channel Currents*

The availability of cloned insect ion channels and functional assays for them are rapidly opening new doors for exploration and development. In critiquing the science fiction movie *Star Ship Troopers* (in which the world is about to be invaded by giant insects), US movie critique Roger Ebert wrote: "You'd think a human race capable of interstellar travel might have developed an effective insecticide, but no...." The method that the human Star Ship Troopers used in this movie was to machine gun the insects to death which, like some of our insecticides, did not work very well. The insects just kept coming. With the rapid advances in molecular cloning and functional expression of insect channels, there is reason to be hopeful that in the future, with a bit of imagination, we will find more effective methods than the Starship Troopers had at their disposal for insect control.

Acknowledgments

Our sodium channel work was supported initially by NIH Jacob Javits Investigator Award NS16204 and subsequently by funding from American Cyanamid. The Drosophila *para* clone was provided by J. Warmke at Merck. Our calcium channel work has been supported by NIH MERIT Award HL39369 and by funding from Rhone Poulenc.

References

1. H. Glossman, C. Zech, J. Striessnig, R. Staudinger, L. Hall, R. Greenberg and B.I. Armah, *Br. J. Pharmacol.*, 1991, **102**, 446.

2. W.A. Catterall, *Annu. Rev. Biochem.*, 1995, **64**, 493.

3. L.L. Isom, D.S. Ragsdale, K.S. De Jongh, R.E Westenbroek, B.F. Reber, T. Scheuer and W.A. Catterall, *Cell*, 1995, 433.

4. K. Loughney, R. Kreber, and B. Ganetzky, *Cell*, 1989, **58**, 1143.

5. F.R. Jackson, S.D. Wilson and L.M. Hall, *J. Neurogenet.*, 1986, **3**, 1.

6. B. Ganetzky, *J. Neurogenet.*, 1986, **3**, 19.

7. G. Feng, P. Deák, D.P. Kasbekar, D.W. Gil and L.M. Hall, *Genetics,* 1995, **139**, 1679.

8. G. Feng, P. Deák, M. Chopra and L.M. Hall, *Cell*, 1995, **82**, 1001.

9. J.W. Warmke, R.A.G. Reenan, P. Wang, S. Qian, J.P. Arena, J. Wang, D., K. Liu, G.J. Kaczorowski, L.H.T. Van der Ploeg, B. Ganetzky and C.J. Cohen, *J. Gen. Physiol.*, 1997, **110**, 119.

10. T.J. Smith, S.H. Lee, P.J. Ingles, D.C. Knipple and D.M. Soderlund, *Insect Biochem. Molec. Biol.*, 1997, **27**, 807.

11. K. Dong, *Insect Biochem. Molec. Biol.*, 1997, **27**, 93.

12. M. Miyazaki, K. Ohyama, D.Y. Dunlap and F. Matsumura, *Mol. Gen. Genet.*, 1996, **252**, 61.

13. M.S. Williamson, D. Martinez-Torres, C.A. Hick and A.L. Devonshire, *Mol. Gen. Genet.*, 1996, **252**, 51.

14. S.H. Heinemann, H. Terlau, W. Stuhmer, K. Imoto, and S. Numa, *Nature*, 1992, **356**, 441.

15. J.R. Thackeray and B. Ganetzy, *J. Neurosci.*, 1994, **14**, 2569.

16. K.P. Campbell, A.T. Leung and A.H. Sharp, *TINS* , 1988, **11**, 425.

17. D.R. Witcher, M. De Waard, J. Sakamoto, C. Franzini-Armstrong, M. Pragnell, S.D. Kahl and K.P. Campbell, *Science*, 1993, **261**, 486.

18. H. Liu, M. De Waard, V.E.S. Scott, C.A. Gurnett, V.A. Lennon and K.P. Campbell, *J. Biol. Chem.*, 1996, **271**, 13804.

19. D. Ren and L. M. Hall, *J. Biol. Chem.*, 1997, **272**, 22393.

20. L.A. Smith, X.-J. Wang, A.A. Peixoto, E.K. Neumann, L.M. Hall and J.C.J. Hall, *Neurosci.*, 1996, **16**, 7868.

21.   W. Zheng, G. Feng, D.Ren, D. F. Eberl, F. Hannan, M. Dubald and L. M. Hall, *J. Neurosci.*, 1995, **15**, 1132.

22.   M. Ashburner, P. Thompson, J. Roote, P.F. Lasko, Y. Grau, M. el Messal, S. Roth and P. Simpson, *Genetics*, 1990, **126**, 679.

23.   D.F. Eberl, D.J. Ren, G.P. Feng, L.J. Lorenz, D. Van Vactor and L.M. Hall, *Genetics*, 1998, **148**, 1159.

24.   M. L. Gielow, G.-G. Gu and S. Singh, *J. Neurosci.*, 1995, **15**, 6085

25.   R. Ren, H. Xu, D.F. Eberl, M. Chopra and L.M. Hall, *J. Neurosci.*, **18**, 2335.

26.   M. De Waard, M. Pragnell and K.P. Campbell, *Neuron*, 1994, **13**, 495.

27.   M. De Waard, D.R. Witcher, M. Pragnell, H. Liu and K.P. Campbell, *J. Biol. Chem.*, 1995, **270**, 12056.

Why Are There So Few Insecticide Resistance-associated Mutations?

R.H. ffrench-Constant, B. Pittendrigh, A. Vaughan and N. Anthony

DEPARTMENT OF ENTOMOLOGY AND CENTER FOR NEUROSCIENCE, UNIVERSITY OF WISCONSIN-MADISON, MADISON, WI 53706, USA

1 INTRODUCTION

The three major targets of conventional insecticides are: 1) the γ-aminobuyric acid (GABA) receptor containing RDL subunits encoded by the gene *Resistance to dieldrin* or *Rdl*, the target for cyclodiene insecticides and the recently introduced fipronils; 2) the PARA voltage gated sodium channel encoded by the gene *para*, the target site for DDT and pyrethroids and 3) insect acetylcholinesterase (AChE) encoded by the gene *Ace*, the target site for organophosphorus (OP) and carbamate insecticides. All three of these target site encoding genes have been cloned in the genetic model *Drosophila melanogaster*, supporting the previously proposed role of this insect as a model in which to study insecticide resistance [1, 2]. However, recently homologs of these *Drosophila* target site genes have also been cloned from a range of pest insects and the underlying resistance-associated mutations compared. Interestingly, despite the wide range of insects studied, and presumed differences in the modes of insecticide selection, the same residues are consistently replaced in the same receptors/enzymes. Namely, a single residue in RDL, two residues in PARA and three or more in AChE.

The purpose of the current chapter is to examine the question: Why are there so few resistance-associated mutations in the genes encoding these receptors/enzymes? This will be achieved by examining our work on receptor/enzyme function in relation to the likely functional constraints placed on these important components of the insect nervous system. In each case a working model or hypothesis is presented to account for the conservation of amino acid replacements observed in the context of what we know about the normal function of the receptor and which residues may interact with the insecticide.

2 CONSERVATION OF RESISTANCE-ASSOCIATED MUTATIONS

2.1 The *Rdl* encoded GABA receptor

The gene, *Rdl*, encoding the GABA receptor subunit RDL was cloned from a *D. melanogaster* mutant resistant to cyclodiene insecticides and picrotoxinin (PTX), a vertebrate GABA$_A$ receptor antagonist [3]. The pharmacology of RDL containing insect receptors and the relationship of these GABA receptors to those found in vertebrates has recently been reviewed elsewhere [4]. In order to determine the resistance-associated mutation(s), we examined worldwide collections of resistant *D. melanogaster*. In these strains we consistently documented the replacement of the same amino acid, alanine302, with a serine [5]. Following functional expression of RDL subunits as homomultimers in a range of heterologous expression systems [6, 7], we also confirmed the functional relevance of this mutation by showing that replacement of alanine302 with a serine results in insensitivity of the resulting GABA gated chloride channels [6]. Importantly, RDL containing GABA receptor subunits are widely expressed in the insect nervous system [8, 9] and, despite the fact that we can document that RDL co-assembles with another unidentified subunit (via observed differences of channel conductance *in vivo* and *in vitro* [10]), RDL expression *in vitro* reconstitutes most of the pharmacology observed in insect GABA receptors *in vivo* [6, 10, 11]. Survey of a wide range of other insect species including several beetles, a mosquito *Aedes aegypti*, the whitefly *Bemisia tabaci* and a cockroach *Blatella germanica* [12-14], showed that this alanine to serine replacement was the most common resistance-associated replacement. Wherease more rarely (in a different fruitfly, *D. simulans* [5] and an aphid, *Myzus persicae* (N. Anthony and R. ffrench-Constant, unpublished) the same residue is replaced with a glycine.

2.2 The *para* voltage gated sodium channel

The gene, *para*, which encodes the PARA voltage gated sodium channel, was cloned from *Drosophila* in the laboratory of Barry Ganetzky on the basis of the *temperature sensitive* paralytic phenotypes displayed by *para^ts* alleles [15]. The PARA sodium channel appears to be the major insect sodium channel and is a large polypeptide composed of four homology domains (I-IV) each containing six proposed hydrophobic membrane spanning domains (S1-6) [15]. Following linkage studies that correlated resistance to DDT and pyrethroids with the location of the *para* homologous sodium channel gene in *knockdown resistant* (*kdr*) house flies [16, 17] and cockroaches [18], *para* homologs were cloned from both species and the underlying resistance-associated mutations examined [19-21]. Again, replacements were confined to a very limited number (two) of different positions. The first, associated with the original *kdr* strain, was in the S6 hydrophobic segment of homology domain II (termed IIS6). The second, associated with another more resistant allele, termed *super-kdr*, was found as a double mutant with both the *kdr* mutation and a second replacement in the intracellular loop between IIS4 and IIS5. The '*kdr*-like' replacement is similar in the house fly [19, 20], the horn fly [22], the cockroach [21], the tobacco budworm *Heliothis virescens* [23], an aphid *M. persicae* [24] and a mosquito *Anopheles gambiae* [25], whereas the second *super-kdr* type mutation has only been found in resistant house flies [19] and horn flies [22]. Interestingly, to date most of these replacements associated with field collected resistance alleles, reside within the second homology domain of the protein.

Recently, the housefly *para* homolog (termed a voltage-sensitive sodium channel α subunit gene or *Vssc1*) has been functionally expressed in *Xenopus* oocytes and the leucine1014 to phenylalanine replacement (*kdr* mutation) has been shown to confer 10-fold insensitivity to cismethrin on the resulting sodium channels [26].

2.3 The acetylcholinesterase encoding locus *Ace*

AChE degrades the neurotransmitter acetylcholine in the insect synapse and is the primary target site for OP and carbamate insecticides which inhibit acetylcholine hydrolysis by binding to the enzyme. The gene, *Ace*, which encodes insect acetylcholinesterase (AChE) was again cloned from *Drosophila* based on the knowledge of its location via isolation of a range of different mutants [27]. Screening of a range of different *D. melanogaster* and house fly strains has identified a range of different amino acid replacements putatively causing resistance (reviewed in [28]). The functional significance of several of these have been tested in the *Drosophila* enzyme following the heterologous expression of different mutants in *Xenopus* oocytes and direct testing of their insensitivity to a range of different insecticide inhibitors [29]. Comparison of the different putative resistance-associated amino acid replacements between the fruitfly and the house fly [28] again suggests that only a limited subset of replacements cause resistance despite the widely differing sizes and structures of different OP and carbamate insecticides. However, many of these resistance-assoicated residues are predicted to lie within or close to the active site gorge of this enzyme, based on superimposition of the insect amino acid sequence upon the three dimensional crystal structure obtained from *Torpedo* [29]. The role of other replacements *linked* to AChE insensitivity in other insects, such as the Colorado potato beetle *Leptinotarsa decemlineata* [30], remains to be functionally proven.

3 IMPLICATIONS FOR RECEPTOR/ENZYME STRUCTURE FUNCTION

3.1 The RDL containing GABA receptor

RDL GABA receptor subunits coassemble in a variety of expression systems to give functional homomultimeric GABA gated chloride ion channels [6, 7]. Further, despite the fact that the conductance of these channels differs from those of RDL containing channels in the insect nervous system [10, 11] (showing that other subunits are present in RDL containing receptors in the insect nervous system), these homomultimers reconstitute much of the GABA receptor pharmacology displayed *in vivo*, notably PTX/cyclodiene sensitivity and bicuculline insensitivity [10]. The observation that replacement of alanine302 with a serine confers insecticide insensitivity leads to the simplest hypothesis that PTX and cyclodienes actually bind within the ion channel pore (as alanine302 is within the second membrane spanning region which is predicted to line the chloride ion channel pore by homology with structural and modelling work performed in the closely related nicotinic acetylcholine receptor [31]). However, our consistent finding of replacements of this same amino acid (either with a serine or a glycine) in a wide range of different insects leads us to examine *why* only this residue is replaced in resistance. Thus, for example, the binding site of PTX and cyclodienes is unlikely to interact with only this single residue, therefore why can't other residues in the binding site be replaced to give resistance?

To examine this question we performed a biophysical analysis of wild type and mutant RDL receptors via the patch clamping of cultured *Drosophila* neurons [11]. Detailed analysis revealed significant but small shifts in a range of channel parameters namely; small changes in the shape of the GABA dose response curves, small changes in both the inward and the outward conductance of the channel and a net stabilisation of the channel's open state. However, the largest change in a single channel parameter was in the rate of receptor desensitization [11, 32]. This can be described as the rate at which the channel returns to its normal activatable state under prolonged exposure to GABA. Thus, channels containing alanine302 to serine replacements desensitized 29 times slower than wild type and desensitization was incomplete. Although these changes are at first difficult to reconcile with the interaction of the receptor with the antagonist, other workers have proposed that PTX binds preferentially to the desensitized state of the vertebrate $GABA_A$ receptor [33]. We have therefore formulated a working model whereby replacements of alanine302 have a dual role in both: 1) interacting directly with the drug binding site within the ion channel pore and 2) allosterically destabilizing the insecticide preferred desensitized state of the RDL containing GABA receptor [11, 32].

Our recent experiments on cultured *Drosophila* neurons have added weight to this hypothesis by demonstrating that replacement of alanine302 with a glycine residue (the alternative resistance-associated replacement found in nature) also confers resistance to PTX and is again (like alanine302 to serine) associated with slower and incomplete receptor densensitization. Further, experiments have been performed to test a corolary of this hypothesis: that replacements of other residues known to affect rates of receptor desensitization should also affect resistance but to a lesser extent. In conclusion, current data is consistent with a model whereby replacements of alanine302 cause resistance by both interacting directly with the insecticide binding site and also allosterically by destabilizing the insecticide preferred (desensitized) conformation of the receptor. This infers that replacements having effects on only one process or the other would not exert sufficient resistance on the whole insect for insecticide selection to be effective in the field.

3.2 The PARA voltage gated sodium channel

We examined DDT resistance in a group of twelve independent *para* mutants, including two that cause dominant temperature-sensitive paralysis, nine showing recessive temperature sensitivity and one that causes a smell-blind phenotype [34]. Of these twelve mutants, we found that six were also associated with DDT insensitivity. As expected, resistance was sex-linked, as *para* is X-linked in *D. melanogaster*, and not responsive to the synergist piperonyl butoxide (PBO) which supresses metabolic resistance [34]. Two general aspects of the overall nature of these mutations are noteworthy. Firstly, exactly half of the temperature sensitive mutants examined conferred resistance, despite the fact that they were not pre-selected with insecticides. This may infer that only a limited number of replacements can be generated in the sodium channel polypeptide which confer a temperature sensitive and/or resistant phenotype. Secondly, although many of them occupy equivalent positions to the *kdr* and *super-kdr* mutations, none reside in domain II. This might infer that replacements in homology domain II are less prone to temperature sensitive phenotypes and this avoidance of a potentially adverse fitness cost may be part of the reason why most resistance-associated replacements appear confined to domain II in natural populations. However, alternatively, we note that a further '*kdr-like* ' replacement (i.e. located in the equivalent secton of S6) correlated with resistance in *Heliothis virescens* lies in homology domain I and not domain II [4]. Thus suggesting that resistance-associated replacements *can* be found in other homology domains and that their previous documentation solely in domain II may just be an artifact of a) the limited number of species examined and b) the emphasis on re-examining the same region i.e. II S6.

Several specific aspects of the relative locations of the different replacements in *D. melanogaster* are also interesting [34]. Thus the replacements fall into three different categories. 1) Those that are '*kdr*-like', such as *para74* which resides in an equivalent position in S6 but in the third rather than second homology domain. 2) Those that are '*super-kdr*-like', such as *paraDN7* and *parats1/parats2* (independent occurences of the same point mutation) which lie within the intracellular S4-S5 linker but in domains III and II respectively. 3) Those that occupy a novel position, such as *paraDTS2/paraDN43* (again independent examples of the same mutation) which lie within the S5-S6 loop that may actually form part of the sodium channel linning. In terms of resistance levels generated, independently, the *kdr*-like or *super-kdr*-like replacements in *D. melanogaster para* both confer low levels of resistance to DDT. Interestingly, similarly to *super-kdr* in the house fly, combination of a *kdr*-like and *super-kdr*-like mutation in *Drosophila* heterozygous for the two alleles also gives increased resistance to the type II (cyano group containing) pyrethroids in the whole fly.

Again the simplest interpretation of these data is that these replacements all denote the binding site for either DDT and type I (*kdr*-like replacements) or additionally type II (*super-kdr*-like replacements) pyrethroids [19]. However, our results suggest the possibility of a different mechanism. The identification of DDT-resistant mutations at nearly equivalent sites to *kdr* and *super-kdr* but in other homology domains suggests that if these mutations do indeed define a binding site, this site is likely to be composed of residues contributed by each of the four homology domains. This possibility seems reasonable given the essentially tetrameric structure of the sodium channel α subunit. However, it is also possible that the sodium channel mutations characterized here, and in previous studies, confer resistance to pyrethroids and DDT by a mechanism other than direct alteration of the binding site. The pharmacological effect of these insecticides is to cause persistent activation of sodium channels by delaying the normal voltage-dependent mechanism of inactivation [35]. Rather than directly affecting the binding of pyrethroids and DDT, the mutations may confer resistance by causing functional changes in sodium channel properties that compensate for or that alleviate the consequences of the insecticide. For example, if the mutations altered the voltage-dependence or kinetics of activation or inactivation, the neurotoxic effects of the insecticide could be reduced or overriden. In this context we note that recent functional analysis of the equivalent of the *kdr* associated amino acid replacement in a rat sodium channel has provided evidence for accompanying changes in voltage dependence [36].

This interpretation is particularly consistent with the resistant mutations that map to the S4-S5 loop in the different homology domains because a variety of evidence from various systems suggests the importance of this region in channel function. Mutations in this loop are known to reduce fast inactivation of potassium channels [37]. Furthermore, mutations in mammalian sodium channels at or near the site defined by the *para*[DN7] mutation are associated with a variety of abnormalities. One form of long QT syndrome, an inherited cardiac arrhythmia, is caused by an amino acid substitution in the SCN5A channel at a site adjacent to the residue affected by *para*[DN7] [38]. At the identical residue as *para*[DN7], an alanine to threonine replacement in the human SCN4A channel causes paramyotonia congenita, a disorder associated with decreased kinetics of sodium channel inactivation [39, 40]. The same replacement in a mouse neuronal sodium channel produces the *jolting* phenotype [41]. Functional studies indicate that this mutation significantly shifts the voltage-dependence of activation in the depolarizing direction. The *para*[ts1] mutation resides at the identical location in homology domain I and may cause functional perturbations analogous to those caused by mutations in the vicinity of *para*[DN7]. The *kdr/para*[74] mutations in S6 transmembrane segments might also alter the gating properties of sodium channel in some distinctive manner.

Our finding of synergistic resistance to pyrethroids in *para*[74]*/para*[DN7] heterozygotes is of particular interest. The lesions in these two mutations in homology domain III are in analogous locations to the two mutant sites in homology domain II in *super-kdr* strains of houseflies and the elevated levels of resistance in the heterozygote approximates the enhanced resistance in *kdr* vs. *super-kdr* strains. But the two circumstances are very different. In *super-kdr* mutants the two lesions reside in the same polypeptide (i.e. they are in *cis*), in *para*[74]*/para*[DN7] heterozygotes the lesions reside in different polypeptides (i.e. in *trans*). The increased resistance in *super-kdr* housefly strains is presumed to reflect a combined deficit on pyrethroid binding by the doubly mutant polypeptide. This explanation seems inadequate to account for the phenotype of *para*[74]*/para*[DN7] heterozygotes. However, this phenotype can be reconciled with the alternative view that resistance is mediated via functional alterations of the encoded sodium channel polypeptides. The particular functional defect associated with one mutation could enhance the perturbation caused by the other. For example, one mutation could alter the inactivation mechanism leading to a slight depolarization of membrane potential and the other could alter the voltage dependence of inactivation. The combined effect in double heterozygotes could be very different from the effect of either mutation alone or when heterozygous with a wild-type allele. This interpretation is also consistent with the observed phenotypic dominance of the double heterozygote in the presence of an extra copy of the *para* locus encoding wild-type sodium channel subunits. This situation is analogous to the dominant effect of mutations causing hyperkalemic periodic paralysis [39, 42, 43] in humans where the misbehavior of a small percentage of mutant sodium channels at the resting membrane potential shifts all the rest of the channels (including wild-type channels) to an inactivated state [44].

3.3 Acetylcholinesterase

To date the functional relevance of potential resistance-associated replacements in insect AChE has only been tested in *D. melanogaster* [29]. Therefore in order to confirm the relevance of putative resistance-associated mutations in a pest insect we have chosen the *Ace* gene from the yellow fever mosquito *A. aegypti* as a model system in which to study the effects of mutations on a pest insect enzyme [45, 46]. This mosquito is a vector of both yellow fever and dengue and in which we have recently found insensitive AChE in populations in Trinidad [47].

Acetylcholinesterase genes (*Ace* homologues) have now also been cloned from a number of insect species including the mosquitoes *Anopheles stephensi* [48] and *Culex pipiens* (C. Malcolm, unpublished). However, although insecticide insensitive AChE has been widely documented biochemically from a range of both *Culex* and *Anopheles* mosquitoes [49-55], no resistance-associated mutations have been described from mosquitoes themselves.

Analysis of insecticide insensitive AChE in mosquitoes has also recently been complicated by the discovery of two AChEs (AChE1 and AChE2) in *Culex pipiens* [56]. These differ in their sensitivity to insecticide inhibition. Thus in susceptible insects, AChE1 can be inhibited by a fixed dose of a carbamate insecticide (propoxur, 5×10^{-4} M) whilst AChE2 is unaffected by this concentration [57]. Linkage mapping of the *Ace* probe cloned from *Culex pipiens* suggest that it is encoded by a sex-linked locus (C. Malcolm, pers. comm.), whereas resistance in *Culex* is not sex-linked. However, detailed analysis of inhibition profiles in a range of other mosquito species, including *A. aegypti*, suggests that most other mosquitoes only bear a single *Ace* locus and that *C. pipiens* may therefore be an exception. Interestingly, linkage mapping of the *A. aegypti* clone discussed here, shows that it maps extremely close to the sex-determining locus [58], suggesting that resistance should be sex linked.

We cloned a section of the *Ace* locus from *A. aegypti* via use of degenerate primers in the polymerase chain reaction and then isolated a full length clone from an adult cDNA library [45]. Functional expression was achieved in baculovirus infected SF21 insect cells [45] and the effects of the resistance associated amino acid replacements found in *Drosophila* and the house fly were tested *in vitro*. Resistance of AChE to OP and carbamate insecticides is due to modifications of the active site (amino acid replacements) and these modifications also appear to alter the catalytic activity of the enzyme towards insecticides and also substrates. Thus the mutant forms of *Aedes* AChE all behaved differently from the wild-type when initial rates of activity were assayed with the synthetic substrates ASCI, PSCI and BSCI. In most cases, the initial rate was highest with ASCI, followed by PSCI and then BSCI. However, in the single mutant F350Y and the double mutant F105S+F350Y, higher rates of activity with PSCI and BSCI when compared to ASCI were observed, for which the rate of activity was approximately 20% of the wild-type enzyme [46]. In *D. melanogaster*, the corresponding F368Y mutant also has higher rates of activity with PSCI and BSCI [59]. Furthermore, decreased rates of reaction with ASCI for insensitive forms of AChE have been documented in both *Anopheles albimanus* and *C. pipiens* [55, 57]. It will therefore be interesting to investigate, if when rates of reaction with ASCI fall, whether replacements equivalent to F368Y are found.

In terms of resistance, mutagenesis of *D. melanogaster Ace* showed a correlation between the number of mutations in the expressed enzyme and the bimolecular constant (k_i) ratio of the mutated versus the wild-type from of the enzyme [29]. In general, the greater the number of resistance-associated amino acid replacements, the higher resistance ratio, although this was not always the case. In the *Aedes* enzyme, a similar pattern of relative insensitivity was found. However, the comparison is complicated by the presence of one of the mutations in the wild-type form of the *A. aegypti Ace* since the Ile199Val mutation in *D.*

melanogaster AChE is already present in *A. aegypti* AChE (Val185). Whereas in *D. melanogaster*, none of the single point mutations gave rise to significant levels of resistance, the G285A mutant gives >20 fold increase in the resistance ratio with the OP paraoxon. For both classes of insecticides, the double mutant G285Y+F350Y and the triple mutant gave substantial increases in the resistance ratio with all the insecticides tested.

The three-dimensional structure of *Torpedo californica* AChE has been determined [60] and it is thus possible to superimpose other AChEs on this. G303 in *D. melanogaster* (G285 in *A. aegypti*) is thought to effect the orientation of the active site serine, which is phosphorylated by OPs and carbamylated by carbamates and F368 (F350 in *A. aegypti*) is near the acyl moiety of the bound substrate [29]. The presence of both these mutations in *A. aegypti* AChE has a profound effect on the binding of insecticide resulting in the high resistance ratios observed.

4 CONCLUSIONS

Despite the potential complexity (e.g. the predicted multi-subunit nature of RDL containing GABA receptors) and/or large size (e.g. the PARA voltage gated sodium channel) of the receptors and enzymes that constitute the primary targets for conventional insecticides, the number of resistance-associated amino acid replacements documented to date are strikingly few. In this paper we have attempted to reconcile this extreme conservation with working hypotheses on the role of these replacements in receptor/enzyme insecticide insensitivity. This was achieved by detailed functional analysis of the insect GABA receptor and also a mutagenesis of the insect voltage gated sodium channel that relies upon phenotypes independent of resistance, namely temperature sensitive paralysis. This latter mutagenesis underscores the potential importance of temperature sensitive phenotypes in isolating toxicologically relevant mutations in insects and in this respect it is also interesting to note in hindsight that *Rdl*$^{alanine302>serine}$, originally isolated on the basis of insecticide resistance, is also itself a temperature sensitive paralytic [61].

To explain this striking degree of conservation in replacements in both the GABA gated chloride channel, and potentially the voltage gated sodium channel, we suggest that the interaction of more than one channel function with insecticide binding sites may be important in constraining the location of resistance-associated replacements. Thus in the RDL containing GABA receptor, alanine302 interacts both directly with the insecticide binding site and also allosterically by destabilizing the insecticide preferred desensitized state of the receptor. In the *para* voltage gated sodium channel, the observation that individual mutations in individual channel polypeptides can combine in *Drosophila* to cause similar effects to mutations found in the same polypeptide, also suggests that each mutation may have a unique role in affecting channel function. For example, one replacement could alter the inactivation mechanism, leading to a slight depolarization of the membrane, and the second could alter the voltage dependence of inactivation. In AChE we need to test the functional relevance of other resistance-associated mutations found in pest insects in order to further test the functional relevance of hypotheses advanced for replacement insecticide interactions in the *Drosophila* enzyme [29].

These types of studies in which the detailed biophysics of the receptors/enzymes associated with insecticide targets not only elucidate potential binding sites but also illustrate that these proteins are dynamic molecules that interact with their antagonists and agonists in a range of different conformations. The effect of resistance-associated replacements may therefore not be easily mimiced by static models based on simple 'lock and key' type binding interactions. Although currently confined to the three historically important targets, such studies will also become important in the face of likely target site insensitivity in new targets such as the nicotinic acetylcholine receptor (nACh), the target for important new compounds such as immidacloprid and spinosad. In the latter case the close structural relationship between GABA receptors and nACh receptors may forewarn us to potential resistance mechanisms to these highly effective compounds.

References

1.   T.G. Wilson. *J. Econ. Entomol.*, 1988, **81**, 22.
2.   R.H. ffrench-Constant, R.T. Roush and F. Carino. in 'Molecular Approaches to Pure and Applied Entomology', Springer-Verlag, Berlin, 1992.
3.   R.H. ffrench-Constant, D.P. Mortlock, C.D. Shaffer, R.J. MacIntyre and R.T. Roush. *Proc. Natl. Acad. Sci. USA*, 1991, **88**, 7209.
4.   A.M. Hosie, K. Aronstein, D.B. Sattelle and R. ffrench-Constant. *Trends Neurosci.*, 1997, **20**, 578.
5.   R.H. ffrench-Constant, J. Steichen, T.A. Rocheleau, K. Aronstein and R.T. Roush. *Proc. Natl. Acad. Sci. USA*, 1993, **90**, 1957.
6.   R.H. ffrench-Constant, T.A. Rocheleau, J.C. Steichen and A.E. Chalmers. *Nature*, 1993, **363**, 449.
7.   H.-J. Lee, T. Rocheleau, H.-G. Zhang, M.B. Jackson and R.H. ffrench-Constant. *FEBS Lets.*, 1993, **335**, 315.
8.   K. Aronstein and R. ffrench-Constant. *Inv. Neurosci.*, 1995, **1**, 25.
9.   K. Aronstein, T. Rocheleau and R.H. ffrench-Constant. *Inv. Neurosci.*, 1996, **2**, 115.
10.   H.-G. Zhang, H.-J. Lee, T. Rocheleau, R.H. ffrench-Constant and M.B. Jackson. *Molec. Pharmacol.*, 1995, **48**, 835.
11.   H.-G. Zhang, R.H. ffrench-Constant and M.B. Jackson. *J. Physiol.*, 1994, **479**, 65.
12.   M. Thompson, J.C. Steichen and R.H. ffrench-Constant. *Insect Mol. Biol.*, 1993, **2**, 149.
13.   R.H. ffrench-Constant, J.C. Steichen and L.O. Brun. *Bull. Ent. Res.*, 1994, **84**, 11.
14.   N.M. Anthony, J.K. Brown, P.G. Markham and R.H. ffrench-Constant. *Pestic. Biochem. Physiol.*, 1995, **51**, 220.
15.   K. Loughney, R. Kreber and B. Ganetzky. *Cell*, 1989, **58**, 1143.
16.   M.S. Williamson, I. Denholm, C.A. Bell and A.L. Devonshire. *Mol. Gen. Genet.*, 1993, **240**, 17.
17.   D.C. Knipple, K.E. Doyle, P.A. Marsella Herrick and D.M. Soderlund. *Proc. Natl. Acad. Sci. USA*, 1994, **91**, 2483.
18.   K. Dong and J.G. Scott. *Ins. Biochem. Mol. Bio.*, 1994, **24**, 647.
19.   M.S. Williamson, D. Martinez-Torres, C.A. Hick and A.L. Devonshire. *Mol. Gen. Genet.*, 1996, **252**, 51.
20.   M. Miyazaki, K. Ohyama, D.Y. Dunlap and F. Matsumura. *Mol. Gen. Genet.*, 1996, **252**, 61.
21.   K. Dong. *Insect Biochem. Molec. Biol.*, 1997, **27**, 93.
22.   F.D. Guerrero, R.C. Jamroz, D. Kammlah and S.E. Kunz. *Insect Biochem. Molec. Biol.*, 1997, **27**, 745.
23.   Y. Park and M.F.J. Taylor. *Insect Biochem. Molec. Biol.*, 1997, **27**, 9.
24.   L.M. Field, A.P. Anderson, I. Denholm, S.P. Foster, Z.K. Harling, N. Javed, D. Martinez-Torres, G.D. Moores, M.S. Williamson and A.L. Devonshire. *Pestic. Sci.*, 1997, **51**, 283.
25.   D. Martinez-Torres, F. Chandre, M.S. Williamson, F. Darriet, J.B. Berge, A.L. Devonshire, P. Guillet, N. Pasteur and D. Pauron. *Insect Mol. Biol.*, 1998, 179.
26.   T.J. Smith, S.H. Lee, P.J. Ingles, D.C. Knipple and D.M. Soderlund. *Insect Biochem. Molec. Biol.*, 1997, **27**, 9.
27.   L.M. Hall and P. Spierer. *EMBO J.*, 1986, **5**, 2949.
28.   R. Feyereisen. *Toxicol. Lets.*, 1995, **82/83**, 83.
29.   A. Mutero, M. Pralavorio, J.-M. Bride and D. Fournier. *Proc. Natl. Acad. Sci. USA*, 1994, **91**, 5922.
30.   K.Y. Zhu and J.M. Clark. *Pestic. Biochem. Physiol.*, 1997, **57**, 28.
31.   R.J. Leonard, C.G. Labarca, P. Charnet, N. Davidson and H.A. Lester. *Science*, 1988, **242**, 1578.

32. R.H. ffrench-Constant, H.-G. Zhang and M.B. Jackson. 'Molecular Action of Insecticides on Ion Channels'., American Chemical Society, San Diego, California, 1995, Volume 591, Chapter 12, p. 192.

33. C.F. Newland and S.G. Cull-Candy. *J. Physiol.*, 1992, **447**, 191.

34. B. Pittendrigh, R. Reenan, R.H. ffrench-Constant and B. Ganetzky. *Mol. Gen. Genet.*, 1997, **256**, 602.

35. D.M. Soderlund and J.R. Bloomquist. *Annu. Rev. Entomol.*, 1989, **34**, 77.

36. Y. Horiguchi, T. Senda, N. Sugimoto, J. Katahira and M. Matsuda. *J. Cell Sci.*, 1995, **108**, 3243.

37. E.Y. Isacoff, Y.N. Jan and L.Y. Jan. *Nature*, 1991, **353**, 86.

38. Q. Wang, J. Shen, Z. Li, K. Timothy, G.M. Vincent, S.G. Priori, P.J. Schwartz and M.T. Keating. *Human Molec. Genetics*, 1995, **4**, 1603.

39. A.I. McClatchey, D. McKennayasek, D. Cros, H.G. Worthen, R.W. Kuncl, S.M. DeSilva, D.R. Cornblath, J.F. Gusella and R.H. Brown. *Nature Genet.*, 1992, **2**, 148.

40. N. Yang, J. Ji, M. Zhou, L.J. Ptacek, R.L. Barchi, R. Horn and A.L. George. *Proc. Natl. Acad. Sci. USA*, 1994, **91**, 12785.

41. D.C. Kohrman, M.R. Smith, A.L. Goldin, J. Harris and M.H. Meisler. *J. Neurosci.*, 1996, **16**, 5993.

42. L.J. Ptacek, A.L. George, R.C. Griggs, R. Tawil, R.G. Kallen, R.L. Barchi, M. Robertson and M.F. Leppert. *Cell*, 1991, **67**, 1021.

43. C.V. Rojas, J.Z. Wang, L.S. Schwartz, E.P. Hoffman, B.R. Powell and R.H. Brown. *Nature*, 1991, **354**, 387.

44. S.C. Cannon, R.H. Brown and D.P. Corey. *Neuron*, 1991, **6**, 619.

45. N. Anthony, T. Rocheleau, G. Mocelin, H.-L. Lee and R.H. ffrench-Constant. *FEBS Lets*, 1995, **368**, 461.

46. A. Vaughan, T. Rocheleau and R. ffrench-Constant. *Exp. Parasitol.*, 1997, **87**, 237.

47. A. Vaughan, D.D. Chadee, and R. ffrench-Constant. *Med. Vet. Entomol.*, **12**, in press.

48. L.M. Hall and C.A. Malcolm. *Cell. Mol. Neurobiol.*, 1991, **11**, 131.

49. Z.H. Tang and S.L. Cammak. *Pestic. Biochem. Physiol.*, 1990, **37**, 192.

50. R. Haas, T.L. Marshall and T.L. Rosenberry. *Biochemistry*, 1988, **27**, 6453.

51. J. Hemingway, C. Malcolm, K. Kissoon, R. Boddington, C. Curtis and N. Hill. *Pest. Biochem. Physiol.*, 1985, **24**, 68.

52. J. Hemingway and G.P. Georghiou. *Pest. Biochem. Physiol.*, 1983, **19**, 167.

53. H. Ayad and G.P. Georghiou. *J. Econ. Entomol.*, 1975, **68**, 295.

54. M. Raymond, D. Fournier, J.-M. Bride, A. Cuany, J. Berge, M. Magnin and N. Pasteur. *J. Econ. Entomol.*, 1986, **79**, 1452.

55. R.H. ffrench-Constant and B.C. Bonning. *Med. Vet. Entomol.*, 1989, **3**, 9.

56. D. Bourguet, M. Raymond, D. Fournier, C.A. Malcolm, J.-P. Toutant and M. Arpagaus. *J. Neurochem.*, 1996, **67**, 2115.

57. D. Bourguet, N. Pasteur, J. Bisset and M. Raymond. *Pest. Biochem. Physiol.*, 1996, **55**, 122.

58. D.W. Severson, N.M. Anthony and R.H. ffrench-Constant. *J. Heredity*, 1997, in press.

59. D. Fournier, S. Berrada and V. Bongibault. in 'Molecular Genetics and Evolution of Pesticide Resistance', American Chemical Society, Washington DC, 1996.

60. J.L. Sussman, M. Harel, F. Frolow, C. Oefner, A. Goldman, L. Toker and I. Silman. *Science*, 1991, **253**, 872.

61. R.H. ffrench-Constant, J.C. Steichen and P. Ode. *Pestic. Biochem. Physiol.*, 1993, **46**, 73.

Functional Genetics of Cholinergic Synaptic Transmission in *Caenorhabditis elegans*

David B. Sattelle and Emmanuel Culetto

THE BABRAHAM INSTITUTE, LABORATORY OF MOLECULAR SIGNALLING, DEPARTMENT OF ZOOLOGY, UNIVERSITY OF CAMBRIDGE, DOWNING STREET, CAMBRIDGE CB2 3EJ, UK

1. INTRODUCTION

In the nervous system, cells communicate at chemical synapses by the regulated discharge and subsequent detection of chemical messengers (neurotransmitters). Our current understanding of chemical synaptic transmission results from the application of techniques including molecular biology, biochemistry and advanced electrophysiology to a variety of nerve terminal preparations. Often work in this field has been led by studies on cholinergic chemical synapses at which acetylcholine (ACh) is the neurotransmitter[1]. Recently progress has been accelerated by powerful new genetic approaches which are also transforming our understanding of human neurogenetic disorders[2,3].

In cholinergic nerve terminals, vesicles generated by endocytosis from the plasma membrane are filled with ACh which is stored until an action potential triggers the release by exocytosis of vesicle contents from the presynaptic nerve terminal into the synaptic cleft. This involves vesicle fusion with the plasma membrane, a sequence of events requiring the co-ordinated actions of many proteins[4]. The released ACh acts on postsynaptic (and presynaptic) ACh receptors. The fast actions of ACh are mediated by ionotropic (nicotinic) receptors containing an integral ion channel; slower actions are mediated by metabotropic (muscarinic) receptors. The actions of ACh are terminated by the hydrolytic enzyme acetylcholinesterase (AChE, EC 3.1.1.7); choline, a product of this hydrolysis is taken up for re-use by a specific, high-affinity choline uptake transporter (HaChUT). The actions on cells of released neurotransmitters such as ACh and other chemical signals result in a diversity of pre- and postsynaptic responses that contribute to the rich array of synaptic interactions in the nervous system.

Genetics offers poweful experimental approaches to the study of chemical synaptic transmission and nowhere is this more evident than in the nematode *Caenorhabditis elegans*. Here we outline the experimental advantages of using *C. elegans* in this way, and review recent genetic, biochemical and molecular analyses of cholinergic synaptic function. First we summarize current knowledge of genes involved in the synthesis and transport of acetylcholine. Secondly, recent data on presynaptic terminal function and the release of ACh are discussed. We then focus on the ongoing characterization in *C. elegans* of two cholinergic gene families, the nicotinic acetylcholine receptors which mediate the fast action of ACh and the acetylcholinesterases which terminate its synaptic action. Members of both gene families are also well established targets for commercial nematode control agents.

2. *CAENORHABDITIS ELEGANS* AS A MODEL ORGANISM FOR STUDIES OF SYNAPTIC TRANSMISSION

Caenorhabditis elegans is a free-living soil nematode. There are 959 somatic nuclei in the mature adult hermaphrodite (1031 in the male) and 302 neurones (381 in the male). The anatomy and the development of this simple animal is essentially invariant, allowing a description of its complete cell lineage[5]. By means of serial section electronmicrographs, the synaptic connections in the nervous system have been described[6]. Molecular genetic studies are facilitated by its small size, ease of culture, rapid generation time (3 days at 25°C) and reproduction by both self-fertilization and cross-fertilization. The ease of obtaining numerous mutants has allowed a very detailed genetic map to be generated. The *C. elegans* hermaphrodite has 6 chromosomes (autosomes 1-5, chromosome X). The haploid DNA content is about 100 megabases and a nearly complete physical map has been produced using overlapping cosmids and YACs (yeast artificial chromosomes)[7]. A genome sequencing project based in Cambridge, UK and St Louis, USA is close to completion[8].

A number of classical genetic methods are applicable to the analysis of gene function in *C. elegans*. These include mutagenesis, mutant screening and selection, genetic mapping and complementation, temperature-shift analysis of temperature-sensitive mutants, mosaic analysis and the study of gene interactions through suppressor selection and epistatic analysis. Transgenic worms are easily produced by injection of DNA into the gonad, thereby extending analysis of gene function by mutant rescue transformation, *in vivo* gene reporter experiments and RNA-mediated gene silencing[9,10].

By offering access to an almost fully sequenced genome, an advanced genetic "toolkit", together with a wealth of neurobiological information, the nematode *Caenorhabditis elegans* is well suited to the functional analysis of genes encoding synaptic proteins.

3. SYNTHESIS OF THE NEUROTRANSMITTER ACETYLCHOLINE

Cholinergic synaptic function relies on two enzymes, choline acetyltransferase (ChAT; EC 2.3.1.6) which synthesizes acetylcholine (ACh) and the vesicle acetylcholine transporter (VAChT) responsible for transporting acetylcholine into synaptic vesicles.

Brenner (1974) first isolated a series of mutants, some with defects in locomotion[11]. One of these, the *unc-17* mutant, was also resistant to an AChE inhibitor. Morover its level of ACh was very low supporting the idea that UNC-17 was involved in ACh synthesis. The *unc-17* gene was cloned by genome walking and found to encode a 12 transmembrane domain protein closely related to the synaptic vesicle monoamine transporter[12]. Using antibody staining, it has been shown that the *unc-17* gene product is closely associated with synaptic vesicles in cholinergic neurons, also consistent with its identity as the *C. elegans* VAChT[12]. A mutant of the *cha-1* gene shows the same locomotion defect *as unc-17*. The *cha-1* gene was cloned by TC1 transposon tagging and encodes the *C. elegans* ChAT[13]. Genetic evidence (non-complementation between some alleles of *cha-1* and *unc-17*) has linked *unc-17* and *cha-1*. Molecular cloning and sequencing of the genomic region in the *cha-1 / unc-17* locus shows that (a) these two genes share the same first untranslated exon and (b) the *unc-17* gene lies in the first intron of *cha-1*[14]. The two genes appear to be part of a single, complex transcription unit and may be under the control of the same promoter resembling a eukaryotic operon structure. Moreover this organization has been shown to be conserved in *Drosophila*[15] and vertebrates[16,17] emphasizing the important role of the genomic organization of the ChAT and VAChT locus in synaptic function.

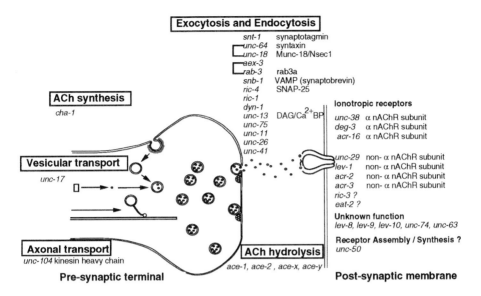

Figure 1 *C. elegans mutants involved in cholinergic transmission. Genes known to act on axonal transport, ACh synthesis and transport are shown; genes involved in exocytosis, endocytosis and the regulation of both mechanisms are also depicted. On the basal lamina and on both membranes the hydrolytic enzyme acetylcholinesterase is active (ace genes). On the postsynaptic element genes encoding nicotinic receptors and others involved in receptor assembly and/or synthesis are indicated. Several mutants involved in one of these process have been isolated based on their resistance to the anthelmintic* **lev***amisole,* **unc***oordinated locomotion, resistance to inhibitors of acetylcholinesterases* (ric) *or defects in pharynx pumping* (**eat***). Other three letter abreviations are deg, neuronal* **deg***eneration; dyn-1,* **dyn***eine; acr,* **ac***etylcholine* **r***eceptor. Based on Ref.* [29].

4. CANDIDATE GENES INVOLVED IN ACETYLCHOLINE RELEASE FROM SYNAPTIC TERMINALS

A genetic screen has been undertaken to isolate additional *C. elegans* mutants involved in synaptic function based on acetylcholinesterase inhibitor resistance[18,19,20]. This mutant selection in combination with screens involving levamisole sensitivity and abnormal behaviour yielded several new classes of mutants known as *ric* mutants (resistance to inhibitors of cholinesterase). We will discuss examples of mutants specific to cholinergic synaptic signalling after briefly considering mutants of synaptic genes expressed in many types of chemical synapses which function in different stages of vesicle release. Mutants with defects in neurotransmitter release have been obtained and characterized at the molecular level. These include the *C. elegans* gene *unc-18*, the product of which resembles the *sec-1* protein that plays a role in vesicle trafficking in yeast. Neurotransmitter release appears to be reduced in *unc-18* mutants of *C. elegans* showing that UNC-18 somehow promotes vesicular release[21]. Two other mutants show a similar phenotype to *unc-18* and may also be involved in vesicle docking; these include *unc-64* and *ric-4*. Recently the *unc-64* gene has been cloned[22]. It is homologous to the human syntaxin I gene and binds UNC-18 with high affinity as in mammals. The *ric-4* gene is the *C elegans* SNAP-25 gene[23]. Small, GTP-binding G proteins are involved in membrane trafficking. A *C. elegans rab-3* mutant has been isolated from among the *ric* phenotypes and shows a slight locomotion defect. It is characterized by the presence of fewer vesicles (40% of the wild type complement) close to the active zone, demonstrating that it acts to recruit vesicles to the release site[24]. One of its interacting partners could be the product of the *aex-3* gene. The *aex-3* mutants are also members of the *ric* class of mutants but with more severe defects in locomotion than those observed for the *rab-3* mutant. This gene codes for a new protein with only one mammalian homologue whose function is unknown[25]. It is involved in the synaptic localization of the RAB-3 protein, but since the *aex-3* mutant defects are more severe than those of the *rab-3* mutant, AEX-3 probably also interacts with other gene products. Genetic evidence shows that products of *unc-31* and *unc-64* are targets for AEX-3 interactions[25]. Synaptobrevin is also involved in neurotransmitter release[4]. The *C. elegans* gene has been cloned and several mutants investigated; it clearly interacts with *unc-64* and SNAP-25 (*ric-4*)[26]. Sequencing of mutants revealed that the amphipathic helical region is one of the interacting domains of the protein[26]. The gene *snt-1* (identical to *ric-2*) is a synaptotagmin-encoding gene[27]. In *C. elegans* synaptotagmin is located in neurones known to employ ACh as a neurotransmitter as well as neurones in which GABA, serotonin, dopamine and FMRFamides are putative neurotransmitters. It appears that *snt-1* is the only gene encoding synaptotagmin in *C. elegans*. A deletion mutant in *snt-1* results in strongly uncoordinated, small and slow-growing animals. The mutants are also impaired in the motor programme required for pharyngeal pumping and defecation. Although synaptotagmin clearly plays a major role in neurotransmitter release, this process is not entirely abolished by the *snt-1* deletion[27]. The primary defect appears to be in endocytotic vesicle regeneration[28]. Jorgensen and Nonet (1995)[29] have pointed out that mutant phenotypes resembling those of *snt-1*, *unc-11*, *unc-26*, and *unc-41* will be of interest in attempts to define the presynaptic role(s) of synaptotagmin.

In the majority of examples available to date, studying *C elegans* has shed new light on the function(s) of genes involved in synaptic transmission and has even been instructive in analysing synaptic genes first cloned in mammals thanks to the ready access to null and hypomorphic mutants.

5. THE NICOTINIC ACETYLCHOLINE RECEPTOR GENE FAMILY: MOLECULAR AND FUNCTIONAL DIVERSITY

The first category of mutants of nicotinic ACh receptors were identified in *C. elegans*. Three mutant genes defective in their responses to the anthelmintic drug, levamisole, *unc-38*, *unc-29*, and *lev-1*[30,31] and another, *deg-3*[32], resulting in neurodegeneration, are among the cloned nicotinic receptor subunit genes described to date. Three of the eleven genes associated with resistance to levamisole are found to encode putative nicotinic receptor subunits[30,32] and the functions of the remaining eight have not all been determined raising the possibility that more subunits may yet be identified in this way. The amino acid sequence of UNC-38 contains the two adjacent cysteines in loop C of the ACh binding site that identify α subunits, whereas *unc-29* and *lev-1* encode non-α subunits. Mutant phenotypes reveal that UNC-38 and UNC-29 subunits are required for function whereas LEV-1 is not. Expression in *Xenopus laevis* oocytes of combinations of these subunits that include the UNC-38 α subunit results in low-amplitude levamisole-induced currents that are suppressed by the nicotinic receptor antagonists mecamylamine, neosurugatoxin and d-tubocurarine, but not α-bungarotoxin[33]. An UNC-29::GFP fusion study has shown that *unc-29* is expressed in body wall and head muscle cells[33]. Two rare dominant mutations of *lev-1* that are highly resistant to levamisole result in a single amino acid substitution or addition in or near transmembrane region 2, in locations important to ion selectivity of the channel and receptor dezensitization[33]. The identification of nAChR mutants in *C. elegans* provides an advantageous system in which receptor expression and synaptic targetting can be manipulated and studied *in vivo*.

By the method of cross-species probing of DNA libraries a nicotinic ACh receptor non-α subunit gene, *acr-2*, has been identified[34]. When its product is co-expressed in *Xenopus* oocytes together with the product of the α subunit gene, *unc-38*, a small but consistent current is observed in response to levamisole. This current is blocked by the nicotinic receptor antagonist mecamylamine[34]. Since then Ballivet and colleagues have described an α7-like subunit, Ce21, which forms a robust functional homomeric receptor when expressed in *Xenopus* oocytes and Ce13, a non-α subunit[35]. Another non-α subunit ACR-3 capable of weak functional co-expression with UNC-38 has been described[36] adding to the growing evidence for an extensive nicotinic ACh receptor gene family in *C. elegans*.

By far the richest source of new nicotinic ACh receptor subunits has been the *C. elegans* Genome Consortium. Many novel putative subunits have been identified. We have used RT-PCR to test whether or not these candidate nicotinic subunits are transcribed. Currently thirteen nicotinic receptor α subunits are known to be transcribed in *C. elegans* and other candidates are under investigation (Table1). This nicotinic ACh receptor α subunit gene family in *C. elegans* is the largest known.

Table1 *Nicotinic ACh receptor subunits of C. elegans.*

deg-3 like	deg-3	(α)	V	cDNA	Treinin and Chalfie, 1995. (Ref. 32)
	acr-4	(α)	V	cDNA	M. Treinin, personal communication
	acr-5	(α)	III	partial cDNA	Mongan et al., 1997. (Ref. 53)
acr-16 like	acr-16	(α)	V	cDNA	Ballivet et al., 1996. (Ref. 35)
	acr-7	(α)	II	partial cDNA	Mongan et al., 1997. (Ref. 53)
	acr-9		X	partial cDNA	Mongan et al., 1997. (Ref. 53)
	acr-10	(α)	X	partial cDNA	Mongan et al., 1997. (Ref. 53)
	acr-11	(α)	I	partial cDNA	Mongan et al., 1997. (Ref. 53)
	acr-14		II	partial cDNA	Mongan et al., 1997. (Ref. 53)
	acr-15	(α)	V	partial cDNA	Mongan et al., 1997. (Ref. 53)
unc-38 like	unc-38	(α)	I	cDNA	Fleming et al., 1997. (Ref. 33)
	acr-6	(α)	I	partial cDNA	J.T. Lewis, personal communication
acr-8 like	acr-8	(α)	X	partial cDNA	Mongan et al., 1997. (Ref. 53)
	acr-12	(α)	X	partial cDNA	Mongan et al., 1997. (Ref. 53)
	acr-13	(α)	X	partial cDNA	Mongan et al., 1997. (Ref. 53)
unc-29 like	unc-29		I	cDNA	Fleming et al., 1997. (Ref. 33)
	lev-1		IV	cDNA	Fleming et al., 1997. (Ref. 33)
	acr-2		X	cDNA	Squire et al., 1995. (Ref. 34)
	acr-3		X	cDNA	Baylis et al., 1997. (Ref. 36)

The question arises - why so many subunits? We can perhaps begin to seek an answer by considering the striking variation in sequences in the channel lining and ACh binding regions. This suggests that *C. elegans* nicotinic ACh receptors expressing different α subunits may differ in their permeability to ions; they may also differ in their affinity for the neurotransmitter and for other ligands. We can recognize pharmacologically-distinct subclasses of nicotinic ACh receptors. In vertebrates and invertebrates nicotinic receptors have been detected at presynaptic, postsynaptic and extrasynaptic locations. Physiological and developmental studies have provided evidence for a diversity of roles of nicotinic receptors. Based on our recent findings from *C. elegans*, this appears to be reflected in an extensive molecular diversity within the nicotinic receptor gene family.

6. THE ACETYLCHOLINESTERASE GENE FAMILY: MOLECULAR AND FUNCTIONAL DIVERSITY

Acetylcholinesterase (AChE) is a key enzyme at the synaptic cleft terminating the actions of ACh. In vertebrates multiple molecular forms of AChE are present in both the peripheral and the central nervous system but only a single AChE gene has been identified. This gene gives rise to two alternative transcripts H and T which differ at their 3'ends resulting in two distinct catalytic subunits possessing different modes of association with each other, the cell membrane and the extracellular matrix[37].

The situation is more complex in *C. elegans* where genetic studies have shown there are at least three genes *ace-1*, *ace-2* and *ace-3* localized respectively on chromosomes X, I and II[38,39,40]. These three genes encode three distinct pharmacological classes of acetylcholinesterase (A, B and C respectively) which differ in their substrate specificities, kinetic parameters, inhibitor sensitivities and molecular forms (see Table 2). Finally, biochemical experiments indicate the existence of at least four AChE classes in *C. elegans*, the additional class (D) being responsible for only 0.1 % total activity (Table 2)[41]. It has been found that the single homozygous mutants *ace-1* and *ace-2* show no visible phenotype, whereas the double mutant *ace-1; ace-2* is uncoordinated and is unable to move backwards[39]. The triple mutant *ace-1; ace-2; ace-3* is developmentally arrested at the L1 larval stage[40]. All these results point to either some genetic redundancy between *ace-1* and *ace-2*, or at least some functional overlap. This also raises the question of the roles of the different *ace* gene in *C. elegans*? In particular, what is the role of each class of AChE at the synaptic cleft?

Biochemical experiments on another rhabditid species *Steinernema carpocapsae* indicate that to some extent the molecular forms generated by multiple *C. elegans* genes are the counterparts of the vertebrate molecular forms. Thus the diversity of molecular forms generated by the alternative splicing of one vertebrate gene is achieved in the nematode by an alternative strategy employing several genes[42]. In order to understand the functional significance of this diversity, the molecular characterization of each *ace* gene has been undertaken. The *ace-1* gene (encoding class A AChE) has been cloned in *C. elegans*[43] and in the related nematode species *C. briggsae*[44]. ACE-1 showed 42% identity at the amino acid level with human AChE and corresponds to the vertebrate hydrophilic catalytic subunit T form. It is mainly expressed in the body wall muscle cells of *C. elegans* and in a few neurones in head ganglia (E. Culetto, unpublished results). Three other AChE partial coding sequences have now been reported in *C. elegans* and *C. briggsae*[44]. Full length cDNAs for each subunit have been cloned and sequenced (M. Grauso and D. Combes, personal communication). The *ace-2* gene shows characteristics of the vertebrate H catalytic subunit as previously suggested[42]. The *ace-2* expression pattern is limited mainly to nerve cells in head and tail ganglia (D. Combes, personal communication).

The two other *ace* sequences are located in very close proximity on chromosome II with only 360 bp between the stop codon of the upstream ORF and the ATG of the downstream ORF. Due to their close proximity it is not possible, at the moment, to know which sequence corresponds to *ace-3* (defined in the literature as encoding a class C type AChE); the other gene is likely to encode the class D type AChE. Thus these third and fourth *ace* genes have been named provisionally *ace-x* (upstream ORF) and *ace-y* (downstream ORF)[44]. So what do we know of their functional roles? At the neuromuscular junction *ace-1* is the major AChE gene expressed; it seems that *ace-2* may be present only in some motor neurones and interneurones in the head and tail ganglia, showing that they are not fully redundant since they are not always expressed at the same synapses. Behavioural assays corroborate this point of view since it has been shown that the single mutants *ace-1* and *ace-2* show a 20% reduction in their speed of locomotion

(E. Culetto, unpublished observations). It may be the case therefore that the required physiological level of AChE can be provided either by the muscles, or by the nerve cells. The class C AChE activity has been detected in the pseudocoelom and an antibody raised against it binds to the nerve ring and to the two canal associated neurones (CAN cells)[41]; this excretory canal plays a role in detoxification[46]. In fact soil nematodes may be in close contact with natural pesticides (ESTHER database)[47]. Thus class C activity may even constitute a detoxification enzyme. Finally, what is currently known of the gene encoding class D (probably encoded by *ace-x* or *ace-y*)? This enzyme may be not involved in cholinergic transmission at all since the triple mutant (with only class D AChE activity remaining) is lethal. This enzyme may have a non-cholinergic function; such functions have been established for vertebrate AChE where a role in neurite growth has been demonstrated[48].

Table 2 *Properties of the four C. elegans AChE classes. Based on refs.[37, 38, 39, 40].*

AChE	Class A	Class B	Class C	Class D
Genes	*ace-1*	*ace-2*	*ace-x/ace-y* ?	*ace-x/ace-y* ?
Chromosomes	X	I	II	II ?
Km (ACSh)	15 mM	80 mM	0.017 mM	1 mM
IC$_{50}$(M) eserine	2.10^{9}	2.10^{7}	5.10^{-3}	5.10^{-3}
% Total activity	~ 50 %	~ 50 %	< 5 %	0.1 %
Molecular forms	14 S	7 S	7 S	3.5 S

7. PESTICIDE TARGETS

Plant parasitic nematodes are devastating pathogens, responsible for an estimated annual $100 billion loss in crops worldwide[49]. Chemical nematicides include carbamates (CXs) and organophophorus compouds (OPs) which inhibit AChE leading to the inhibition of neuromuscular transmission. Although *C. elegans* is a free-living nematode it can serve as a useful model to understand aspects of the biology of plant and animal parasitic nematodes and may assist in the development of new plant protection chemicals and anthelmintics. The cloning of all the *ace* genes in *C. elegans* will facilitate the cloning of AChE genes in agriculturally-important species such as those of the genus *Meloidogyne*. Comparing these sequences may then enable us to understand the unusual pharmacological properties of the class C and class D types of AChE. For example, the plant parasite *Heterodera glycina* has only two classes of AChEs, class A and class C[50]. Class C is resistant to eserine (Table 2) and to OPs; in fact, when plant cultures are infected with *H. glycina* OP treatment is stopped. The *ace-x* sequence (probably encoding class C or D) around the active-site center could explain this naturally occuring resistance. The FGESAG motif present in *ace-1* and *ace-2* is changed to FGQSAG in *ace-x* (M. Grauso and D. Combes, personal communication). In fact such mutations have been generated for mouse AChE[51], lowering the inhibitor affinity and reducing the ageing of the enzyme which is then more easily reactivated. Such findings could be useful for managing the use of OPs in the control of plant parasitic nematodes. *In vitro* expression would enable us to purify and thereby characterize more fully the pharmacology of each AChE class. The elucidation of the 3-D structure of each AChE class would also constitute a major step forward in defining more specifically anti-cholinesterase nematicidal actions. Moreover the 3-D structure of a *C. elegans* AChE would make a fascinating comparison with the recently elucidated 3-D structure of *Drosophila melanogaster* AChE.

The nicotinic ACh receptors of nematodes are now well established targets for anthelmintic drugs. Using a genetic screen for resistance to the anthelmintic drug, levamisole, it has been possible to identify, from the wealth of nicotinic subunits, a particular subset. One of our current goals is to determine the right combination of the many subunits constituting native nicotinic ACh receptors. The expression patterns of these subunits are currently being investigated using GFP constructs and *in situ* hybridization analysis. The *in vivo* combination will be reproduced *in vitro* by nuclear injection of appropriate cDNAs into *Xenopus* oocytes in order to study the physiology and pharmacology of the nicotinic receptor subtypes and their interactions with new anthelmintics From genomics we now know much more about the molecular diversity of nicotinic receptor subunits and it appears that some *C. elegans* nicotinic subunits have no known counterpart in mammals. Once host and parasite genomes have been fully sequenced, there may be the opportunity to use this advanced understanding of molecular diversity to generate new and highly selective anthelmintic drugs. Perhaps most exciting of all is the finding that in contrast to a single gene responsible for the synthesis of ACh, there is extensive diversity in the genes encoding fast-acting nicotinic receptors that detect ACh and also in the enzymes that inactivate it, thereby extending our horizons of the functional spectrum of the neurotransmitter acetylcholine. Now that advanced physiological methods such as patch-clamp electrophysiology can be applied to *C. elegans* cells[52], we can look forward to major advances in understanding of cholinergic synaptic function as this model organism leads neurobiology into the postgenome era.

8. REFERENCES

1. B. Katz, "The release of neuronal transmitter substances" Liverpool: Liverpool University Press, 1969.

2. X. O. Breakfield, "An introduction to molecular neurobiology" edited by Hall, Z. Sunderland, MA: Sinauer Associates Inc, 1992, p496.

3. R. Nawrotzki, D. J. Blake and K. E. Davies, *Trends in Genetics*, 1996, **12**, 294.

4. T. C. Sudhof, *Nature*, 1995, **375**, 645.

5. J. Sulston and H. R. Horwitz, *Dev. Biol.*, 1977, **56**, 110.

6. J. G. White, E. Southgate, J. N. Thompson and S. Brenner, *Philos. Trans. R. Soc. Lond. B Biol Sci.*, 1986, **314**, 1.

7. A. R. Coulson, J. Sulston, S. Brenner and J. Karn, *Proc. Natl. Acad. Sci. U.S.A*, 1986, **83**, 7821.

8. J. E. Sulston, K. Du, K. Thomas, R. Wilson, L. Hillier, R. Staden, N. Halloran, P. Green, J. Thierry-Mieg, L. Qiu, S. Dear, A. Coulson, M. Craxton, R. Durbin, M. Berks, M. Metzstein, T. Hawkins, R. Ainscough and R. Waterston, *Nature*, 1992, **335**, 37.

9. C. Mello and A. Fire, "*Caenorhabditis elegans*: Modern Biological Analysis of an Organism" ed H. F. Epstein and D. C. Shakes, San Diego: Academic Press, 1995, p452.

10. A. Fire, S. Xu, M. K. Montgomery, S. A. Kostas, S. E. Driver and C. C. Mello, *Nature*, 1998, **361**, 806.

11. S. Brenner, *Genetics*, 1974, **77**, 71.

12. A. Alfonso, K. Grundahl, J. S. Duerr, H.-P. Han and J. B. Rand, *Science*, 1993, **261**, 617.

13. A. Alfonso, K. Grundahl, J. McManus and J. B. Rand, *J. Neurosci.*, 1994, **14**, 2290.

14. A. Alfonso, K. Grundahl, J. R. McManus, J. M. Asbury and J. B. Rand, *J. Mol. Biol.*, 1994, **241**, 627.

15. T. Kitamoto, W. Y. Wang and P. M. Salvaterra, *J. Biol. Chem.*, 1998, **273**, 2706.

16. S. Bejanin, R. Cervini, J. Mallet and S. Berard, *J. Biol. Chem.*, 1994, **269**, 21944.

17. J. Erichson, H. Varochi, M. Schafer, W. Modi, M. Diebler, E Weihe, J. Rand, L. Eiden, T. Bonner and T. Usdin. *J. Biol. Chem.*, 1994, **269**, 21929.

18. J. T. Fleming, C. Tornoe, H. A. Riina, J. Coadwell, J. A. Lewis and D. B. Sattelle, "Comparative Molecular Neurobiology" edited by Pichon, Switherland: Birkhauser Verlag, 1993, p45.

19. M. Nguyen, A. Alfonso, C. D. Johnson and J. B. Rand, *Genetics*, 1995, **140**, 527.

20. K. G. Miller, A. Alfonso, M. Nguyen, J. A. Crowell, C. D. Johnson and J. B. Rand, *Proc. Natl. Acad. Sci.* USA, 1996, **93**, 12593.

21. K. Gengyo-Ando, Y. Kamiya, A. Yamakawa, K.-I. Kodaira, K. Nishiwaki, J. Miwa, I. Hori and R. Hosono, *Neuron*, 1993, **11**, 703.

22. H. Ogawa, S. Harada, T. Sassa, H. Yamamoto and R. Hosono, *J. Biol. Chem.*, 1998, **273**, 2192.

23. J. B. Rand and M. L. Nonet, "*C. elegans* II", Cold Spring Harbor Laboratory Press, 1997, Chapter 22, p611.

24. M. L. Nonet, J. E. Staunton, M. P. Kilgard, T. Fergestad, E. Hartwieg, H. R. Horvitz, E. M Jorgensen and B. J. Meyer, *J. Neurosci.*, 1997, **17**, 8061.

25. K. Iwasaki, J. Staunton, O. Saifee, M. L. Nonet and J.H. Thomas, Neuron, 1997, **18**, 613.

26 M. L. Nonet, O. Saifee, H.J. Zhao, J. B. Rand and L.P. Wei, *J. Neurosc.*, 1998, **18**, 70.

27. M. L. Nonet, K. Grundahl, B. J. Meyer and J. B. Rand, *Cell*, 1993, **73**, 1291.

28. E. M. Jorgensen, E. Hartwieg, K. Schuske, M. L. Nonet, Y. Jin and H. R. Horvitz, *Nature*, 1995, **378**, 196.

29. E. M. Jorgensen and M. L. Nonet, *Sem. Dev. Biol.*, 1995, **6**, 207.

30. J. A. lewis, C. H. Wu, J. H. Lewine and H. Berg, *Genetics*, 1980, **95**, 905.

31. J. A Lewis, J. T. Fleming, S. McLafferty, H. Murfy and C. Wu, *Mol. Pharmacol.*, 1987, **31**, 185.

32. M. Treinin and M Chalfie, *Neuron*, 1995, **14**, 871.

33. J. T. Fleming, M. D. Squire, T. M. Barnes, C. Tornoe, K. Matsuda, K. Ahnn, A. Fire, J. E. Sulston, E. A. Barnard, D. B. Sattelle and J. A Lewis, *J. Neurosci.*, 1997, **17**, 5843.

34. M. D. Squire, C. Tornoe, H. A. Baylis, J. T. Fleming, E. A. Barnard and D. B. Sattelle, *Receptors and Channels*, 1995, **3**, 107.

35. M. Ballivet, C. Alliod, S. Bertrand and D. Bertrand, *J. Mol. Biol.*, 1996, **258**, 261.

36. H. A. Baylis, K. Matsuda, M. D. Squire, J. T. Fleming, R. J. Harvey, M. G. Darlison, E. A. Barnard and D. B. Sattelle, *Receptors and Channels*, 1997, **5**, 149-158.

37. J. Massoulié, L. Pezzementi, S. Bon, E. Krejci and F. M. Vallette, *Prog. Neurobiol.*, 1993, **41**, 31.

38. C.D. Johnson, J.G. Duckett, J.G. Culotti, R.K. Herman, P.M Meneely and R.L Russell, *Genetics*, 1981, **97**, 261.

39. J. G. Culotti, G. Von Ehrenstein, M. R. Culotti and R. L. Russell, *Genetics*, 1981, **97**, 281.

40. C. D. Johnson, J. B. Rand, R. K. Herman, B. D Stern and R. L. Russell, *Neuron*, 1988, **1**, 165.

41. B. D. Stern, Ph.D. Thesis dissertation. University of Pittsburgh, PA, USA, 1986.

42. M. Arpagaus, P. Richier, J.-B. Bergé and J.-P. Toutant, *Eur. J. Biochem.*, 1992, **207**, 1101.

43. M. Arpagaus, Y. Fedon, X. Cousin, A. Chatonnet, J.-B. Bergé, D Fournier and J.-P. Toutant, *J. Biol. Chem.*, 1994, **269**, 9957.

44. M. Grauso, E. Culetto, J.-B. Bergé, J.-P. Toutant and M. Arpagaus, *DNA Sequence* 1996, **6**, 217.

45. M. Grauso, E. Culetto, Y. Fedon, D. Combes, J.-P. Toutant and M. Arpagaus, *FEBS Lett.*, 1998, **424**, 279.

46 A. Broeks, H. W. R. M. Janssen, J. Calafat and R. H. A. Plasterk, *EMBO J.*, 1995, **14**, 1858.

47. X. Cousin, T. Hotelier, K. Giles, J.-P. Toutant and A. Chatonnet, *Nucleic Acid Res.*, 1998, **26**, 226.

48. M. Sternfeld, G. C. Ming, H. J. Song, K. Sela, R. Timberg, M. M. Poo and H. Soreq, *J. Neurosci.*, 1998, **18**, 1240.

49. D. Cai, M. Kleine, S. Kifle, H. J. Harloff, N. N. Sandal, K. A. Marcker, R. M. Klein-Lankhorst, E. M. J. Salentijn, W. Lange, W. J. Stiekema, U. Wyss, F. M. W. Grundler and C. Jung, *Science*, 1997, **275**, 832.

50. S. Chang and C. H. Opperman, *J. Nematol.*, 1992, **24**, 148.

51. P. Taylor and Z. Radic, *Ann. Rev. Pharmacol. Toxicol.*, 1994, **34**, 281.

52. M. B. Goodman, D. H. Hall, L. Avery and S. R. Lockery, *Neuron*, 1998, **20**, 763.

53. N. Mongan, H. A. Baylis and D. B. Sattelle, *Soc. Neurosci. Abs.*, 1997, **23**, 392.

Natural Products

Pharmacological Studies of Delphinium Alkaloids at the Nicotinic Acetylcholine Receptor

K.R. Jennings[1,2], A.N. Starratt[3], P. Penaranda[1] and B.G. Loughton[1]

[1] DEPARTMENT OF BIOLOGY, YORK UNIVERSITY, 4700 KEELE ST., NORTH YORK, ON, M3J 1PS, CANADA
[2] CYANAMID, 88 MCNABB ST., MARKHAM, ON, L3R 6E6, CANADA
[3] AGRICULTURE & AGRI-FOOD CANADA, 1391 SANDFORD ST., LONDON, ON, N5V 4T3, CANADA

1 INTRODUCTION

Currently available therapies for the treatment of Alzheimer's disease target acetylcholinesterase, the acetylcholine-degrading enzyme integral to cholinergic neurotransmission. Organophosphorus and carbamate acetylcholinesterase inhibitors have long been used as insecticides in agriculture and public health, and organophosphorus insecticides are currently in clinical trials as treatments for Alzheimer's[1]. The acetylcholine receptor has also been exploited as an insecticide target using nicotine, imidacloprid, cartap and delphinium alkaloids. With cholinergic neurotransmission as a common target, it is not surprising that interest in medicinal and agricultural applications of delphinium alkaloids has led to much of the research on these potent neurotoxins.

The norditerpenoid alkaloids from Delphinium spp. were identified as nicotinic cholinergic agents by medicinal researchers isolating physiologically active natural products and agricultural scientists investigating cattle poisoning from larkspur[2]. The delphinium alkaloids can be classified into two categories[3], lycoctonine and aconitine types based on the presence or absence of an oxygenated substituent at C-7 (Scheme 1). Methyllycaconitine (MLA) was identified as the major cholinergic toxicant in larkspur[2] and found to be a potent nicotinic ligand by studies on an insect (dipteran) neural preparation[4] and subsequently, mammalian nervous system receptors[5].

Pharmacological analysis of the nicotinic activity in insects demonstrated that MLA was over 1,000-fold more potent at this receptor than previously reported for muscle endplate in rats. Physiological studies in the cockroach[6] indicated that MLA antagonized cholinergic transmission in a cercal nerve preparation and Sattelle et al.[7] definitively established this alkaloid as a nicotinic receptor antagonist.

Further study in mammalian systems showed MLA to be most effective as a ligand of central α_7- and α_8-containing nicotinic receptors, having only moderate activity at other nicotinic receptor types. Delphinium alkaloids represent the most potent nicotinic cholinergic ligands identified to date, with effects being seen as low as 1fM[8] with MLA.

Due to its potency and reversibility, MLA has become a valuable neurobiological tool for the study of nicotinic receptor function, especially the α_7 subunit type. Until relatively recently while the physiological role of the alphabungarotoxin (α-BGTx) binding site was well established in insects, it was unclear whether the analogous binding site in mammalian neural tissue was a true receptor. It was only with the realization of the rapid desensitization of the mammalian α-BGTx binding site that the identification of the α-BGTx binding site as a true nicotinic receptor generally accepted[9]. This article extends previous studies on the comparative pharmacology/ toxicology of the delphinium alkaloids including both naturally occuring alkaloids and semi-synthetic derivatives of MLA.

2 MATERIALS AND METHODS

2.1 Housefly receptor and Southern armyworm insecticidal testing:

Musca domestica α-BGTx receptor binding and *Spodoptera eridania* bioassay were as previously described[4,10].

2.2 Rat and Locust Experiments

Male Sprague-Dawley and Wistar rats were retrieved from laboratories at York University, Toronto, ON. Adult male *Locusta migratoria* were taken from colonies reared at York University. All of the chemicals were prepared and diluted in a multipurpose buffer as described. ^{125}I-labelled α-BGTx, with a specific activity of 200 Ci/mmol, was purchased from Amersham Canada. Methyllycaconitine citrate was purchased from Research Biochemicals International, Natick, MA. Dehydromethyllycaconitine, dehydrolycacontine, dehydropuberaconitine, and dehydrocashmiradelphine were synthesized as described.

2.2.1 Preparation of Rat Neural Membrane. Rats (approx. 300 g) were anaesthetized and the brain, minus the cerebellum, was dissected out and placed on ice. Using a Polytron homogenizer, the brain tissue was homogenized for 10 s in chilled (4°C) pH 7.4 buffer containing 10 mM Tris HCl; 0.1 mM Phenylmethylsulphonylfluoride; 3 mM Ethylene glycol-bis(β-aminoethyl ether)N,N',N'-tetracetic acid; 0.2% Sodium azide. The homogenate was centrifuged at 45,000 x g for 10 min at 4 °C. The remaining pellet was resuspended in 16 volumes of buffer and stored at -80°C.

2.2.2 Preparation of Locust Ganglia Membrane. Adult male *Locusta migratoria* were decapitated and the brains and suboesophogeal ganglia dissected out and immediately placed on ice. The tissue was homogenized in 5 ml buffer in a ground glass homogenizer for 30 min on ice. The homogenate was centrifuged at 3200 x g for 10 min at 4°C. The supernatant was homogenized further in a ground glass homogenizer for 30 min on ice. The homogenate was re-centrifuged at 30,000 x g for 25 min at 4 °C and the resulting pellet resuspended in 3 ml of buffer solution and stored at -80°C. Protein concentrations were determined by the Bradford Assay with bovine serum albumin as the standard.

2.3 Competitive Binding Studies

2.3.1 Rat. Aliquots (100µL) of membrane suspension (approx. 250 µg protein) were incubated with 10 µL buffer and 50 µL aliquots of the test ligand (final concentrations ranging from 10^{-4} to 10^{-11} M) in Eppendorf tubes. Incubation was carried out for 30 Min at room temperature on a shaker. 40 µL of ^{125}I α-BGTx (1nM final concentration) was then added to the tubes and the resulting mixture was incubated, with agitation, for an additional 30 Min After the incubation period, 1mL of 0.2 M NaCl was added to each tube to terminate further binding. The preparations were centrifuged at 11,000 x g for 2 min at 4°C, supernatant removed, and the resulting pellet washed with 1 mL 0.2M NaC1.

2.3.2 Locust. 100 µL aliquots of membrane suspension (approx. 250 µg protein) were incubated with 10 µL buffer, 50 µL aliquots of the test ligand (final concentrations ranging from 10^{-4} to 10^{-11} M), and 40 µL of ^{125}I α-BGTx (1 nM final concentration) in Eppendorf tubes. Incubation was conducted with continuous agitation for 45 Min at room temperature. Assay tubes were then centrifuged at 40,000 x g for 20 Min at 4°C, supernatant was removed and the resulting pellet washed with 200 µL buffer solution. The radioactivity of the pellet was counted in a Packard scintillation counter.

2.3.3 Binding Analysis. Each assay was conducted a minimum of three times. For each assay duplicate samples were prepared. Values shown are the means of 6 samples.

2.4 Chemical Synthesis

For the investigations reported here, four novel analogues of MLA were prepared from lycoctonine (see Scheme 1): dehydrolycaconitine (dLA), dehydropuberaconitine (dPA), dehydrocashmiradelphine (dCD) and dehydromethyllycaconitine (dMLA).

Hydrolysis of MLA citrate by stirring in 5% potassium hydroxide in methanol for 18 h at room temperature in an atmosphere of nitrogen yielded lycoctonine. Thin layer chromatography of the product, obtained by extraction into chloroform after dilution with water, indicated that hydrolysis was complete. Treatment of this material with isatoic anhydride as described by Blagbrough *et al.*[11] afforded inuline which was purified by reverse phase HPLC.

The half acid amide dPA was prepared by reacting inuline in methylene chloride with maleic anhydride (3.4 equiv.). After 18 h at room temperature, HPLC indicated that the reaction was nearly complete. Unreacted inuline and maleic acid, formed from the anhydride, were removed by washing a chloroform solution of the product with water. dLA was synthesized by direct treatment of a reaction mixture containing dPA with PyBOP (1.1 equiv.) and N,N-diisopropylethylamine (2.5 equiv.) at room temperature for 1.5 h. The product, dLA, was purified by reverse phase HPLC. Heating dLA in refluxing methanol for 18 h yielded dCD which was similarly purified by HPLC. Yields of dPA and dCD were estimated by comparison of UV absorption at 312 nm of these compounds with that of the crystalline half acid amide obtained when methyl anthranilate was reacted with maleic anhydride.

dMLA was prepared by a procedure similar to that described for the partial synthesis of MLA[12]. Inuline in methylene chloride was treated with excess citraconic anhydride to afford a mixture of unreacted inuline and half acid amides. The latter were cyclized using carbonyldiimidazole and the product dMLA was separated from reagents, inuline, and unreacted half acid amides by HPLC. The amounts of purified dMLA and dLA were estimated by comparison of UV absorption of these compounds at 277 nm with that of MLA.

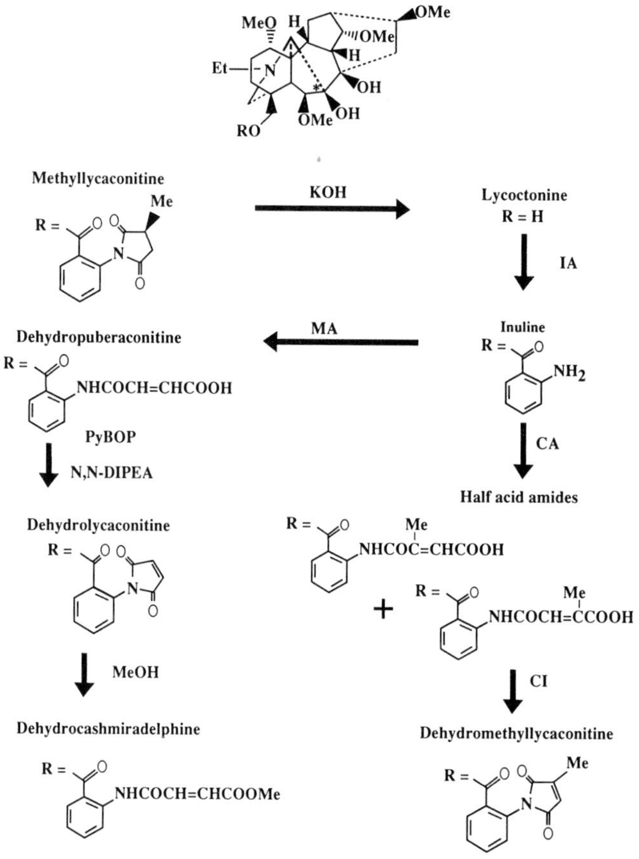

Scheme 1

Synthesis of dehydromethyllycaconitine, dehydrolycaconitine, dehydropuberaconitine and dehydrocashmiradelphine from methyllycaconitine. C-7 is indicated by*. KOH = Potassium hydroxide; UA = Isatoic anhydride; CI = Carbonyldiimidazole; PyBOP = benzotriazole-1-yl-oxy-tris-pyrrolidino-phosphonium hexafluorophosphate; N,N-DIPEA = N,N-diisopropyl ethylamine; MeOH = Methanol.

3 RESULTS AND DISCUSSION

A study was conducted to compare the insecticidal and insect nicotinic activity of 110 previously identified delphinium alkaloids. Insecticidal activity was measured by use of the leaf dip bioassay in *Spodoptera eridania* at a series of doses (100-1000 ppm) while nicotinic receptor activity was measured by use of α-BGTx binding inhibition in *Musca domestica* head membrane preparations[10]. The results (Figure 1) demonstrated a correlation between insecticidal potency and nicotinic receptor activity, with an apparent threshold observed at IC_{50} of $\leq$5nM.

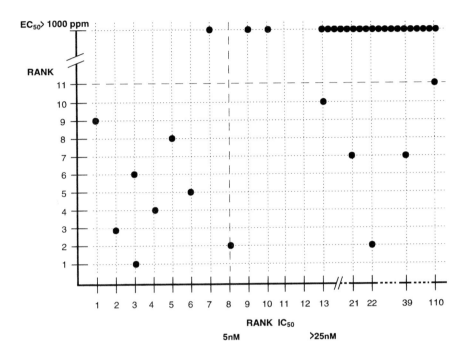

Figure 1 *Correlation of* Spodoptera eridania *insecticidal activity and* Musca domestica *receptor inhibition for 110 alkaloids   X: Rank ordered IC_{50} values from nicotinic receptor assay Y: Rank ordered EC_{50} values from insecticidal bioassay*

From 110 delphinium alkaloids tested, of the 9 alkaloids with an IC_{50} of 5nM or less 8 were insecticidal, with a clear trend towards the rank order of the most potent cholinergic ligands being the most insecticidal. Of the 101 other alkaloids tested, 5 had some insecticidal activity, but 3 of these alkaloids were of the aconitine rather than lycoctonine type. The insecticidal activity observed for the aconitine type is likely due to a different mechanism of toxic action, namely voltage-sensitive sodium channels. In this study, the lycoctonine type alkaloids were more potent insecticides than the aconitine-types. In rodent studies there have been a number of investigations that correlate *in vivo* toxicity with *in vitro* receptor activity. Table 1 presents some of these published data from a number of different investigators, comparing intravenous toxicity in mice to inhibition of α-BGTx binding in rat central nervous system tissue.

Table 1 *Toxicity Comparison of Aconitine (A) and Lycoctonine (L) Alkaloids*

ALKALOID	TYPE	Mouse Acute Toxicity (IV)mg/kg [13,14,15]	Rat αBGTx IC_{50}M [10,14,17]
Aconitine	A	~0.15	1.9×10^{-5}
Delphinine	A	1.50	$> 10^{-5}$
Nudicauline	L	2.7	1.7×10^{-9}
Methyllycaconitine	L	3.20/7.5	1.2×10^{-9}
Elatine	L	5.20/9.2	$4.3 \times 10^{-9}/6.1 \times 10^{-9}$
Lycaconitine	L	15	$Ki = 8 \times 10^{-8}$ (est IC_{50}:2×10^{-7})
Delsemine	L	6(est)	3.6×10^{-7}
Anthranoyllycoctonine (inuline)	L	20.8	1.6×10^{-6}
Condelphine	A	35(est)	$8 \times 10^{-7}/1.6 \times 10^{-6}$
Karakoline	L	52	$3.4 \times 10^{-7}/1.8 \times 10^{-6}$
Lycoctonine	L	350/443.5	$1.1 \times 10^{-5}/1.0 \times 10^{-5}$

Aconitine-type alkaloids are among the most toxic in the rodents when delivered by this route. Lycoctonine-type alkaloids display an increased toxicity with increased receptor potency. Some of these alkaloids may also possess mixed cholinergic and sodium channel activity, as has been reported for N-desacetyllappaconitine.

Limited structure-activity information is available on the factors contributing to nicotinic potency in the delphinium alkaloid family. The methyl succinimido moiety was identified early as an important element of nicotinic binding for both invertebrates[4] and vertebrates[16] by the relative potency of MLA versus the alcohol lycoctonine and this has been confirmed by evaluation of inuline[17] which contains the ester linkage, but not the succinimide ring. Studies of bicyclic and tricyclic analogues of MLA[18] have shown that the homocholine-like motif of the ester carbonyl with the nitrogen atom of the norditerpenoid in isolation is insufficient for nicotinic activity and further components of the diterpenoid structure are necessary for potency. Other structure-activity observations include the finding[10] that alkaloids such as elatine which have the methylenedioxy bridging C-7 and C-8 are potent ligands at the α-BGTx nicotinic receptor, indicating that hydrogen bonding is not necessary for receptor binding[17].

The studies reported here were undertaken to further investigate the effect of structural alterations of the methylsuccinimide moiety on nicotinic potency in both vertebrates and invertebrates. The synthesis of the maleimido analogues was based on the similarity in structure to maleimidobenzyl-trimethylammonium, an alkylating agent[19] subunit, interfering with receptor-ligand binding. Ring-open forms of the maleimido analogues were also synthesized to determine if the intact ring was necessary for activity.

Analogues dMLA and dLA were evaluated in ^{125}I α- BGTx ligand binding assays conducted on rat and nerve tissue using unlabelled α- BGTx and MLA as standards for comparison. Both dehydro analogues were inhibitors of α- BGTx binding in vertebrate and invertebrate neural tissue with somewhat greater activity in the rat brain.

A dissociation study conducted under non-reducing conditions with dMLA, dLA and MLA demonstrated the reversibility of ligand competition by these agents. Neural membranes of rat or locust exposed to saturating concentrations of ligand for 30-60 minutes washed three times with buffer and challenged with ^{125}I αBGTx displayed normal binding. It has previously been demonstrated[13,14] that elimination of the methyl group on the succinimide ring of MLA (resulting in lycaconitine) results in a 5 to 20-fold loss in activity. Comparable receptor binding activity was observed in this study with both methyl and demethyl analogues. All data presented in Figures 2,3,4,5 and 6 are specific binding $\pm$ Standard Error.

The open ring analogues dPA and dCD displayed greater potency at the rat receptor. Previously, the open ring forms delavaine A and B have been shown to be 3-fold more toxic than MLA[15]. In a study[10] of 17 delphinium alkaloids, activity was found to be comparable or less on vertebrate (rat) nAChR compared to invertebrate (housefly) preparations.

Analogues of dMLA and dPA were further evaluated for nicotinic receptor activity. Screening at a dose of 10^{-5}M against the rat cortex $α_4$ receptor using [^{3}H] cytisine[20], dMLA demonstrated 51% inhibition (N=4), dPA 31% (N=2) and MLA 41% (N=2). These results are consistent with the inhibitory constant previously reported[5] for MLA at the rat brain nicotine receptor. Investigation of *in vivo* activity was conducted by administering dMLA intraperitoneally (20 mg/kg) to a group of two ICR derived male mice weighing 22 ± 2g and observing for the presence of acute toxic symptoms (mortality, convulsions, tremors, muscle relaxation, sedation) and autonomic effects (diarrhea, salivation, lacrimation, vocalization, piloerection) during the first 30 minutes. No behavioural changes or autonomic signs were observed in the test animals. There was no mortality observed at the termination of the experiment, 72 hours after treatment.

Table 2 *Comparison of Inhibition Concentrations for Test Compounds in Rat and Locust α-Bungarotoxin Binding*

COMPOUND	INHIBITION CONCENTRATION (IC$_{50}$):	
	Rat Brain	Locust Brain
α-Bungarotoxin	2.0×10^{-9}M	6.0×10^{-9}M
Nicotine	4.0×10^{-6}M	1.0×10^{-5}M
Methyllycaconitine	2.0×10^{-9}M	5.0×10^{-9}M
Dehydromethyllycaconitine	3.5×10^{-8}M	1.0×10^{-7}M
Dehydrolycaconitine	4.4×10^{-8}M	5.6×10^{-8}M
Dehydropuberaconitine	$<1.0 \times 10^{-7}$M	1.5×10^{-7}M
Dehydrocashmiradelphine	$<1.0 \times 10^{-7}$M	1.8×10^{-7}M

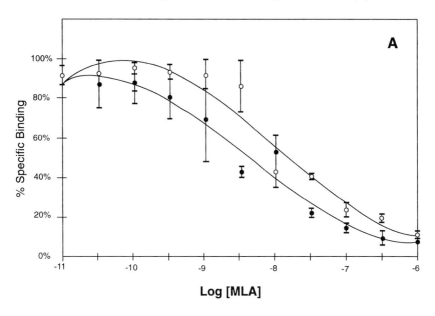

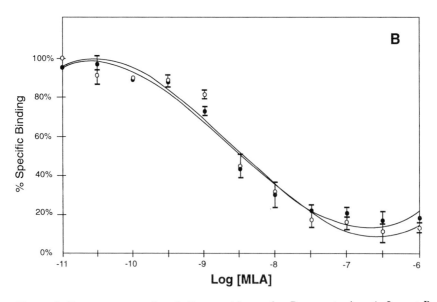

Figure 2 *Dose-response of methyllycaconitine and α-Bungarotoxin. A. Locust B. Rat (o) α-bungarotoxin, (●) methyllycaconitine*

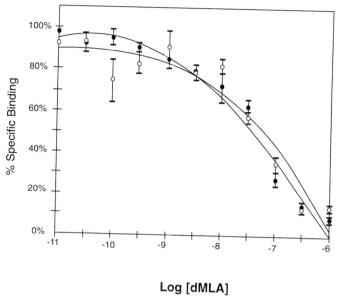

Figure 3 *Dose-response curve for dehydromethyllycaconitine* (●) *Rat;* (o) *Locust*

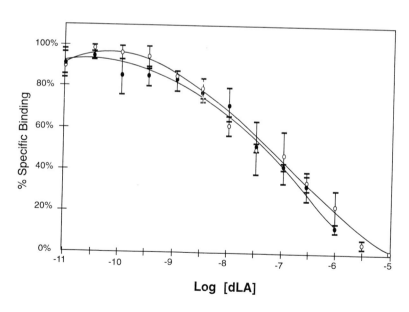

Figure 4 *Dose-response curve for dehydrolycaconitine* (●) *Rat;* (o) *Locust*

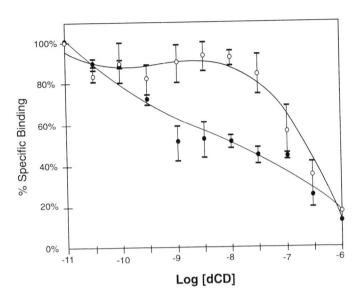

Figure 5 *Dose-response curve for dehydrocashmiradelphine (●) Rat; (o) Locust*

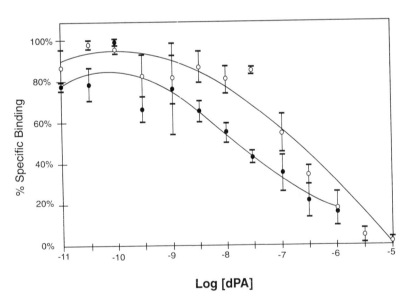

Figure 6 *Dose-response curve for dehydropuberaconitine (●) Rat; (o) Locust*

Plant extracts containing lycoctonine alkaloids have been used for millenia as insecticides[21] and in this century as the isolated alkaloids for medicinal purposes[22]. Research on delphinium alkaloids has led to an increased understanding of cattle toxicosis, a major problem on the rangelands of North America. It has also contributed to research on nicotinic cholinergic receptor function, targets for both insecticides and medical applications. The nicotinic receptor targeted by delphinium alkaloids of the MLA type have been implicated[23,24] in a wide range of neural functions such as memory, schizophrenia, neuroprotection, vestibular/auditory function, and is present on non-neural cells such as bronchial epithelium.

The development of selective α_7 agents based on delphinium alkaloid structure-activity information could lead to novel therapies for Alzheimer's that act by modulating cholinergic function either directly or through upregulation of nicotinic receptors[25]. Similarly, insect selective cholinergic neurotoxins offer the promise of developing a new class of insecticides to supplement those products currently available, most of which were derived from initial natural product leads[26].

Acknowledgment: The valuable technical assistance of Ms. Loretta Ross and the valuable contribution of Ms. Marny Morris in the preparation of this manuscript are appreciated.

References

1.   H.M. Lamb and D. Faulds, *Drugs and Aging*, 1997, **11**, 490.
2.   V. N. Aiyar, M.H. Benn, T. Hanna, J. Jacyno, S.H. Roth and J.L. Wilkens, *Experientia,* 1979, **35** 1367.
3.   J.D. Olsen and G.D. Manners, 'Toxicants of Plant Origin', CRC Press, Boca Raton, 1989, Chapter 12, p.291.
4.   K.R. Jennings, D.G. Brown, and D.P. Wright Jr., *Experientia,* 1986, **42,** 611.
5.   D.R.E. Macallan, G.G. Lunt, S. Wonnacott, K.L. Swanson, H. Rapoport, and E.X. Albuquerque, *FEBS Lett.,* 1988, **226,** 357.
6.   K.R. Jennings, D.G. Brown, D.P. Wright and A.E. Chalmers, Sites of Action for Neurotoxic Pesticides, ACS, Washington, 1987, Chapter 20, p.274.
7.   D.B. Sattelle, R.D. Pinnock and S.C.R. Lummis, *J. Exp. Biol.,* 1989, **142**, 215.
8.   M. Alkondon, E.F.R. Pereira, S. Wonnacott, and E.X. Albuquerque, *J. Pharm. Exp. Therap.,* 1992, **41**, 802.
9.   L.W. Role and D.K. Berg, *Neuron,* 1996, **16**, 1077.
10.   C.F. Kukel and K.R. Jennings, *Can. J. Physiol. Pharmacol.,* 1994, **72,** 104.
11.   I.S. Blagbrough, P.A. Coates, D.J. Hardick, T. Lewis, M.G. Rowan, S. Wonnacott, and B.V.L. Potter, *Tetrahedron Lett.,* 1994, **35,** 8705.
12.   D.J. Hardick, I.S. Blagbrough, S. Wonnacott and B.V.L. Potter, *Tetrahedron Lett.,* 1994, **35**, 3371.
13.   S. Sakai, *Gendai Toyo Igaku,* 1981, **2**, 50.
14.   J.M. Jacyno, J.S. Hardwood, N-H Lin, J.E. Campbell, J.P. Sullivan and M.W. Holladay, *J. Nat. Prod.,* 1996, **59**, 707.
15.   G.D. Manners, K.E. Panter and S.W. Pelletier, *J. Nat. Prod.,* 1995, **58**, 863.

16. D.J. Hardick, G. Cooper, T. Scott-Ward, I.S. Blagbrough, B.V.L. Potter and S. Wonnacott, *FEBS Lett.*, 1995, **365**, 779.
17. D.J. Hardick, I.S. Blagbrough, G. Cooper, B.V.L. Potter, T. Critchley and S. Wonnacott, *J. Med. Chem.*, 1996, **39**, 4860.
18. A.R.L. Davies, D.J. Hardick, I.S. Blagbrough, B.V.L. Potter, A.J. Wolstenholme and S. Wonnacot. *Bioch. Soc. Trans.*, 1997, **25**, 180.
19. P.N. Kao, and A. Karlin, *J. Biol. Chem.*, 1988, **261**, 8085.
20. L.A. Pabreza, S. Dhawan and K.J. Kellar, *Molec. Pharmacol.*, 1991, **39**, 9.
21. G. Plinius, Naturalis Historia, **23**, Ch. 13.
22. M.D. Mashkovsky and V.V. Churyukanov, *Handbook of Experimental Pharmacology*, 1986, **79**, 391.
23. M.A. Holladay, M.J. Dart and J.K. Lynch, *J. Med. Chem.*, 1997, **40**, 4169.
24. E.M. Meyer, E. T. Tay, J.A. Zoltewicz, C. Meyeres, M.A. King, R.L. Papke and C.M. De Fiebre, *J. Pharm. Exp. Therap.*, 1998, **284**, 1026.
25. E.J. Molinari, O. Delbono, M.L., Messi, M. Renganathan, S.P., Arneric, J.P. Sullivan, and M. Gopalakrishnan, *European Journal of Pharmacology*, 1998, **347**(1), 131.
26. R.W. Addor, 'Agrochemicals from Natural Products', Marcel Decker, New York, 1995, Chapter 1, p.1.

Nicotinic Receptors in Parasitic Nematodes and Anthelmintic Resistance

Richard J. Martin[1], Alan P. Robertson[1] and Henrik E. Bjorn[2]

[1] DEPARTMENT OF PRECLINICAL VETERINARY SCIENCES, R.(D.)S.V.S., SUMMERHALL, UNIVERSITY OF EDINBURGH, EDINBURGH, EH9 1QH, UK
[2] DEPARTMENT OF PHARMACOLOGY AND TOXICOLOGY, AND DANISH CENTRE FOR EXPERIMENTAL PARASITOLOGY, ROYAL VETERINARY AND AGRICULTURAL UNIVERSITY, BULOWESVEJ 13 DK-1870, FREDERIKSBERG C, DENMARK

1. INTRODUCTION

Nematode parasites are a common problem faced by man and animals. In man, particularly in developing countries, diseases like filariasis, ascariasis and river blindness inflict tremendous suffering, and even loss of life. In animals similar problems occur but the economic pressure for control relates to the loss of production in the western world. So it has been animal nematode parasites that have created the economic pressure for the development of modern anthelmintic drugs for the control of these parasites.

Most modern drugs used for the control of animal nematode parasites fall into one of three groups: 1) the benzimidazoles, like thiabendazole, which bind to β-tubulin of nematodes to prevent the formation of microtubules[1] and act at the colchicine binding site; 2) the nicotinic agonists, like levamisole, that have a selective effect on nicotinic receptors of nematodes, and produce spastic paralysis of the parasite with little effect on the host;[2] and 3) the avermectins, like ivermectin, that gate glutamate chloride channels[3] only present in invertebrates. All of the drugs in the groups above have been used regularly and resistance to therapy has appeared in many nematodes species in most parts of the world.[4] The mechanism of resistance to the benzimidazoles is understood at the molecular level[5] but we have still little understanding of the mechanism of resistance to the other two groups of anthelmintic.

Because the last two groups of anthelmintic have effects on nematode ion-channels, it is important to study these receptors using electrophysiological techniques. In this paper we focus on the nicotinic receptors and the actions of nicotinic anthelmintics levamisole and pyrantel. We also consider properties of receptors in anthelmintic resistant nematode parasites.

2. MATERIALS AND METHODS

We have developed a single-channel recording technique for recording levamisole activated channels from extrasynaptic nicotinic receptors on muscle cells of *Ascaris suum,* the large nematode parasite recovered from the pig intestine. Figure 1 illustrates

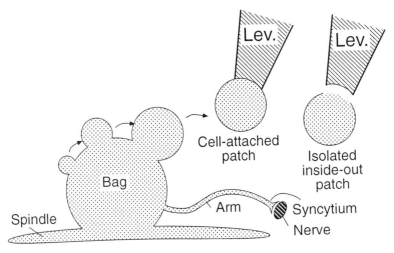

Figure 1 *Diagram of the preparation of muscle membrane vesicle and patch-clamp recording. Vesicle 'bud-off' the muscle cells following collagenase treatment. Levamisole (LEV) is added to the patch-pipette solution*

the preparation of membrane vesicles we use for making cell-attached and isolated-inside out patch recordings. Briefly, a 10 minute application of collagenase to a muscle flap preparation followed by incubation in a Ringer solution at 37°C leads to the production of muscle vesicles which may be harvested and viewed under phase contrast for patch-clamp.[6] Nicotinic anthelmintics (levamisole and pyrantel) are added to the patch-pipette solution and single-channel currents recorded onto DAT tape via a List or Axon instruments patch-clamp amplifier. Channel mean open-times, probabilities of the channels being open, and mean closed-times are determined using Pclamp 6.0 software or Pat software (Dempster, Strathclyde University) from the observed channel events. The conductances of the channels are measured by determining the slope of the single-channel current against the patch-potential. Different concentrations of levamisole are applied in the patch solution. The solutions contain Cs as the main cation to block K channels and low-Ca to prevent Ca-dependent Cl channels.

We have also carried out similar experiments on isolates of a smaller nematode parasite of the pig, *Oesophagostomum dentatum,* which were sensitive (SENS) and resistant (LEVR) to normal therapeutic concentrations of levamisole. The methods we used for this preparation were similar to that used in *Ascaris.*

3. RESULTS

3.1 Properties of levamisole and pyrantel activated currents in *Ascaris*

Figure 2 shows representative channel recordings and the distributions of the open-times of receptor channels activated by 3μM levamisole (top) and by 0.1μM pyrantel (bottom) from patches of *Ascaris* muscle. Both produced brief (~1 ms) inward current pulses at -75mV, and openings of channels which had conductances between 20-45 pS.

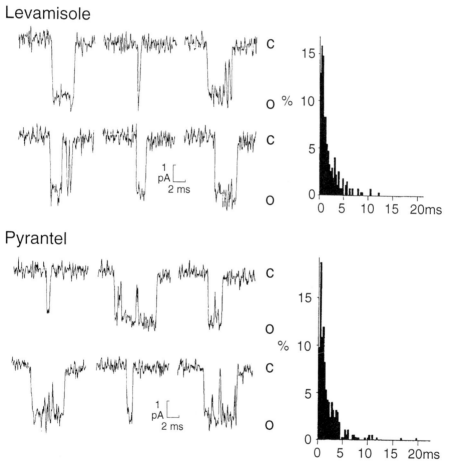

Figure 2 *Top: levamisole-activated channels currents from* Ascaris *muscle membrane and open-time histogram; mean open-time 1.34 ms, -75mV, 3μM levamisole. Bottom: pyrantel-activated channels currents and open-time histogram; mean open-time 1.09 ms -75mV, 0.1μM pyrantel.*

The levamisole-activated channels had a corrected mean open-time of 1.47 ms ±0.11 ms (n=12) while the pyrantel-activated channels had a corrected mean open-time of 1.73 ± 0.2 ms (n=17).

At higher concentrations of agonists we observed flickering open-channel block, which was voltage-sensitive, and increased with a more negative patch-potential. Figure 3 illustrates an example of the flickering channel-block produced at a membrane potential of -75 mV with 30 μM levamisole. A similar channel-block was also observed with pyrantel. We were able to estimate the dissociation constant, K_D for the channel block using a simple closed↔open↔blocked model[7]. The forward block rate constant, k_{+b}, was estimated from the slope of the plot 1/mean open-time *vs.* drug concentration. The unblocking rate constant, k_{-b}, was estimated as 1/mean blocked-time. K_D was then k_{-b}/k_{+b}. At -75mV we determined K_D to be 46μM for levamisole and 20μM for pyrantel.

We also observed that at higher concentrations of the nicotinic agonists that there were long closed times (many seconds) between bursts of openings. This behaviour resembles that seen in vertebrate nicotinic receptors[8] and was therefore interpreted as desensitization. We can summarize our observations at this stage by saying that the *Ascaris* nicotinic receptors have similarities to the biophysical properties of vertebrate nicotinic receptors.

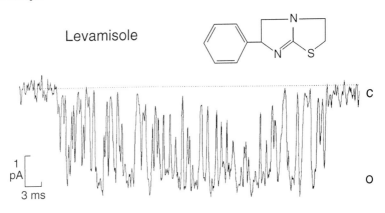

Figure 3 *Flickering open-channel block produced in a cell-attached patch form Ascaris produced by 30μM levamisole at -75mV. The comb effect is characteristic of the block.*

3.2 Changes in properties of nicotinic receptors in levamisole resistance

Unfortunately, resistance studies on *Ascaris* are limited because anthelmintic-resistant strains are not available. To overcome this problem we have selected the nodular worm of the pig, *Oesphagostomum dentatum,* for further study. *O. dentatum* may be maintained by cryopreservation of l_3 larvae and experimental infection of pigs, and anthelmintic-resistant isolates of *O. dentatum* are available.[9]

We made recordings from levamisole-activated channels using vesicle preparations prepared from levamisole-sensitive and levamisole-resistant parasites. We used cell-attached patches with 10, 30 or 100μM levamisole present in the patch pipette. The channel currents were similar in behaviour to those activated by levamisole in *Ascaris.*

Figure 4A illustrates representative open-time histograms from levamisole-sensitive (SENS) and levamisole-resistant (LEVR) isolates obtained with cell-attached patches at -75mV with 30μM levamisole as the agonist.   The mean open-time (τ) for the SENS isolate was 1.0 ms but the LEVR patch had a shorter τ, 0.6 ms.   Figure 4B is a histogram

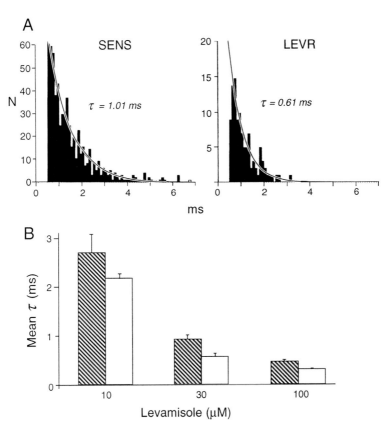

Figure 4 *A: Open-time distributions produced by 30μM levamisole from levamisole-sensitive (SENS) and levamisole-resistant (LEVR) isolates of* O. dentatum *obtained with cell-attached patches at -75mV with 30μM levamisole as the agonist. B: mean ±S.E. τ values at -75mV and effect of levamisole concentration. Cross-hatched: SENS isolate. Open: LEVR isolate.*

showing mean τ values at -75 mV for SENS and LEVR at 10, 30 and 100 μM levamisole: it can be seen that the mean τ values for SENS, at each concentration, are bigger than for LEVR, despite the dose-dependent reduction in τ produced by open channel-block. When we tested the statistical significance using ANOVA to compare the SENS and LEVR isolates, we found that there was a highly significant (F test, P<0.001) difference between the two isolates. The reduced τ was also associated with a reduced probability of the channels being open and a highly significant (F test, P<0.001) difference between P_{open} values of SENS and LEVR isolates was observed.

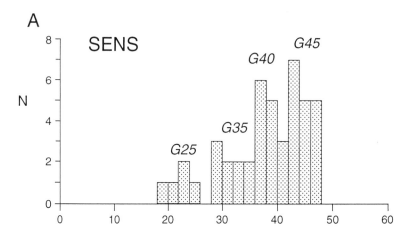

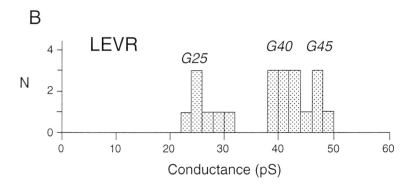

Figure 5 *Histograms of the conductance distributions obtained from the SENS isolate (A) and from the LEVR isolate (B). The peaks in the conductance distributions are labelled using a G notation near the mean of the individual peaks. Note that G35 is missing from the resistant isolate*

3.3 Conductance changes associated with development of resistance

We were able to measure the conductance of the nicotinic channels with a degree of precision from the slope of the current-voltage plots between ±75mV. The standard error of our individual estimates was often less than ± 1.0 pS. In the sensitive isolate, the conductance of the levamisole-activated channels ranged from 18.1 pS to 48.0 pS with a mean ± S.E. of 37.7 pS ± 1.1 pS, N = 45 In the resistant isolate the conductance values ranged from 15.2 pS to 47.8 pS with a mean ± S.E of 36.6 pS ± 2.0 pS, N= 21. The mean conductance values of SENS and LEVR were not significantly different (t-test, p > 0.05). The variation in the slope conductances observed between channels was interesting because it was much greater than could be accounted for by experimental technique. Figure 5A is a histogram of the conductances observed from the SENS isolate obtained with the concentrations 10-100 μM levamisole. The distribution has four peaks, was skewed towards the higher conductances, and was significantly different from a normal distribution (Anderson-Darling test for normality, P < 0.01) so that the conductance histogram is not consistent with a single population of levamisole receptors

We described the data in Figure 5A by fitting the conductance distribution to the sum of 4 Gaussian distributions with peaks means ± S.D. at: 21.4 ± 2.3 pS, labelled *G25*; 33.0 ± 4.8 pS, labelled *G35*; 38.1 ± 1.2 pS, labelled *G40*; and 44.3 ± 2.2 pS, labelled *G45*. We have used the *G* labelling for convenience to refer to peaks in the conductance distribution. These peaks appear to represent subtypes of levamisole receptor. In support of the existence of different receptor subtypes we have occasionally observed levamisole-activated channels with different conductances in the same patch. We have observed in one of our patches, at least three levamisole channel subtypes. This observation suggests that each nematode muscle has a range of levamisole receptor subtypes.

Figure 5B shows the distribution of channel conductances obtained from our LEVR isolate. Again the LEVR distribution was significantly different from a normal distribution (Anderson-Darling test for normality, P < 0.01) and could not be described by a single normal distribution. The LEVR distribution had similar peaks to the SENS conductance distribution but lacked the *G35* peak. When the conductance distribution was fitted by the sum of 3 Gaussian distributions the peaks (mean ± S.D.) were: 25.2 pS ± 4.5 pS, labelled *G25*; 41.2 ± 1.7 pS, labelled *G40*; and 46.7 pS ± 1.1 pS, labelled *G45*.

4. DISCUSSION

4.1 Types of resistance

Four general types of acquired drug resistance are recognised.[10]

Type 1, site exclusion, the first type of resistance to be recognised[11] is due to the therapeutic drug failing to get to its site of action because of some change in the transport of the drug by the organism.

Type 2, DNA amplification, probably the most common mechanism of resistance, involves increases in production of the drug receptor in the pathogen or an increase in drug destroying enzymes produced by the pathogen;

Type 3, receptor modification, a form of 'withdrawal of receptor' resistance[12] includes receptor loss and reduction of the receptor affinity for the drug;

Type 4, post receptor modification is a form of resistance associated with modifications of pathways that follow receptor activation and which can accommodate the effects of excessive receptor stimulation.

We have observed that the levamisole receptor channels in the LEVR isolate of *Oesophagostomum dentatum* have on average shorter mean open-times and reduced mean P_{open} values compared to the SENS isolate. However we did not observe a significant difference in the average channel conductances. We are able to explain a reduction in the sensitivity of the parasite to the therapeutic action of levamisole as a receptor modification, *Type 3*.   We observed that the channels were able to carry less current in the resistant isolate making the drug less potent.

It is interesting and important to recognise that receptor changes associated with the development of resistance are not the only mechanisms available to the parasite for the development of resistance.   We are not able to exclude other mechanisms of resistance also being present but it seem unlikely that *Type 1, site exclusion*, is involved because levamisole has a pKa of 8.0 so that at a pH of 7.0 10% is unionized and levamisole redistributes well across membranes,[13] making site exclusion difficult.   *Type 2, DNA amplification*, did not occur in the form of increased receptor because we counted the proportion of patches of membranes which contained active receptors.   We did not observe an increase in levamisole receptor numbers.   In addition an increase in levamisole receptor numbers would be expected to increase the sensitivity of the parasite to the drug.   We did not observe any evidence for or against the presence of *Type 4, post receptor modification*.   An example of post receptor modification might have included a reduction in the sensitivity to calcium of the contractile machinery of the muscle cell.

4.2   Origin of receptor subtypes

We have observed evidence of receptor subtypes which may be separated on the basis of channel conductances. We suggest that an explanation for the presence of multiple receptor subtypes within an individual parasite[14] is based on variations in the pentameric subunit composition of the nAChR ion-channel in the parasite which is the target site of levamisole.   It appears likely that there are 3 genes in *Oesphagostomum dentatum* analogous to the *C. elegans* genes (*Unc-39*, coding an α subunit; *lev-1* and *Unc-39*, coding for different β subunits),[15] and that each may contribute one or more of the subunits of the pentameric levamisole nAChR ion-channel.[16,17]   Although *C. elegans* and *O. dentatum* have widely different life-styles (free-living in contrast to parasitic), recent molecular studies have demonstrated that they are very closely related phylogenetically.[18]   So it is likely that our extrapolation of genetic information from *C. elegans* to *O. dentatum* is appropriate and informative.   This approach is further supported by the 91% similarity of the α-subunit *Tar 1* gene in the sheep nematode parasite, *Trichostrongylus colubriformis* with the *Unc-38* gene of *C elegans*.[19] Variation in the stochiometry and subunit composition is likely to occur and to give rise to variations in the conductance and agonist sensitivity of the pentameric nicotinic channel that is formed.[16]   Variation of the subunit structure may be under genetic control and explain the disappearance of the *G35* subtype from the LEVR isolate.

To conclude we have been able to compare the properties of individual levamisole receptors from sensitive and resistant isolates using the patch-clamp technique.   We have observed changes in the average properties of the receptors that can explain a reduced sensitivity to the therapeutic actions of the nicotinic anthelmintic, levamisole. The molecular mechanisms underlying these changes have yet to be elucidated

Acknowledgments

R. J. Martin is pleased to acknowledge the financial support of the Wellcome Trust. H. E. Bjorn is pleased to acknowledge the support of the Danish National Research Foundation.

References

1. Sangster, N. C., Prichard, R. K. & Lacey, E. *J. Parasitol.*, 1985, **71**, 645.
2. Aceves, J., Erliji, D. & Martinez-Marnon, R. *Brit. J. Pharmacol.*, 1970, **38**, 602.
3. Cully, D. F., Vassilatis, D. K., Liu, K. K., Paress, P. S., Vanderploeg, L. H. T. & Schaeffer, J. M. *Nature*, 1994, **371**, 707.
4. Prichard, R. K. *Vet. Parasitol.*, 1994, **54**, 259.
5. Roos, M. H., Kwa, M. S. G. & Grant, W. N. *Parasitol. Today*, 1995, **11**, 148.
6. Martin, R. J., Kusel, J. R. & Pennington, A. J. *J. Parasitol.*, 1990, **76**, 340-348
7. Neher, E. & Steinbach, J. H.. *J. Physiol.*, 1978, **277**, 153.
8. Sakmann, B., Patlak, J. & Neher, E. *Nature*, 1980, **286**, 71-73
9. Verady, M., Bjorn, H., Craven, J. & Nansen, P. *Internat J. Parasitol.*, 1996, **27**, 77.
10. Albert, A. 'Selective Toxicity *The physico-chemical basis of therapy'*. Seventh Edition. Chapman and Hall. London and New York, 1985.
11. Yorke, W, Murgatroyd, F, and Hawking, F. *Ann., Trop., Med., Parasitol.*, 1931, **25**, 351.
12. Erlich, P. *Ber, dtsch. Chem. Ges.*, 1909, **42**, 17.
13. Robertson, S. J. & Martin, R. J. *Pest. Sci.*, 1993, **37**, 293.
14. Martin, R. J., Robertson, A. P., Bjorn, H. & Sangster, N. C. *Eur. J Pharmac.*, 1997, .**322**, 249.
15. Fleming, J. T., Squire, M. D., Barnes, T. M., et al. *J. Neurosci.*, 1997, **17**, 5843.
16. McGehee, D. S. & Role, L. W. *Ann. Rev, Physiol.*, 1995, **57**, 521.
17. Changeau, J.-P., Devillers-Thiery, A. & Chemouilli, P., *Science*, 1996, **225**, 1335.
18. Blaxter, M. L., DeLey, P., Garey, J. R., et al. *Nature*, 1998, **392**, 71.
19. Wiley, L. J., Weiss, A. S., Sangster, N. C. & Li, Q. *Gene*, 1996,. **182**, 97.

Strategies for Developing Natural Products as Crop Protection Agents Employing Neurotoxicological and Other Neurophysiological Modes of Action

M.A. Birkett, B.P.S. Khambay, J.A. Pickett, L.J. Wadhams and C.M. Woodcock

BIOLOGICAL AND ECOLOGICAL CHEMISTRY DEPARTMENT, IACR-ROTHAMSTED, HARPENDEN, HERTFORDSHIRE AL5 2JQ, UK

1 INTRODUCTION

Natural products offering prospects for use in pest control continue to be identified. With the success of recombinant DNA technologies in genetic modification of crop plants, novel approaches are thereby emerging for incorporation into Integrated Pest Management strategies. As a result, a wider range of neurophysiological interactions, including toxicological and behavioural effects resulting from neurophysiological activities, can be exploited in the future, and will enable the more efficient manipulation of beneficial arthropods.

2 NEUROTOXICOLOGICAL MECHANISMS

2.1 Animal-derived toxins

A great deal of work has been directed at amphibians, in particular "neotropical" frogs of the family Dendrobatidae, e.g. *Phyllobates* spp.[1] These contain toxicants typically active as agonists of acetylcholine and which are providing lead structures, e.g. epibatidine (1), for new analgesics, and are closely related to new pesticides such as the nicotinoid (= chloronicotinyl) imidacloprid (2). One of the typical compounds from *P. aurotaenia* is homobatrachotoxin (3).[2] Another group of vertebrates known to contain toxicants, but which have received comparatively little attention, are the birds, e.g. pitohui birds (Pachycephalidae) such as the hooded pitohui, *Pitohui dichrous*, from Papua New Guinea, which also contains homobatrachotoxin.[3] Although the toxins of this genus have been studied, there are others, such as the golden oriole, *Oriolus oriolus* (Oriolidae), which are relatively uninvestigated.

Although it is very exciting to study exotic animals such as poison frogs and the birds described above, other animals are commonly found in our midst which contain structurally-related toxins with equal potency. Not least amongst these are the ladybirds, or ladybird beetles (Coccinellidae). These insects provide a range of toxic compounds and it was recently found that 2-methoxy-3-(1-methylethyl)pyrazine (4), identified unequivocally for the first time in the seven-spot ladybird, *Coccinella septempunctata*, acts as an aggregation pheromone for this species.[4] Currently, attempts are being made to use the aggregation behaviour to conserve these beneficial insects in the autumn and winter for use against aphids on high value crops such as Christmas trees in the spring. It was considered, before this pheromonal role was discovered, that these compounds were merely part of the system warning predators that the ladybirds contain highly toxic alkaloids, typified by their bright red and black aposematic coloration. Coccinelline (5), the *N*-oxide of the free base precoccinelline (6), which has also been isolated from poison frogs,[1] has an extremely high mammalian toxicity. The ladybird eggs also contain these materials and only a few are needed to achieve a lethal dose by intravenous application to a mammal. The two-spot ladybird, *Adalia bipunctata*, contains (-)-adaline (7) and (-)-adalinine (9) and when presented to a range of insects, the former proved to be highly toxic, whereas its mammalian toxicity is substantially less than for the seven-spot ladybird toxicants. The adaline provided for these experiments was from *de novo* synthesis, also giving rise to the unnatural (+)-isomer (8) which was even more insecticidal, with an LC_{50} of 3 ppm in the whitefly vial test.[5] This test gives *ca* 10 ppm for the LC_{50} of the pyrethroid cypermethrin against cotton whitefly, *Bemisia tabaci* (Aleyrodidae), a major target for development of new insecticides, particularly those involving mechanisms to which resistance has not yet developed (M.A. Birkett and B.P.S. Khambay, unpublished data).

Another exciting discovery relating to toxicants of the seven-spot ladybird has been made in that the free base precoccinelline (6) is highly active at the electrophysiological level with the ladybird parasitoid *Dinocampus* (= *perilitus*) *coccinellae* (Braconidae), and thereby acts as a semiochemical in its host location.[6]

2.2 Insect Neuropeptides

Major physiological processes in insects are regulated by neurohormones, many of which are peptidic in nature. These can often have very high intrinsic activities, are involved in fundamental biological processes, and present targets that might be amenable to combinatorial chemistry and allow toxicants to be developed for high selectivity.[7,8] Recently, a C-terminal pentapeptide (10) of the nonapeptide achetakinin AK-I, first obtained from the house cricket, *Acheta domesticus* (Gryllidae), was taken as a target molecule for structure-activity studies. Compared with the full sequence, the core peptide (10) retains most of the diuretic activity at 8.7×10^{-12} molar. The objective was to examine the dependence on structure of measured and predicted lipophilicity and metabolic stability, and to attempt to correlate this with effects on cuticle penetration and, of course, biological activity.[9] Structural changes were made as shown in the diagram and one of the best compounds (11), in terms of increased lipophilicity and reduced decomposition by proteinase attack, is when R_1 = $PhCH_2CH_2CH_2CH_2$, R_2 = methyl and R_3 = *O*-methyl. It has a log K_{ow} nearly 10 times larger than the core peptide and a metabolic stability of over 24 hours. Such studies demonstrate that many regions are amenable to modification and that activity can be higher for some analogues. However, changes in polarity (log K_{ow}) may not always correlate with cuticle penetration or metabolic stability. In the latter case, results can depend upon the source of proteinases employed in the assays. None the less, although analogues with cuticle-penetrating properties have been identified where activity could be shown *in vitro*, this could not be reproduced when injected into the whole organism, suggesting that other processes are responsible for metabolism, or that physiological processes (e.g. hind gut contraction) occur which counter their effect.

2.2.1 Novel Toxic Peptides. The neuropeptides discussed above mainly have

(1)

(2)

(3)

(4)

(5)

(6)

(7)

(8)

(9)

primary metabolic amino acids in the amino acid sequences of the lead compound, However, some insect-produced toxicants incorporating non-protein amino acids could, as neuropeptides, be developed by combinatorial chemistry. An insect fungal pathogen, the hyphomycete *Metarhizium anisopliae*, produces cyclic peptides, the destruxins, during the pathogenesis process. These readily accessible compounds are highly cytotoxic but provide interesting leads for the development of selective pest control agents.[10] However, a very simple dipeptide (12) with one non-protein amino acid is obtained from a coleopterous pest, the Colorado potato beetle, *Leptinotarsa decemlineata* (Chrysomelidae).[11] Although the natural product was known to be toxic to ants by ingestion, insufficient material was available for full investigation of its insecticidal activity. The total synthesis has now been achieved in seven steps (S. Cameron, unpublished data) from the known pinacol propene boronate. The non-protein amino acid product (13), protected as the methyl ester with BOC on the amino group, is then joined with the protected glutamic acid to give the Colorado potato beetle toxicant (12). To date, the compound has shown poor activity against mosquito larvae (*Aedes aegypti*, Culicidae) and by injection into waxmoth larvae (*Galleria mellonella*, Pyralidae). However, toxicological studies against ants are under way and combinatorial structure-activity relationship studies are planned.

3 NON-TOXIC NEUROPHYSIOLOGICAL MECHANISMS

Signalling between organisms of the same species and also across different trophic levels is mediated by chemical signals, termed "semiochemicals" from the Greek "semeion" (σημεῖον), meaning "sign" or "signal". It is well known that the sex pheromones of lepidopterous pests, which comprise a major group of semiochemicals, can be utilised directly in crop protection by disrupting mating. Indeed, even in nature, different species producing the same sex pheromones, but normally separated spatially or temporally, can occasionally be seen to mate, although fertile offspring are not produced.[12] Semiochemicals can be identified by coupling highly sensitive spectroscopic and chromatographic techniques with electrophysiological recordings from the sensory neurons involved in their perception. In the 1970s, it became clear that some semiochemicals detected by contact chemosensory perception could interfere with feeding. These so-called antifeedants were demonstrated to have potential in crop protection.[13,14,15,16] There is now even more demand for such materials, not simply as adjuncts or alternatives to pesticide use, but to provide agents with which to protect the highly valuable genes transferred to crop plants by recombinant DNA techniques for direct generation of toxicants against herbivorous pests. The antifeedant is thus directed against initial colonisation by the pest so that, if individuals break through this first line of defence, the toxicant is then encountered, thereby reducing the selection pressure for resistance on this aspect of the crop protection package. Indeed, the clerodane antifeedants can be highly effective against lepidopterous and coleopterous pests, and plants in the *Ajuga* genus (Lamiaceae) are now being cultivated as a potential commercial source of these valuable products.

3.1 Non-Host Repellents

In evolutionary terms, it is more advantageous to detect unsuitability of a host

(10)

(11)

(12)

(13)

(14)

before contact rather than to sample the tissues and either waste energy or risk ingestion of toxicants. New discoveries are leading to a rational search for repellent agents derived from non-host or otherwise unsuitable plants. The discoveries that led to this were, first of all, that location of suitable hosts by insects involves the detection of volatile compounds via highly specific mechanisms. It is well known that insects detect pheromonal components by such specific mechanisms, with there usually being individual olfactory neurons for each component, e.g. as for the sex pheromones of aphids (Aphididae).[17] When it was shown, in a number of laboratories, that insects colonising particular plant taxa also used specific olfactory cells in their response to characteristic volatile chemical components, this was of no great surprise. For example, the cabbage seed weevil, *Ceutorhynchus assimilis* (Curculionidae), a pest of oilseed rape, *Brassica napus* (Brassicaceae), has neurons responding to 3-butenyl and 4-pentenyl isothiocyanates which give only a weak response to 2-phenylethyl isothiocyanate, and none to allyl (2-propenyl) isothiocyanate, even at high stimulus concentrations; another cell type responds only to the 2-phenylethyl isothiocyanate.[18] However, this insect also responds to *ca* 20 other compounds found in oilseed rape, one of which is 1-octen-3-ol. The cell responsible gives a response to homologues such as octan-3-ol, (*Z*)-3-octen-1-ol, octan-3-one and 1-octen-3-one only when they are presented at orders of magnitude higher stimulus concentrations.[18] Such specificity for ubiquitous plant components is now shown to be a general phenomenon. For example, a specific cell for the green leaf volatile (*Z*)-3-hexen-1-ol can readily be found on the antenna of the pea and bean weevil, *Sitona lineatus* (Curculionidae).[19] The polyphagous peach-potato aphid, *Myzus persicae*, has a specific cell for another common green leaf volatile, (*E*)-2-hexenal, which must be stimulated by concentrations several orders of magnitude higher to respond to the related compounds (*Z*)-3-hexen-1-ol, (*Z*)-3-hexen-1-yl acetate, hexanal and 2-ethylhexan-1-ol.[20] Carnivorous or haematophagous insects can exhibit similar abilities. The mosquito disease vector *Culex quinquefasciatus* (Culicidae) has an olfactory neuron specific for 3-methylindole, a common component of the polluted water used for oviposition, which shows no response to indole or other oviposition site related compounds.[21] Such discoveries contradicted the accepted theory that insects respond to ubiquitous host components using generalist receptors.

During this research, certain neurons, although clearly of an olfactory nature, were found which could not be stimulated either by host volatiles or the insects' own metabolites, e.g. pheromones. A number of insects displaying these so-called "redundant" cells were tested using volatiles from plants which were either non-hosts or unsuitable because of aspects related to taxonomy or conditions of stress. For the black bean aphid, *Aphis fabae*, two compounds stimulated cells that were not associated with host location: (1*R*,5*S*)-myrtenal (14), an isoprenoid common to members of the Lamiaceae and generally present in gymnosperms, and methyl salicylate, typical of non-host taxa but having other roles, as will be elaborated.[22] These compounds were shown to interfere with the normal attractiveness of host plants such as broad bean, *Vicia faba* (Fabaceae), in a behavioural assay[22] and also at higher levels acted as repellents. In addition, it was found that cereal aphids such as the bird-cherry-oat aphid, *Rhopalosiphum padi*, and the grain aphid, *Sitobion avenae*, possess specific cells for methyl salicylate.[23] In field trials in Sweden, this compound at extremely low release rates reduced aphid populations by approximately 50%. These experiments have been repeated, with similar results, in Scandinavia and in the United Kingdom.[19] Such effects can be sufficient to reduce aphid populations to below the economic threshold for pesticide treatment but, more particularly, are finding use in combination with other means of control, including attraction of parasitoids.[19] Over 30 insect species from four Orders have now been shown to respond to methyl salicylate (C.M. Woodcock, unpublished data). In 1995, we advanced the theory that the role of methyl salicylate may be to indicate the level of induction of the phenylalanine ammonialyase defence pathway, known to be induced and associated with a flux of salicylic acid in the plant.[23] It has subsequently been shown that methyl salicylate can be used as a signal by plants in switching on defence against pathogen attack.[24]

A non-host repellent has also been discovered for the pine shoot beetles, *Tomicus* (= *Blastophagus* = *Myelophilus*) *destruens* and *T. piniperda* (Scolytidae). These major pests of *Pinus* species (Pinaceae) avoid deciduous trees, since they represent unsuitable hosts, and again by using electrophysiological preparations of olfactory cells having no clearly defined role, other non-host plant indicators were demonstrated. Thus, by using volatiles from fennel, *Foeniculum vulgare* (Apiaceae), benzyl alcohol was identified as an electrophysiologically active compound which, in field trials, significantly reduced attacks by *T. destruens* on *Pinus pinea* logs.[25]

3.2 Repellency and Stress

In the course of developing an intercropping programme against lepidopterous stem borers attacking subsistence cereal crops such as maize and sorghum, a repellent has been identified which has other beneficial uses. In this programme, as well as planting trap crops to attract pests away from the main crop, plants shown to be repellent were placed between the rows of cereals. One such repellent plant is the molasses grass, *Melinis minutiflora* (Poaceae). Electrophysiological studies on pests such as the maize stalk borer, *Busseola fusca* (Noctuidae), using volatiles from *M. minutiflora*, revealed active compounds additional to those normally attracting these insects to cereals and grasses (Poaceae), including various hydrocarbons and the homomonoterpene (*E*)-4,8-dimethyl-1,3,7-nonatriene. It was also found that increased parasitisation of stem borer larvae was occurring in the maize plants intercropped with *M. minutiflora* and it was subsequently shown that the nonatriene, as well as repelling adult stem borers, promotes foraging by the parasitoid *Cotesia sesamiae* (Braconidae). This monoterpene is typical of stress signals released from plants being attacked by herbivores, which are then subsequently used by parasitoids in locating their hosts. Boland's group has shown that the nonatriene and the related homosesquiterpene are produced by oxidative cleavage of the corresponding higher isoprenoid alcohol,[26,27] which in the case of the homoterpene is the sesquiterpenoid nerolidol. We now know from feeding studies with aphids and caterpillars that the volatiles released by plants under such stress are typical of the species causing the damage. For example, the volatiles produced when the pea aphid, *Acyrthosiphon pisum*, infests a bean plant are slightly different from those produced when, for example, the black bean aphid, *Aphis fabae*, colonises the same plant. This allows parasitoids which have a specific host, e.g. *Aphidius ervi* that attacks only *A. pisum*, to locate particular host species.[28] For the major caterpillar pest *Spodoptera exigua* (Noctuidae), the beet armyworm, the chemical responsible for systemic release of these stress compounds has been identified as *N*-(17-hydroxylinalenoyl)-L-glutamine.[29,30]

The search is now on for other systemically active cues that herbivores introduce into plants and which have the potential to induce release of compounds repelling herbivorous pests while, at the same time, attracting in parasitoids to attack the herbivores, all of this achieved by non-toxic neurophysiological mechanisms underlying the behavioural changes.

Acknowledgements

IACR receives grant-aided support from the Biotechnology and Biological Sciences Research Council of the United Kingdom. This work was in part supported by the United Kingdom Ministry of Agriculture, Fisheries and Food.

References

1. J. W. Daly, *J. Nat. Prod.*, 1998, **61**, 162.
2. T. Tokuyama, J. W. Daly and B. Witkop, *J. Am. Chem. Soc.*, 1969, **91**, 3931.
3. J. P. Dumbacher, B. M. Beehler, T. F. Spande, H. M. Garraffo and J. W. Daly, *Science*, 1992, **258**, 799.
4. S. Al Abassi, M. A. Birkett, J. Pettersson, J. A. Pickett and C. M. Woodcock, *CMLS*, 1998, **54**, 876.
5. M. R. Cahill and B. S. Hackett, *Proc. Brighton Crop Prot. Conf. - Pests and Diseases*, 1992, **1**, 251.
6. M. A. Birkett, J. A. Pickett, L. J. Wadhams and C. M. Woodcock, *Ninth IUPAC Congress of Pesticide Chemistry, August 2-6, 1998*.
7. M. Altstein, O. Ben-Aziz, I. Schafler, I. Seltzer and C. Gilon, *Abstract, Third Int. Symp. on Mol. Insect Sci., Snowbird, Utah, U.S.A., June 5-19, 1998*.
8. P. E. A. Teal and R. J. Nachman, *Abstract, Third Int. Symp. on Mol. Insect Sci., Snowbird, Utah, U.S.A., June 5-19, 1998*.
9. S. Cameron, G. M. Coast, M. G. Ford, G. Goldsworthy, B. P. S. Khambay, J. V. Stone and P. Watson, 'Proceedings of the 1st International Conference on Insects: Chemical, Physiological and Environmental Aspects, September 26-29, 1994, Ladek Zdroj, Poland', D. Konopińska, G. Goldsworthy, R.J. Nachman, J. Nawrot, I. Orchard, G. Rosiński and W. Sobótka (eds.), University of Wrocław, Poland, p. 248.
10. F. Cavelier, J. Verducci, F. Andre, F. Haraux, C. Sigalat, M. Traris and A. Vey, *Pestic. Sci.*, 1998, **52**, 81.
11. D. Daloze, J. C. Braekman and J. M. Pasteels, *Science*, 1986, **233**, 221.
12. C. A. Clarke, A. Cronin, W. Francke, P. Philipp, J. A. Pickett, L. J. Wadhams and C. M. Woodcock, *Experientia*, 1996, **52**, 636.
13. J. A. Pickett, G. W. Dawson, D. C. Griffiths, A. Hassanali, L. A. Merritt, A. Mudd, M. C. Smith, L. J. Wadhams, C. M. Woodcock and Z-n. Zhang, 'Pesticide Science and Biotechnology', R. Greenhalgh and T. R. Roberts (eds), Blackwell Scientific Publications, Oxford, 1987, p. 125.
14. D. C. Griffiths, A. Hassanali, L. A. Merritt, A. Mudd, J. A. Pickett, S. J. Shah, L. E. Smart, L. J. Wadhams and C. M. Woodcock, *Proc. Brighton Crop Prot. Conf. - Pests and Diseases*, 1988, 1041.
15. D. C. Griffiths, J. A. Pickett, L. E. Smart and C. M. Woodcock, *Pestic. Sci.*, 1989, **27**, 269.
16. D. C. Griffiths, S. P. Maniar, L. A. Merritt, A. Mudd, J. A. Pickett, B. J. Pye, L. E. Smart and L. J. Wadhams, *Crop Prot.*, 1991, **10**, 145.

17. G. W. Dawson, D. C. Griffiths, L. A. Merritt, A. Mudd, J. A. Pickett, L. J. Wadhams and C. M. Woodcock, *J. Chem. Ecol.*, 1990, **16**, 3019.
18. M. M. Blight, J. A. Pickett, L. J. Wadhams and C. M. Woodcock, *J. Chem. Ecol.*, 1995, **21**, 1649.
19. J. A. Pickett, L. J. Wadhams and C. M. Woodcock, *Agr. Ecosyst Environ.*, 1997, **64**, 149.
20. N. Agelopoulos, M. A. Birkett, A. J. Hick, A. M. Hooper, J. A. Pickett, L. E. Smart, D. W. M. Smiley, L. J. Wadhams and C. M. Woodcock, *Pestic. Sci.* (in press).
21. J. A. Pickett and C. M. Woodcock, 'Olfaction in Mosquito-Host Interactions', G. Cardew (ed.), John Wiley & Sons Ltd., Chichester, 1996, CIBA Foundation Symposium No. 200, p. 109.
22. J. Hardie, R. Isaacs, J. A. Pickett, L. J. Wadhams and C. M. Woodcock, *J. Chem. Ecol.*, 1994, **20**, 2847.
23. J. Pettersson, J. A. Pickett, B. J. Pye, A. Quiroz, L. E. Smart, L. J. Wadhams and C. M. Woodcock, *J. Chem. Ecol.*, 1994, **20**, 2565.
24. V. Shulaev, P. Silverman and I. Raskin, *Nature*, 1997, **385**, 718.
25. A. Guerrero, J. Feixas, J. Pajares, L. J. Wadhams, J. A. Pickett and C. M. Woodcock, *Naturwissenschaften*, 1997, **84**, 155.
26. A. Gäbler and W. Boland, *Helv. Chim. Acta*, 1991, **74**, 1773.
27. J. Donath and W. Boland, *Phytochemistry*, 1995, **39**, 785.
28. Y. Du, G. M. Poppy, W. Powell, J. A. Pickett, L. J. Wadhams and C. M. Woodcock, *J. Chem. Ecol.*, 1998, **24**, 1355.
29. T. C. J. Turlings and J. H. Tumlinson, *Proc. Natl. Acad. Sci. USA*, 1992, **89**, 8399.
30. H. T. Alborn, T. C. J. Turlings, T. H. Jones, G. Stenhagen, J. H. Loughrin and J. H. Tumlinson, *Science*, 1997, **276**, 945.

Neurotoxicity

Effects of Heptachlor Exposure on Neurochemical Biomarkers of Parkinsonism

J.R. Bloomquist[1], M.L. Kirby[1], K. Castagnoli[1] and G.W. Miller[2]

[1] DEPARTMENTS OF ENTOMOLOGY (JRB & MLK), AND CHEMISTRY (KC), VIRGINIA POLYTECHNIC INSTITUTE AND STATE UNIVERSITY, BLACKSBURG, VA 24061, USA
[2] DEPARTMENT OF CELL BIOLOGY, DUKE UNIVERSITY, DURHAM, NC 27710, USA

1 INTRODUCTION

Idiopathic Parkinson's Disease (PD) is a neurodegenerative condition with a unique set of motor symptoms including bradykinesia, muscle rigidity, altered posture, shuffling gait, and a rhythmic tremor of 2-6 Hz.[1] PD usually has its onset late in life, but in certain individuals manifests itself as Young Onset Parkinson's Disease (YOPD) when it occurs between the ages of 21-40 years.[2] Symptomatic progression in YOPD occurs more slowly than in PD, but is qualitatively similar in other respects.[2] Both types of PD eventually cause serious motor disability, mental decline, and death.

The motor symptoms of PD are accompanied by degeneration of neurons in the dopaminergic nigro-striatal pathway of the brain.[1] Because the substantia nigra is the origin of the pathway innervating the striatal nuclei, the degeneration of these neurons results in severe striatal dopamine (DA) loss, which is the primary neurochemical abnormality in the Parkinsonian brain.[3] Other indices of dopaminergic neurons are also reduced, including tyrosine hydroxylase activity, levels of the DA metabolites 3,4-dihydroxyphenylacetic acid (DOPAC) and homovanillic acid, and the density of dopamine uptake sites.[3]

Among the possible factors contributing to idiopathic PD, the leading candidates are mitochondrial dysfunction, genetic predisposition, and exposure to environmental toxins. A dysfunction in energy metabolism, evidenced by a 37% deficiency in complex I activity, is observed in nigral mitochondria of the Parkinsonian brain.[4] There is also evidence of oxidative stress specific to the substantia nigra of PD patients, as suggested by the presence of increased levels of mitochondrial superoxide dismutase and lipid hydroperoxides.[5] Free radical-mediated oxidative stress could be a consequence of defective or increased complex I activity, but might also be a symptom of toxin exposure.[5] Recent studies have also linked a defect in the synaptic protein α-synuclein with a family history of YOPD[6], although there is little information available on the function of this protein.

A number of environmental agents have also been implicated in the development of PD. Unique evidence for a role of environmental agents in PD comes from the Parkinsonian syndrome generated by the neurotoxin 1-methyl-4-phenyl-1,2,3,6-tetrahydropyridine, or MPTP (Figure 1). This compound was injected by drug addicts who quickly developed a syndrome nearly indistinguishable from idiopathic PD.[7] Extensive research efforts revealed that MPTP is bioactivated by brain monoamine oxidase-B (MAO-B) to the toxic pyridinium, MPP^+,[8] which is sequestered within nigral neurons by the dopamine uptake transporter.[9] Once inside the dopaminergic terminals, it destroys the cells,[10] apparently via inhibition of mitochondrial respiration.[11] Related toxins hypothesized to play a role in idiopathic PD are certain dietary and metabolism-generated tetrahydroisoquinolines and β-carbolines. These compounds are metabolized to the corresponding quaternary species (Figure 1) and have neurotoxic properties similar to those of MPP[+].[12]   The observed effects of MPTP stimulated new hypotheses of how endogenous factors such as defective energy metabolism and oxidative stress, along with environmental toxins, might contribute to a multifactorial etiology for PD. Overall, there seems to be an emerging consensus that the etiology of PD is related to a combination of genetic predisposition and exposure to an environmental toxin trigger.[13]

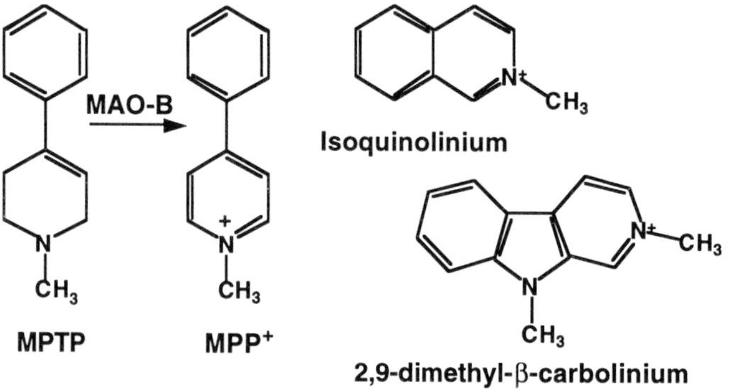

Figure 1 *Neurotoxic compounds thought to play a role in environmental parkinsonism.*

Another possible environmental trigger for PD is exposure to pesticides. Epidemiological studies have shown a consistent linkage between rural populations and PD.[14]   Among the specific factors found to pose an increased risk for PD and YOPD within rural populations were drinking well water[15], exposure to herbicides[15], and in other cases, exposure to insecticides.[16,17]   A recent study specifically linked exposure to organochlorine and organophosphorus compounds with the incidence of PD in Germany.[18]   Case history studies have identified individuals exposed to mixtures of pesticides who suffered from YOPD.[19]   Exposure to the herbicide diquat has also been associated with the development of a Parkinsonian syndrome and nigro-striatal lesions.[20] Analysis of finger tremor frequencies in grain elevator workers exposed to the fumigant carbon disulfide found that they were around 5-7 Hz, which is similar to the tremor frequency found in idiopathic PD.[21]   Post mortem brain tissue from individuals afflicted with PD was analyzed for the presence of organochlorine pesticides.[22]   The authors found that the occurrence of PD was significantly correlated ($p = 0.03$) with the presence of brain residues of the insecticide dieldrin (mean = 13 ppb).   Thus, Fleming *et al.*,[22] concluded that residues of organochlorines such as dieldrin may contribute to the development of PD. We chose heptachlor for this study because it is an environmentally persistent cyclodiene similar to dieldrin.[23]   Moreover, there was widespread human exposure to heptachlor and heptachlor epoxide in contaminated milk products that occurred in the state of Hawaii in 1981 and 1982[24], perhaps rendering the population at increased risk for PD.

Although previous studies have linked exposure to specific pesticides with Parkinsonism, they are generally supported by little or no mechanistic investigation. Accordingly, we have initiated studies on neurochemical biomarkers of parkinsonism in an animal model of PD.   We evaluated the effects of the persistent organochlorine insecticide heptachlor in the MPTP-treated, C57BL6 mouse. When treated with MPTP, adult C57 mice show neuronal cell loss and reductions in dopamine content and dopamine transport that correlate with a reduced motor activity and impaired coordination.[25,26]   Thus, this system shows many of the hallmarks of idiopathic PD, and appears to be a valid rodent model for the investigation of toxicant-induced Parkinsonism.[27]   It is, therefore, an ideal model system for studying the possible role of insecticide exposure in the etiology of PD.

2 MATERIALS AND METHODS

C57BL/6 mice were treated by intraperitoneal injection with either vehicle or vehicle containing toxicant as shown in Figure 2. Heptachlor was given alone and also in combination with MPTP to test its ability to synergize the actions of MPTP. This latter experimental paradigm was used to model the ability of insecticide exposure to accelerate or intensify idiopathic disease processes. This treatment paradigm was used based on studies that showed a single dose of MPTP depressed levels of dopamine in the striatum 2 weeks later (Figure 3).

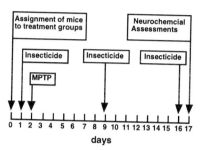

Figure 2 *Treatment regime for C57BL/6 mice given insecticide and/or MPTP.*

We determined DA and DOPAC levels in the striata of treated mice using HPLC with electrochemical detection, according to the method of Hall *et al.*[28]

Kinetics of dopamine transport was determined in *ex vivo* synaptosomes isolated from treated mice. Striatal synaptosomes were isolated according to the methods of Bloomquist *et al.*,[29] and kinetic parameters (K_m and V_{max}) of uptake were determined by the method of Kreuger.[30] Data were analyzed using Prism® software (GraphPad Software, San Diego, CA, USA). Levels of dopamine transporter (DAT) were measured in synaptosomal samples from heptachlor-treated mice. Monoclonal antibody labeling of DAT was performed according to established methods.[31]

At the end of the treatment period, striata for nerve terminal respiration studies were excised from treated mice and the synaptosomes isolated using the methods described above.[29] For assessing mitochondrial function, the thiazolyl blue (MTT) assay kit from Sigma Chemical Co. (St. Louis, Missouri, USA) was used. This assay reports on the amount of dehydrogenase activity at mitochondrial complex one[32] and is a common measure of cytotoxicity.[33]

Neurotransmitter release studies were performed in synaptosomes from untreated male ICR mice. The final synaptosomal pellets[29] were pooled and resuspended in incubation buffer containing [³H]neurotransmitters (5 min, 37°C). Membranes were then centrifuged at 10000x*g* for 10 minutes. Labelled pellets were resuspended in buffer and incubated with toxicants for 10 minutes at 37 °C. Incubates were diluted, filtered, and washed 3 times with 37 °C buffer. Treatment means were compared by ANOVA and a Student-Newman-Keuls means separation test.

For evaluating interaction of heptachlor with the vesicular monoamine transporter, SK-N-MC cells, a human neuroblastoma line, were stably transfected with human vesicular monoamine transporter 2 cDNA (VMAT2).[34] Assay of vesicular dopamine uptake was performed as described by Erickson and coworkers.[34]

3 RESULTS

Initial dose-response studies with MPTP measured the dopamine content of the striatum two weeks after a single intraperitoneal dose. A typical dose-response curve for MPTP-induced depletion of dopamine is given in Figure 3. In these studies, doses of 10-40 mg/kg gave 20-80% depletion of DA. The ED_{50} (effective dose that depletes 50% of striatal DA) was about 25 mg/kg.

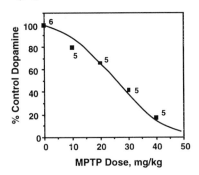

Figure 3. *Dose-response curve for a typical experiment on MPTP-dependent depletion of striatal dopamine in C57 black mice. The numbers next to the points indicate the number of mice tested at each dose.*

In contrast, 25 mg/kg heptachlor given three times over a two week period (Figure 2), caused a 20% decline in DA levels, similar to that observed for 20 mg/kg MPTP, but neither effect was not statistically significant (Figure 4). There was no change in DOPAC levels in mice given heptachlor, but there was a significant 21% reduction of DOPAC in mice given MPTP. There was no evidence of synergism when the two toxicants were injected together (Figure 4)

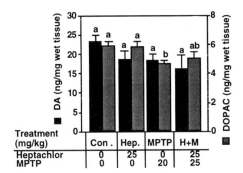

Figure 4 *Striatal dopamine and DOPAC levels following Control (Con.), heptachlor (Hep.), MPTP, or heptachlor + MPTP (H + M) treatment. Bars represent the mean (±SEM) levels of DA and DOPAC averaged over 4-6 mice/treatment group. Letters above bars are the results of ANOVA and Student-Newman-Keuls means separation test, where bars not labeled by the same letter differ significantly at p < 0.05 level..*

Because idiopathic PD and the effects of the Parkinsonian toxin MPTP appear to involve compromised mitochondrial function, we analyzed the respiratory capacity of striatal synaptosomes isolated from mice treated with heptachlor and/or MPTP (Figure 5). These results show a significant effect of 50 mg/kg heptachlor on synaptosomal respiration (a 31% reduction). A similar reduction (37%) followed treatment with MPTP. When given together, the reduction was 53%, less than the 68% reduction expected, if the effects of these compounds were additive. Because MPP^+ (the active metabolite of MPTP), is a known complex 1 inhibitor, heptachlor epoxide (the more toxic metabolite of heptachlor) was tested for its ability to inhibit synaptosomal respiration when incubated with synaptosomes prepared from untreated mice. In these studies, heptachlor epoxide did not consistently reduce synaptosomal respiration at concentrations up to 100 µM (data not shown).

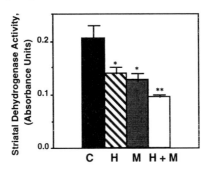

Figure 5 *Respiration in striatal synaptosomes following treatment with vehicle (C), 50 mg/kg heptachlor (H), 20 mg/kg MPTP (M), or heptachlor and MPTP (H + M). Bars indicate mean ± SEM. Asterisks indicate statistical significance (ANOVA, *p < 0.05, **p < 0.01).*

Regulation of dopamine transporters, as well as overall nerve terminal integrity, are reflected in the ability of synaptosomes to sequester dopamine. We performed studies on the kinetics of DA uptake by striatal synaptosomes from heptachlor-treated mice. A representative experiment comparing control and 50 mg/kg heptachlor-treated mice is shown in (Figure 6). In these studies, the effect of heptachlor treatment on transporter K_m values was small, but statistically significant, as judged from non-overlap of the 95% confidence limits (given in parentheses). Control K_m was 138 nM (111-165 nM). For heptachlor, K_m was 191 nM (171-210 nM). Maximal uptake rates (V_{max}) were significantly increased. Control V_{max} was 178 pmoles/min/mg (169-186) and Heptachlor was 276 pmoles/min/mg (268-283). This level represents a 55% increase over the control. These results suggested that there was an upregulation of DAT expression in heptachlor-treated mice. This hypothesis was confirmed in Western blots of synaptosomal protein, where monoclonal antibody labeling of DAT was increased 46% compared to controls, in mice given 9 mg/kg heptachlor.

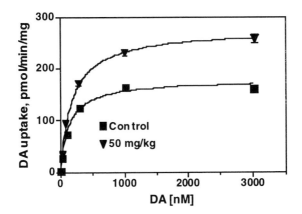

Figure 6 *Increased dopamine uptake in mice treated with 50 mg/kg heptachlor.*

We hypothesized that increased DAT expression in vivo reflected increased synaptic levels of DA caused by insecticide exposure. Thus, in a search for a possible mechanism, we evaluated the ability of heptachlor to release [^{3}H]neurotransmitters loaded into synaptosomes prepared from untreated ICR mice (Figure 7) These experiments were performed on cortical synaptosomes for serotonin and striatal synaptosomes for the other transmitters. There was no induced release of serotonin by 3 μM heptachlor. Similarly, this concentration released only about 20% of preloaded GABA and glutamate. Release of dopamine, in contrast, was nearly complete, with over 90% of the label released by 3 μM heptachlor. A similar specificity for dopamine was observed in release studies with heptachlor epoxide.

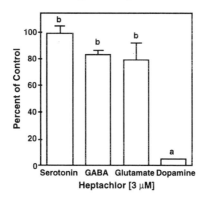

Figure 7 *Heptachlor-evoked release of neurotransmitters from synaptosomes. Data are expressed as percent of control retention of label. Bars represent the mean (±SEM) of two separate experiments, performed with different membrane preparations. Letters above bars are the results of a Student-Newman-Keuls means separation test, where bars not labeled by the same letter differ significantly at p < 0.05 level.*

4 DISCUSSION

Although in the past, many studies of chronic exposure to organochlorine insecticides have been performed, an extensive literature search found none that looked specifically for biomarkers of PD. They do, however, provide evidence for organochlorine-induced polyneuropathies and also for effects on dopamine neurochemistry in nigro-striatal neurons, which is discussed below. Chronic exposures to cyclodienes such as dieldrin in humans and animals show persistent neurological impairments (> 1 yr), along with a sensitization to subsequent acute exposures, and an increased responsiveness to epileptogenic stimuli.[35] Moreover, these effects of dieldrin can occur at low doses, since Ecobichon and Joy[35] reviewed data that as little as 30 μg/kg/day of dieldrin could cause convulsions in some people. Thus, even a small percentage of sensitive individuals suffering from insecticide exposure can be significant: if 0.1% of the U.S. population would prove to be hypersensitive to these compounds, it would include a cohort of over 200,000 individuals. These considerations support an analysis of the possible role of organochlorines in the development of PD.

Our results on the dose-dependent depletion of striatal DA following MPTP treatment are similar to those reported previously[10] and validated our treatment regime as being sufficient to detect toxicant-induced DA depletion. In contrast, doses of heptachlor which produced measurable impacts on other biomarkers failed to yield significant changes in concentration of either DA or the primary DA metabolite, DOPAC. DOPAC is a product of MAO metabolism of DA and is considered a general index of dopamine turnover.[1] However, *O*-methylated metabolites (*e.g.*, 3-methoxytyramine) are considered by other researchers to specifically represent metabolism of released dopamine.[36] Previous studies with organochlorines, using different exposure routes or doses, have shown depletion of brain DA. Rats fed 50 ppm dieldrin for 10 weeks showed small reductions in whole brain DA after 4 weeks, but no change in the amount of striatal DA, even though striatal serotonin and norepinephrine levels were depressed.[37] Mallard ducks[38] and ring doves[39] fed dieldrin suffered 70% and 41% reduction, respectively, in brain DA; but the significance of these findings for mammalian brain is unclear. All of these studies employed longer exposure times than that used here. Future studies with organochlorines should include experiments having a longer duration of treatments.

Exposure to heptachlor caused a significant reduction in synaptosomal respiration, consistent with the mitochondrial impairment observed in PD.[4] Heptachlor epoxide did not consistently reduce respiration in untreated synaptosomes, even at concentrations up to 100 µM, indicating that its inhibition of respiration in *ex vivo* striatal synaptosomes was probably secondary to other toxic effects. Both heptachlor[40,41] and endosulfan[42,43] are reported to inhibit state 3 (ADP-stimulated) respiration rates at concentrations of 50-100 µM in liver mitochondria using succinate as an energy substrate. The lower activity in our studies may stem from the use of a synaptosomal preparation instead of free mitochondria.

Under these experimental conditions, no synergism with heptachlor and MPTP was detected. The lack of synergism was surprising, given the heptachlor-dependent increase in DAT expression and the known role of active transport for sequestering MPP$^+$ into the interior of dopaminergic nerve terminals.[9] However, MPTP was given on day 2, and the increase in DAT expression by heptachlor may not develop until later. Giving MPTP after the insecticides may alleviate this potential problem. Alternatively, the presence of heptachlor may alter the bioactivation or other aspects of the disposition of MPTP, so that less MPP$^+$ is ultimately produced. For example, if cyclodienes inhibited MAO, they would reduce production of MPP$^+$. Inhibition of MAO-A by pyrethroids has been documented[44], although we are unaware of any similar findings with cyclodienes.

Significant changes in the kinetics of striatal DA transport (especially V_{max}) was observed following heptachlor treatment. Increased V_{max} was associated with an increase in DAT protein expression. Whether this increase in DAT protein results from increased synthesis or decreased degradation remains to be determined. The only other toxicant we are aware of that produces an upregulation of dopamine transport is cocaine, which blocks dopamine uptake[45] and causes a 50% upregulation of dopamine transport in mice treated intermittently for 5 days by i.p. injection.[46] Changes in striatal dopamine uptake evoked by heptachlor treatment also resemble changes in the kinetics of the striatal dopamine transporter observed in postmortem studies of schizophrenics, where an average 74% increase in maximal uptake of dopamine in the caudate nucleus of 12 schizophrenics was observed.[47] Schizophrenia is essentially a mirror image of PD, where there is a hyperactivity in dopaminergic systems.[1] Our results do not directly suggest that organochlorines, specifically heptachlor, cause schizophrenia. However, the two diseases can be interrelated as reported in several studies.[48-50] Moreover, symptoms of dementia and hallucinations resembling schizophrenic states are reported in individuals with advanced Parkinson's disease and a history of insecticide exposure.[51] Further, humans exposed to organochlorines have been reported to experience manic states, dementia and visual and auditory hallucinations.[52,53] It is possible, therefore, that an initial augmentation of dopaminergic transmission may be related to these organochlorine-induced central effects, and over time may overwhelm these pathways, leading to the depleted dopamine condition that is a hallmark of the Parkinson's disease process.

DAT upregulation would be consistent with increased synaptic levels of DA *in vivo*, and we observed a specific release of preloaded DA *in vitro* by heptachlor. The specificity of the release effect matches the specific involvement of DA in Parkinson's disease. The exact mechanism underlying release of transmitters by heptachlor in *ex vivo* synaptosomes is not known. Early studies on the mode of action of cyclodienes focused on their ability to release neurotransmitters,[54,55] which was later attributed to a rise in intracellular calcium.[56] Subsequent studies clearly demonstrated that blockage of the GABAa receptor plays a decisive role in the lethal action of these compounds.[57] However, preliminary evidence shows that release of dopamine *in vitro* does not involve an action at the GABAa receptor, since picrotoxinin and bicuculline are inactive in this system.[58] Another possible mechanism would involve interaction of organochlorines with the VMAT, which packages DA into presynaptic vesicles.[59] A number of insecticides are potent displacers of [^{3}H]tyramine binding from the VMAT in synaptic vesicle preparations.[60] The K_i value of dieldrin for blocking [^{3}H]tyramine binding was about 3 μM. We have observed that 10 μM heptachlor blocks uptake of dopamine about 50% in cultured neuroblastoma cells expressing a VMAT2 clone, confirming an action at this site for other cyclodienes. Thus, interaction of organochlorines with VMAT and its role in their ability to release DA from presynaptic terminals merits further study.

Acknowledgements

This work was supported by grant HHHERP 94-01 from the Hawaii Heptachlor Research and Education Foundation to J.R.B. and National Institute of Health grants NIEHS-09248 and NINDS-09930 to G.W.M. The authors would also like to thank Becky Barlow, Shannon Penland, and Jason Holt for their excellent technical assistance.

References

1. W. Bowman and M. Rand, 'Textbook of Pharmacology', 2nd Ed., Blackwell, Oxford, 1980, Chapter 18, p. 17.
2. L. I. Golbe, *Neurology*, 1991, **41**, 168.
3. O. Hornykiewicz and S. Kish, *Adv. Neurol.* ,1987, **45** 19.
4. H. Schapira, J. Cooper, D. Dexter, J. Clark, P. Jenner, and C. Marsden, *J. Neurochem.*, 1990, **54**, 823.
5. P. Jenner, H. Schapira, and C. Marsden, *Neurology*, 1992, **42**, 2241.
6. M. Polymeropoulos, C. Lavedan , E. Leroy, S. Ide, A. Dehejia, A. Dutra, B. Pike, H. Root, J. Rubenstein, R. Boyer, E. Stenroos, S. Chandrasekharappa, A. Athanassiadou, T. Papapetropoulos, W. Johnson, A. Lazzarini, R. Duvoisin, G. Di Lorio, L. Golbe, R. Nussbaum, *Science* , 1997, **276**, 2045.
7. P. Ballard, J. Tetrud, and J. Langston, *Neurology* , 1985, **35**, 949.
8. K. Chiba, A. Trevor, and N. Castagnoli, *Biochem. Biophys. Res. Comm.*, 1984, **120**, 574.
9. J. Javitch, R. D'Amato, S. Strittmatter, and S. Synder, *Proc. Natl. Acad. Sci. USA*, 1985, **82**, 2173.
10. R. Heikkila, A. Hess, and R. Duvoisin, *Science* , 1984, **224**, 1451.
11. W. Nicklas, I. Vyas, and R. Heikkila, *Life Sci.*, 1985, **36**, 2503.
12. N. Castagnoli, J. Rimoldi, J. Bloomquist, and K. Castagnoli, *Chem. Res. Toxicol.*, 1997, **10**, 924.
13. H. Schapira, A. Hartley, M. Cleeter, and J. Cooper, *Biochem. Soc. Trans.*, 1993, **21**, 367.
14. C. Marsden and M. Sandler, The MPTP story: an introduction. In : 'MPTP and the aetiology of Parkinson's disease: clinical implications', Springer-Verlag. New York, D. Parkes, Ed. 1986, p. 214.
15. K. Semchuk, E. Love, and R. Lee, *Neurology,* 1993, **43**, 1173.
16. P. Butterfield, B. Valanis, P. Spencer, C. Lindeman, and J. Nutt, *Neurosci. Behav.*, 1993, **43**, 1150.
17. C. Tanner and J. Langston, *Neurology*, 1990, **40**, 17.

18. A. Seidler, W. Hellenbrand, B. Robra, P. Vieregge, P. Nischan, J. Joerg, W. Oertel, G. Ulm, and E. Schneider, *Neurology* , 1996, **46**, 1275.
19. A. Bocchetta and G. Corsini, *Lancet* , 1986, **2**, 1163.
20. G. Sechi, V. Agnetti, M. Piredda, M. Canu, F. Deserra, H. Omar, M. and Rosati, *Neurology* , 1992, **42**, 261.
21. L. Chapman, S. Sauter, R. Henning, R. Levine, C. Matthews, and H. Peters, *Arch. Neurol.*, 1991, **48**, 866.
22. L. Fleming, J. Mann, J. Bean, T. Briggle, and J. Sanchez-Ramos, *Ann. Neurol.*, 1994, **36**, 100.
23. G. T. Brooks, 'Chlorinated Insecticides', CRC Press, Cleveland, Vol. 2, 1974.
24. D. Baker, S. Loo, and J. Barker, *Hawaii Med. J.*, 1991, **50**, 108.
25. N. Arai, K. Misugi, Y. Goshima, and Y. Misu Y, *Brain Res.*, 1990, **515**, 57.
26. E. Sundstrom, A. Fredriksson, and T. Archer, *Brain Res.*, 1992, **528**, 181.
27. R. Heikkila RE and P. Sonsalla, *Neurochem. Int.*, 1992, **20**, 299S.
28. 28. L. Hall, S. Murray, K. Castagnoli, and N. Castagnoli, *Chem. Res. Toxicol.*, 1992, **5**, 625.
29. J. Bloomquist, E. King, A. Wright, C. Mytilineou, K.Kimura, K. Castagnoli, and N. Castagnoli, *J. Pharm. Exp. Ther.*, 1994, **270**, 822.
30. B. Kreuger, *J. Neurochem.*, 1990, **55**, 260.
31. G. Miller, C. Heilman, J. Perez, J. Staley, D. Mash, D. Rye, and A. Levey, *Ann. Neurol.*, 1997, **41**, 530.
32. T. Slater, B. Sawyer, and U. Strauli, *Biochim. Biophys. Acta*, 1963, **77**, 383.
33. J. Fang, D. Zuo, and P. Yu, *Biogenic Amines*, 1996, **12**, 125.
34. J. Erickson, L. Eiden, B. Hoffman *Proc. Natl. Acad. Sci. USA*, 1992; **89**, 10993.
35. D. Ecobichon and R. Joy, 'Pesticides and Neurological Diseases', 2nd Ed., CRC Press, Boca Raton, 1994, Chapter 3, p. 81
36. F. Karoum, S. Chrapusta, and M. Egan MF *J. Neurochem.*, 1994, **63**, 972.
37. S. Wagner, and F. Greene, *Toxicol. Appl. Pharmacol.*, 1974, **29**, 119.
38. R. Sharma, *Life Sci.*, 1973, **13**, 1245.
39. G. Heinz, E. Hill, and J. Contrera, *Toxicol. Appl. Pharmacol.*, 1980, **53**, 75.
40. M. Ogata, F. Izushi, K. Eto, R. Sakai, B. Inoue, and N. Noguchi, *Toxicol. Lett.*, 1989, **48**, 67.
41. T. Meguro, F. Izushi, and M. Ogata, *Ind. Health* , 1990, **28**, 151.
42. R. Dubey, M. Beg, and J. Singh, *Biochem. Pharmacol.*, 1984, **33**, 3405.
43. R. Mishra, *Pestic. Biochem. Physiol.*, 1994, **50**, 240.
44. G. Rao and K. Rao, *Mol. Cell. Biochem.*, 1993, **124**, 107.
45. J. Kilty, D. Lorang, and S. Amara, *Science*, 1991, **254**, 578.
46. L. Miller, J. Koff, J. Byrnes, *Clin. Pharmacol. Therap.*, 1993, **53**, 199.
47. N. Haberland and L. Hetey, *J. Neural Transm.*, 1987, **68**, 303.
48. M. Carlsson and A. Carlsson, *Trends Neurol. Sci.*, 1990, **13**, 272.
49. M. Caligiuri, J. Lohr, and D. Jeste *Am. J. Psychiatry* , 1993, **150**, 1343.
50. W. Danielczyk, *J. Neural Transm. Suppl.*, 1992, **38**, 115.
51. C. Hertzman, M. Wiens, D. Bowering, B. Snow, and D. Calne, *Am. J. Ind. Med.*, 1990, **17**, 349.
52. S. Pradhan, N. Pandey, R. Phadke, A. Kaur, K. Sharma, and R. Gupta, *J. Neurol. Sci.*, 1997, **147**, 209.
53. J. Taylor, J. Selhorst, S. Houff, and A. Martinez, *Neurology*, 1978, **28**, 626.
54. D. Shankland and M. Schroeder, *Pestic. Biochem. Physiol.*, 1973, **3**, 77.
55. L. Akkermans J. van den Bercken, J. van der Zalm, and H. van Straaten, *Pestic. Biochem. Physiol.*, 1974, **4**, 313.
56. I. Yamaguchi, F. Matsumura, and A. Kadous, *Biochem. Pharmacol.*, 1980, **29**, 1815.
57. J. Bloomquist, *Comp. Biochem. Physiol.*, **106C**: 301-314 (1993b).
58. M. Kirby and J. Bloomquist, *Soc. Neurosci. Abstr.*, 1996, **22**, 1910.
59. J. Henry, C. Sagne, C.. Bedet, and B. Gasnier, *Neurochem. Int.*,1998, **32**, 227
60. A. Vaccari and P. Saba, *Eur. J. Pharmacol.*, 1995, **292**, 309.

A New Basis for Therapy against Type-II Pyrethroid Poisoning

D.E. Ray, T. Lister and P.J. Forshaw

MRC TOXICOLOGY UNIT, UNIVERSITY OF LEICESTER, LANCASTER ROAD, LEICESTER, LE1 9HN, UK

1. ABSTRACT

We have previously shown that low concentrations of the type II pyrethroid, deltamethrin, decrease voltage-gated chloride conductance in neuroblastoma cells. This effect would be expected to amplify the sodium channel-mediated signs of poisoning produced by this compound. In the present study we have looked at ivermectin and two barbiturates, pentobarbitone and phenobarbitone, which have the potential to act on chloride conductance since they been shown to bind in varying degree to voltage-gated chloride channels in *Torpedo* membranes. *In-vitro* patch clamp experiments were carried out to test the effects of ivermectin, pentobarbitone and phenobarbitone on the open channel probability (P_o) of voltage-dependent maxi chloride channels in excised, inside-out patches from mouse NIE 115 neuroblastoma cells. In these experiments ivermectin (10^{-7}M) and pentobarbitone (10^{-6}M) significantly increased P_o ($p \leq 0.03$ and 0.02 respectively) whereas phenobarbitone did not at any concentration tested (10^{-6}M to 10^{-4} M). This result suggested that ivermectin and pentobarbitone might antagonise pyrethroid poisoning *in-vivo* by nullifying the action on chloride channels. In order to test this hypothesis male F344 rats were pretreated with glycerinformal solvent (0.5ml/kg i.v.) as controls, ivermectin (4mg/kg i.v.), or equi-sedative dose of either pentobarbitone (15mg/kg i.p.) or phenobarbitone (45mg/kg i.p.). This was followed after 10-40 minutes by deltamethrin (1.5 or 2mg/kg i.v). The animals were observed for up to 1 hour after deltamethrin and scored for the severity of motor signs of poisoning and for the presence of salivation. Although ivermectin reduced salivation in these rats, of the two barbiturates, only pentobarbitone significantly reduced the motor signs score ($p \leq 0.01$). In another study, using rats anaesthetised with urethane, ivermectin (4mg/kg i.v.) reduced the effects of deltamethrin (2.5mg/kg i.v.) on both repetitive firing in the electromyogram and increased time to peak muscle tension ($p \leq 0.01$ and 0.05 respectively). Ivermectin therefore appears to protect only against the peripheral signs of poisoning and pentobarbitone against both central and peripheral signs. Thus these studies support the idea that the voltage-gated chloride channel is a toxicologically significant site of action of deltamethrin and that chloride channel agonists can form the basis for an innovative approach to the problem of effective therapy for type II pyrethroid poisoning.

2. INTRODUCTION

The synthetic pyrethroid insecticides are used on a world-wide scale, their chief advantages over other types being high insecticidal potency but low mammalian toxicity coupled with rapid metabolism and freedom from terrestial bioaccumulation. Inevitably, there have been cases of accidental or occupational human exposure involving contact with the skin or eyes but there have also been reports of acute pyrethroid poisoning generally following accidental ingestion of the type II pyrethroids deltamethrin or fenvalerate.[1] Skin contact with pyrethroids causes transient local symptoms (paresthesia), particularly in facial areas,[2,3] whereas the diagnostic signs of acute poisoning following ingestion of deltamethrin include muscle fasciculations and convulsions which may lead to death in a few cases.[1] In animals salivation followed by opisthotonus and seizures are the most prominent signs of systemic deltamethrin poisoning.[4]

Although cases of systemic poisoning have been rare it would be desirable to have available antidotes capable of alleviating poisoning as the majority recover within a few days with effective supportive therapy.[1] Atropine controls salivation but phenytoin and diazepam have been found to be relatively ineffective at preventing symptoms such as opisthotonus in humans, although animal experiments have shown that diazepam does have some activity against the convulsions which are a feature of lethal doses of pyrethroids.[5] In animal experiments the motor signs, but not the salivation, can be controlled by the administration of muscle relaxants of the mephenesin class.[6,7]

Although the major site of action of deltamethrin has been shown to be the voltage-dependent sodium channel,[8] we have shown that a significant additional component of deltamethrin's action on nerve and muscle is the inhibition of the voltage-dependent chloride channel.[9,10,11] Therefore it seemed possible that compounds acting as agonists at this site would be capable of at least partially antagonising the signs of hyperexcitability in the nervous system of poisoned animals. One such compound is ivermectin which we have previously found to antagonise the action of deltamethrin in ex-vivo isolated vagus nerve.[9] Duce and Scott[12] found that ivermectin produced an increase in GABA-insensitive chloride conductance which presumably was due to prolonged opening of the voltage-dependent chloride channel. Unfortunately the central actions of ivermectin are severely limited by active multidrug receptor pump activity at the blood-brain barrier which largely excludes ivermectin from the brain.[13]

Abalis *et al.*,[14] and Matsumoto *et al.*,[15] have shown that the *Torpedo* electric organ membranes, which are a rich source of chloride channels, contain a binding site for the convulsant ligand [^{35}S]-t-butyltricyclophosphorothionate (TBPS). This binding site may be the voltage-dependent chloride channel since GABA receptor ligands such as bicuculline, muscimol and the benzodiazepine, flunitrazepam, do not inhibit binding of TBPS. The binding of TBPS was found to be inhibited by some barbiturates and it is possible that the barbiturates (which readily penetrate the central nervous system) may act as more effective antagonists to deltamethrin in-vivo. Pentobarbitone was found to be a strong inhibitor and phenobarbitone a weak inhibitor of TBPS binding.[15] Although the binding of drugs to a voltage-dependent chloride channel does not necessarily indicate an effect on chloride flux, it has also been shown that barbiturates activate chloride flux in hippocampal slices.[16] Therefore the following experiments were designed to test the hypothesis that ivermectin and chloride channel-acting barbiturates would antagonise type II pyrethroids. Thus the compounds were tested as possible antidotes to deltamethrin in-vivo and also tested to see if they modify the function of voltage-dependent chloride channels in-vitro using excised membrane patches from mouse neuroblastoma (NIE 115) cells. In addition, four other barbiturates were assessed for their ability to act as chloride channel openers.

3. METHODS

3.1 In-vivo Protection Experiments.

Male rats (200-220g) of the F344 strain were anaesthetised with isoflurane (2%) and the dorsal tail artery, as well as one lateral vein, cannulated to enable small volumes of blood (0.2-0.5ml) to be withdrawn and used to wash in intravenous (i.v.) doses of deltamethrin (Roussel-Uclaf) to minimise the chance of precipitation occurring. Preliminary experiments were carried out with the barbiturates alone in order to find the intraperitoneal (i.p.) doses of each compound which would just abolish the eye blink reflex. These doses, which were found to be 60mg/kg for pentobarbitone (Sigma) and 180mg/kg for phenobarbitone (Sigma) respectively, were then regarded as equivalent with respect to the depth of anaesthesia. For protection against deltamethrin poisoning an equal fraction, 1/4, of these doses was used; i.e. 15mg/kg for pentobarbitone and 45mg/kg for phenobarbitone. Following cannulation rats were placed in a restrainer and predosed i.v. with ivermectin (Merck), glycerinformal (Fluka) or with one of the barbiturates (i.p.). Deltamethrin, at a dose level of 2 or 1.5mg/kg (i.v.) in the case of ivermectin treated animals and 1.5mg/kg in the case of barbiturate treated animals, was administered 10, 15-20 and 40-50min after ivermectin, pentobarbitone or phenobarbitone respectively (see Table 1). The animals were observed for an hour following deltamethrin administration and the incidence of salivation noted together with signs of CNS poisoning scored on a scale of 1-4 (see Table 1).

3.2 In-vivo Muscle Experiments.

Experiments were also carried out to assess the effectiveness of ivermectin as an antidote to the peripheral actions of deltamethrin. Repetitive firing in the electromyogram (EMG) and enhancement of muscle contraction are characteristic effects of deltamethrin in animals.[17] Two groups of 200-220g male rats (F344 strain) were anaesthetised with urethane (15mmol/kg i.p.) and the gastrocnemius muscle tension in one leg recorded by means of an isometric transducer. The electromyogram was recorded with needle electrodes inserted into the ventral surface of the foot. The responses to supramaximal stimulation (1-5volts, 0.100msec at 1Hz) of the tibial branch of the sciatic nerve were digitized and recorded onto disc using Axotape software (Axon Instruments) and the parameters described in Table 2 measured. One group of rats was treated with ivermectin (4mg/kg i.v.) 10min before deltamethrin and the other group (controls) received glycerinformal (0.5ml/kg i.v.) 10min before deltamethrin (Table 2).

3.3 Patchclamp Experiments.

To test the effectiveness of ivermectin, pentobarbitone and phenobarbitone as potential antidotes to deltamethrin on membrane chloride channels, experiments were carried out using *inside-out* excised patches from mouse NIE 115 neuroblastoma cells.[10] Control of patch membrane potential and signal recording were carried out using an Axopatch 1d amplifier (Axon Instruments); data acquisition and analysis for open channel probability (P_o) were done with PClamp 6.2 software (Axon Instruments). The intracellular solution had the following composition (in mM):- NaCl 144; CsCl 5; EGTA 1 and Hepes 5. The pH was adjusted to 7.3 with NaOH and the solution was essentially Ca2+-free. The extracellular (pipette) solution contained (mM):- NaCl 143; $CaCl_2$ 2; $MgCl_2$ 1 and Hepes 5. The pH was again 7.3. The experiments were carried out at room temperature (22-25°C). Deltamethrin and ivermectin were made up as stock solutions ($10^{-3}M$) in glycerinformal and aliquots of these added to the intracellular patch clamp solution. The final concentration of glycerinformal did not exceed 0.03%; this concentration had no effect on mean (P_o) The barbiturates thiopentone, hexobarbitone, mephobarbitone and barbituric acid as well as pentobarbitone and phenobarbitone, were dissolved in patchclamp intracellular solution to give the desired final concentration The drug-containing solution was contained in a glass reservoir pressurised by means of an infusion pump so that the drug reached the patch at a rate of 0.04ml/min via a glass tube with a 20μm tip orifice diameter placed within 50μm of the patch pipette tip.

3.4 Statistical Analysis.

In the conscious rat experiments and the muscle experiments a Chi-square or Student's t-test for unpaired data was used to evaluate the significance of the means for the ivermectin- and glycerinformal-treated groups; the motor signs scores for the pentobarbitone/phenobarbitone plus deltamethrin groups were compared with the scores for the glycerinformal plus deltamethrin groups using the Wilcoxon two sample test for unpaired data (see Tables 1 and 2). In the patchclamp experiments pre- and post-dose groups were compared using Student's t-test for paired data.

4. RESULTS

4.1 In-vivo Protection Experiments.

The most effective agent at reducing deltamethrin-induced salivation was ivermectin but this compound was much less effective than pentobarbitone at reducing the centrally-generated toxicity of deltamethrin as shown by comparing the reductions in the motor signs score, particularly in the case of animals given 1.5mg/kg of deltamethrin following ivermectin (Table 1). Although phenobarbitone was ineffective at reducing the motor signs it appeared to be as effective as pentobarbitone at preventing terminal seizures and deaths.

Table 1. *The effects of pretreatment with ivermectin, pentobarbitone and phenobarbitone on the signs of deltamethrin poisoning in adult rats.*[a]

Treatment Group	Response Measured: Salivation	Motor Signs Score[b]	Deaths
Glycerinformal + Deltamethrin (high dose)	8/9	3.89 ± 0. 11 (n=9)	7/9
Ivermectin + Deltamethrin (high dose)	4/16 [d]	3.19 ± 0.03 [c] (n=16)	7/16 [e]
Glycerinformal + Deltamethrin (low dose)	6/6	3.00 ± 0.37 (n=6)	2/6
Ivermectin + Deltamethrin (low dose)	2/6	2.42 ± 0.20 (n=6)	0/6
Pentobarbitone + Deltamethrin (low dose)	5/8 [f]	1.25 ± 031 [c] (n=8)	0/8 [g]
Phenobarbitone + Deltamethrin (low dose)	8/9	2.39 ± 0.16 (n=9)	0/9 [h]

[a] 200-220g male rats received either glycerinformal (0.5ml/kg i.v.) as controls, ivermectin (4mg/kg i.v.), pentobarbitone (15mg/kg i.p.) or phenobarbitone (45mg/kg i.p.) 10, 10, 15-20 or 40-50 minutes respectively prior to the administration of deltamethrin (2mg/kg i.v. = 'high dose' or 1.5mg/kg i.v. = 'low dose').

[b] Motor signs of poisoning were scored as follows:- 1. no chorea but may have other mild signs 2. splayed hindlimbs or intermittent chorea. 3. continuous chorea but no seizures or death. 4. severe chorea with seizures or death. Scores presented as mean ± s.e; number of animals = n.

[c] $p \leq 0.01$ compared with the respective glycerinformal controls.

[d] $p \leq 0.001$ compared with the glycerinformal+deltamethrin (high dose) group.

[e] $p \leq 0.01$ compared with the glycerinformal+deltamethrin (high dose) group.

[f] $p \leq 0.02$ compared with the glycerinformal+deltamethrin (low dose) group.

[g] $p \leq 0.05$ compared with the glycerinformal+deltamethrin (low dose) group

[h] $p \leq 0.05$ compared with the glycerinformal+deltamethrin (low dose) group.

4.2 Antagonism of the Peripheral Effects of Deltamethrin.

Ivermectin significantly reduced the deltamethrin-enhanced time to peak muscle tension and the degree of repetitive firing in the EMG compared with the GF controls (Table 2). However ivermectin was not found to be very effective when given after deltamethrin. In contrast pentobarbitone appeared equally effective when given before or after deltamethrin (results not shown).

Table 2 *Effects of pre-treatment with ivermectin on the subsequent responses of skeletal muscle to deltamethrin in the rat.*[a]

Treatment Group	Response Measured	
	Time to peak muscle tension (msec)	**EMG score** [b]
Glycerinformal+ Deltamethrin	147.2 ± 6.5 (n=9)	0. 179 ± 0.03 (n=9)
Ivermectin+ Deltamethrin	109.5 ± 18.0 [c] (n=9)	0.086 ± 0.02 [d] (n=9)

[a] 200-2208 male F344 rats were anaesthetised with urethane (15mmol/kg i.p.) and a lateral tail vein cannulated for the intravenous administration of drugs. Glycerinformal (0.5ml/kg), as controls, or ivermectin (4mg/kg) were given 10 minutes before deltamethrin (2.5mg/kg). Time to peak gastrocnemius muscle tension and the EMG responses to supramaximal stimulation of the sciatic nerve were recorded before and for up to 1hour after deltamethrin administration.
[b] EMG score = amplitude of the first repetitive potential in the EMG divided by the amplitude of the compound action potential.
Statistical evaluations were made with Student's *t*-test.
[c] $p \leq 0.05$ compared with the glycerinformal control group.
[d] $p \leq 0.01$ compared with the glycerinformal group.

4.3 Patchclamp Experiments.

Ivermectin (10^{-7}M) significantly increased the chloride channel P_o when given alone from the pre-dose value of 0.632 ± 0.09 (n=4) to 0.799 ± 0.11 (n=4) within 30 min of starting the drug perfusion. In contrast previous experiments[11] have shown that deltamethrin significantly reduces P_o at concentrations ranging from 10^{-10}M to 10^{-4}M. However when patches were exposed to ivermectin and deltamethrin at the same time the decrease in P_o (0.789 ± 0.04 to 0.608 ± 0.08; n=7) was not significantly different from that produced by deltamethrin (10^{-6}M) alone as shown in Fig.1A.

In the experiments with the barbiturates, changes in the number of conducting channels after treatment were seen as well as changes in P_o. However channel numbers were not affected by pyrethroids or ivermectin. The barbiturates phenobarbitone and pentobarbitone showed differential effects on the P_o of the chloride channel. Whereas phenobarbitone caused only a non-significant reduction of P_o, at both 10^{-5} and 10^{-6}M, pentobarbitone at 10^{-6}M significantly increased P_o as shown in Fig 1B and Table 3. However when the dose of pentobarbitone was increased to 10^{-5}M or 10^{-4}M, P_o showed a decrease (Fig 1B). The results of treatment with pentobarbitone, phenobarbitone and thiopentone are summarised in Table 3. Pentobarbitone and thiopentone at 10^{-6}M both caused a significant increase in the number of conducting channels as well as a significant increase in P_o. None of the other barbiturates had any significant effect on either the number of channels or on P_o when tested at a concentration of 10^{-6}M.

Table 3 *Effect of some barbiturates on chloride channels in excised inside-out patches from NIE 115 neuroblastoma cells.*

Treatment	Number of Channels			P_{open}		
	pre-dose	post-dose	% change	pre-dose	post-dose	% change
Pentobarb. 10^{-7}M	1.86±0.34 n=7	1.86±0.34 n=7	0.00	0.72±0.06 n=7	0.75±0.06 n=7	4.9±5.40
Pentobarb. 10^{-6}M	2.56±0.32 n=8	3.31±0.37 n=8	40.4 ±20 **p≤0.04**	0.60±0.04 n=8	0.74±0.07 n=8	25.2±9.27 **p≤0.02**
Pentobarb. 10^{-5}M	2.17±0.54 n=6	2.67±0.33 n=6	50.0 ±22	0.68±0.10 n=6	0.64±0.10 n=6	-4.9±7.65
Pentobarb. 10^{-4}M	1.67±0.33 n=6	1.67±0.33 n=6	0.00	0.79±0.05 n=6	0.65±0.08 n=6	15.1±12.5
Phenobarb. 10^{-6}M	2.25±0.63 n=4	2.25±0.63 n=4	0.00	0.83±0.03 n=4	0.75±0.09 n=4	-9.4±10.6
Phenobarb. 10^{-5}M	2.00±0.45 n=5	2.00±0.45 n=5	10.0±24.5	0.82±0.08 n=5	0.70±0.12 n=5	-16±11.6
Thiopent. 10^{-6}M	1.86±0.34 n=7	2.86±0.52 n=7	57.1±17.4 **p≤0.01**	0.83±0.04 n=7	0.83±0.03 n=7	0.65±3.32 **p≤0.04**
Control	2.18±0.30 n=9	2.26±0.33 n=9	5.11±8.72	0.80±0.05 n=9	0.80±0.06 n=9	0.31±4.21

5. DISCUSSION

Our results clearly show that agents which increase chloride channel activity can reduce the severity of deltamethrin poisoning. This confirms our proposals that chloride channels play a practical role in the generation of the type II poisoning syndrome[10, 11] and has therapeutic implications. Although the relatively selective chloride channel opener, ivermectin, was effective against peripheral signs (salivation and repetitive EMG discharges), it had only limited central effects. Of centrally acting agents, pentobarbitone was effective, but that action would have been expected to be due to both a chloride channel and membrane-stabilising actions. Our own and other findings show that several aspects of the hyperexcitability seen in deltamethrin poisoning can be attenuated by central nervous system depressants. However not all general anaesthetics and muscle relaxant drugs share this property. Thus urethane, the anaesthetic used in our muscle experiments, did not prevent choreoathetosis, even at the anaesthetic dose, and phenobarbitone was much less effective than pentobarbitone at equi-anaesthetic doses.The use of muscle relaxants of the mephenesin class is of limited value as therapy in cases of human poisoning by deltamethrin due to their short duration of action, which necessitates a continuous infusion system.[6,7] Drugs that have been used to try and control the muscle fasciculations and convulsions with little success include benzodiazepines, chlorpromazine and phenytoin.[1] Although barbiturates have also been used, apparently without much success,[1] these were not specified. In animal experiments it has been reported that phenobarbitone slightly delayed the development of

FIG. 1. *Effects of various treatments on the open channel probability (P$_o$) of maxi chloride channels in excised inside-out patches from mouse NIE 115 neuroblastoma cells.*

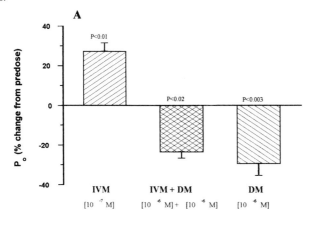

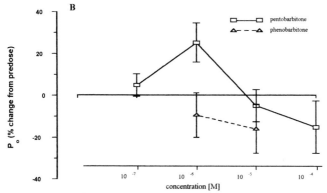

In the upper part (A) the treatment was ivermectin (IVM) alone, combined with deltamethrin (DM), or DM alone. In the lower part (B) the treatment was phenobarbitone or pentobarbitone *pre-* and postdose means for P$_o$, were compared. Numbers of patches were 10^{-6}M (n=4); 10^{-5}M (n=5); 10^{-4}M (n=6). * *indicates p $\leq$ 0.05.* ** *indicates p $\leq$ 0.01*

deltamethrin poisoning signs,[5] however pentobarbitone does not appear to have been previously tested as a pyrethroid antidote.

Our results suggest that pentobarbitone is a potentially useful antidote in clinical cases of deltamethrin poisoning. Although both barbiturates appeared to prevent deaths by suppressing seizure activity only pentobarbitone caused a significant reduction in the motor signs score. This difference between the two barbiturates cannot be explained on the basis of anaesthetic potency since the doses used were an equal fraction of the doses needed to block the eyeblink reflex; also the protected animals did not show signs of anaesthesia such as loss of the righting reflex. Pentobarbitone also caused some reduction in deltamethrin- induced salivation although it was less effective in this respect than ivermectin.

Ivermectin was less effective than pentobarbitone in reducing motor signs and deaths, probably because of its rapid removal from the CNS following entry via the blood-brain barrier.[18,13] Thus although our rats were treated with large doses of ivermectin they were only moderately sedated and still reacted to mild stimulation. Ivermectin was found to be an antagonist of deltamethrin at peripheral sites. Thus besides reducing the incidence of salivation, other signs of deltamethrin poisoning such as repetitive firing in the EMG and the prolonged muscle contraction time were also reduced. The latter effects have been shown previously to be associated with an increase in muscle input resistance which is chloride dependent.[9] However it is not clear to what extent peripheral actions of deltamethrin contribute to the signs of poisoning in the whole animal.

A unifying hypothesis for the effectiveness of ivermectin as a peripheral antagonist and pentobarbitone as a central antagonist of deltamethrin could be that in both cases the effects are due to increased chloride conductance reducing the spread of the depolarising membrane sodium current which is prolonged by deltamethrin.[8] Ivermectin has been shown to prolong both GABA-sensitive and non GABA-sensitive chloride currents.[12] Deltamethrin has not been found to block GABA-dependent chloride currents in spinal neurones[19] or $GABA_A$-mediated hippocampal inhibition[20] nor does it antagonise the binding of benzodiazepines to the $GABA_A$ receptor; also baclofen had no antidote properties in deltamethrin-poisoned rats.[7] These findings suggest that the voltage-dependent rather than the ligand-gated chloride channel is more likely to be the site of action of ivermectin as a deltamethrin antagonist. This idea is supported by our patchclamp experimental results which show that ivermectin is a potent voltage-dependent chloride channel opener. Although we do not have enough data for ivermectin to know whether 10^{-6}M for these two compounds represents similar multiples of their respective ED50 values, it seems probable that ivermectin is not a competitive antagonist of deltamethrin but acts at a different site on the channel. Ivermectin has been found to prolong the action of diazepam in genetically epileptic chickens.[21] Although this protective effect could result from an action at GABA-gated chloride channels, Bloomquist[22] has shown that ivermectin is no more effective when given directly into the brain than by the intra-peritoneal route (i.p.) which suggests that another target site mediates the protective action of ivermectin.

Our patchclamp experimental results have shown that pentobarbitone, at a concentration of 10^{-6}M, significantly increases the duration of opening of the voltage-dependent chloride channel and also increases the number of available channels significantly whereas phenobarbitone did not. However at higher anaesthetic levels chloride channel current was progressively decreased by pentobarbitone. Concentrations of barbiturates sufficient to cause full anaesthesia would be expected to have a non-specific membrane stabilising effect which would probably involve a reduced chloride as well as cation conductance.

Thus although both pentobarbitone and phenobarbitone directly activate GABA-gated chloride channels in rat hippocampal neurones at concentrations of approximately 0.3 and 3mM (for pentobarbitone and phenobarbitone respectively) but at concentrations of one order of magnitude higher the channels were blocked.[23] The difference between the two barbiturates in this and in our present experiments may be related to their different potencies for binding to the putative voltage-dependent chloride channel in the *Torpedo* electric organ.[15] Although the barbiturates are also known to potentiate the affinity of the $GABA_A$ receptor for GABA[24] it seems unlikely that the protective action of pentobarbitone in our whole animal experiments can be explained on the basis of an enhancement of GABA-gated chloride conductance since the concentration of pentobarbitone we used to protect against deltamethrin- induced chorea is estimated to be only about one quarter of that necessary to activate GABA-gated chloride currents in rat central neurones.[23] Furthermore in our patchclamp experiments pentobarbitone activated voltage-dependent chloride channels at only 10^{-6}M which equates to more than two orders of magnitude lower than that found to activate GABA-gated channels.[23] Of the other barbiturates we have assessed for their ability to potentiate chloride channel opening only thiopentone significantly increased the number of available channels and P_o. It may be of interest that this compound, like pentobarbitone, does not have a ring substituent in the basic barbiturate structure.

In summary, we believe our results form the basis of a novel approach to the problem of effective therapy for type II pyrethroid poisoning. Thus pentobarbitone appears to hold promise as a potential antidote to the central signs of deltamethrin poisoning and ivermectin may also be useful in controlling the peripheral symptoms. The ideal compound would have a higher therapeutic index than pentobarbitone and be capable of effectively antagonising signs of poisoning due to deltamethrin and other type II pyrethroids after they have developed.

6. REFERENCES

1. F. He, S. Wang, L. Liu, S. Chen, Z. Zang and J. Sun, Clinical manifestations and diagnosis of acute pyrethroid poisoning. *Arch. Toxicol.*, 1989, **63**, 54-58.
2. J. M. Knox, S. B. Tucker, and S. A. Flannigan, Paresthesia from cutaneous exposure to a synthetic pyrethroid insecticide. *Arch. Dermatol.*, 1984, **120**, 744-746.
3. P. M. Le Quesne and I. C. Maxwell, Transient facial sensory symptoms following exposure to synthetic pyrethroids: a clinical and electrophysiological assessment. *Neurotoxicol.*, 1980, **2**, 1-11.
4. R. D. Verschoyle and W. N. Aldridge, Structure-activity relationships of some pyrethroids in rats. *Arch. Toxicol.* 1980, **45**, 325-329.
5. D. W. Gammon, L. J. Lawrence and J. E. Casida, Pyrethroid toxicology: protective effects of diazepam and phenobarbital in the mouse and cockroach. *Toxicol. Appl. Pharmacol.*, 1982, **66**, 290-296.
6. J. E. Bradbury, A. J. Gray and P. J. Forshaw, Protection against pyrethroid toxicity in rats with mephenesin. *Toxicol. Appl. Pharmacol.*, 1981, **60**, 382-384.
7. J. E. Bradbury, P. J. Forshaw, A. J. Gray, and D. E. Ray, The action of mephenesin and other agents on the effects produced by two neurotoxic pyrethroids on the intact and spinal rat. *Neuropharmacol.*, 1983, **22**, 907-914.
8. K. Chinn and T. Narahashi, Stabilization of sodium channel states by deltamethrin in mouse neuroblastoma cells. *J. Physiol.*, 1986, **380**, 191-207.
9. P. J. Forshaw and D. E. Ray, A novel action of deltamethrin on membrane resistance in mammalian skeletal muscle and non-myelinated nerve fibres. *Neuropharmacol.*, 1990, **29**, 75-81.
10. P. J. Forshaw, T. Lister and D. E. Ray, Inhibition of a neuronal voltage-dependent chloride channel by the Type II pyrethroid, deltamethrin. *Neuropharmacol.*, 1993, **32**, 105-111.

11. D. E. Ray, S. Sutharson, and P. J. Forshaw, Actions of pyrethroid insecticides on voltage-gated chloride channels in neuroblastoma cells. *Neurotoxicol.*, 1997, **18**, 755-760.

12. I. R. Duce and R. H. Scott, Actions of dihydroavermectin B, on insect muscle. *Brit. J. Pharmacol.*, 1985, **85**, 395-401.

13. A. H. Schinkel, E. Wagenaar, C. A. A. M. Mol, and L. Van Deemter, P-glycoprotein in the blood-brain barrier of mice influences the brain penetration and pharmacological activity of many drugs. *J. Clin. Investig.*, 1996, **97**, 2517-2524.

14. I. N. Abalis, M. E. Eldefrawi, and A. T. Eldfrawi, Binding of GABA receptor channel drugs to a putative voltage-dependent chloride channel in Torpedo electric organ. *Biochem Pharmacol.*, 1985, **34**, 2579-2582.

15. K. Matsumoto, M. E. Eldefrawi, and A. T. Eldefrawi, Action of polychloro-cycloalkane insecticides on binding of [35S]t-butylbicyclophosphorothionate to Torpedo electric organ membranes and stereospecificity of the binding site. *Toxicol. Appl. Pharmacol.*, 1988, **95**, 220-229.

16. E. J. F. Wong, L. M. Leeb-Lunberg, V. L. Teichberg, and R. W. Olsen, χ-aminobutyric acid activation of 36C1- flux in rat hippocampal slices and its potentiation by barbiturates. *Brain Res.*, 1984, **303**, 267-275.

17. C. D. P. Wright, P. J. Forshaw, and D. E. Ray, Classification of the actions of ten pyrethroid insecticides in the rat using the trigeminal reflex and skeletal muscle as test systems. *Pestic. Biochem. Physiol.*, 1988, **30**, 79-86.

18. A. D. Didier and F. Loor, Decreased biotolerability for ivermectin and cyclosporin-a in mice exposed to potent P-glycoprotein inhibitors. *Int. J. Cancer*, 1995, **63**, 263-267.

19. N. Ogata, S. Vogel, and T. Narahashi, Lindane but not deltamethrin blocks a component of GABA-activated chloride channels. *Faseb J.*, 1988, **2**, 2895-2900.

20. R. M. Joy, T. Lister, D. E. Ray and M. P. Seville, Characteristics of the prolonged inhibition produced by a range of pyrethroids in the rat hippocampus. *Toxicol. Appl. Pharmacol.*, 1990, **103**, 528-538.

21. E. C. Critchlow, P. R. Mishra, and R. D. Crawford, Anticonvulsant effects of ivermectin in genetically-epileptic chickens. *Neuropharmacol.*, 1986, **25**, 1085-1088.

22. J. R. Bloomquist, Intrinsic lethality of chloride channel-directed insecticides and convulsants in mammals. *Toxicol. Lett.*, 1992, 60, 289-298.

23. J. M. Rho, S. D. Donovan, and M. A. Rogawski, Direct activation of GABAA receptors by barbiturates in cultured rat hippocampal neurones. *J.Physiol.*, 1996, **497**, 509-522.

24. R. W. Olsen and A. M. Snowman, Chloride-dependent enhancement by barbiturates of GABA receptor binding. *J. Neurosci.*, 1982, **2**, 1812-1823.

Subject Index

SCI

CONNECTING SCIENCE &
INDUSTRY WORLDWIDE
http://sci.mond.org

Journals from the SCI...

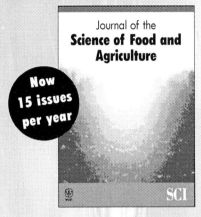

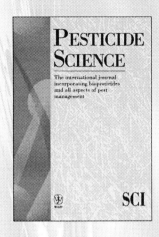

Take this opportunity to discover the latest international developments in applied scientific research. Send for a FREE Evaluation Copy of either or both of these high quality, peer-reviewed journals and stay at the leading edge.

Journal of the Science of Food and Agriculture
ISSN: 0022-5142
Volume 79
1999 15 issues per year
www.wiley.com/journals/jsfa

Pesticide Science
ISSN: 0031-613X
Volume 55
1999 Monthly
www.wiley.com/journals/ps

For Your FREE Evaluation Copy

Fax: +44 (0) 1243 770154
E-mail: phys-sci@wiley.co.uk
Or write to: Physical Sciences Marketing Department,
John Wiley & Sons, Baffins Lane, Chichester, PO19 1UD, UK

If you are interested in submitting an article to an SCI journal, contact
the Society of Chemical Industry, 14/15 Belgrave Square, London, SW1X 8PS, UK
for our helpful Guide to Authors booklet.

WILEY

...Science from the Leading Edge

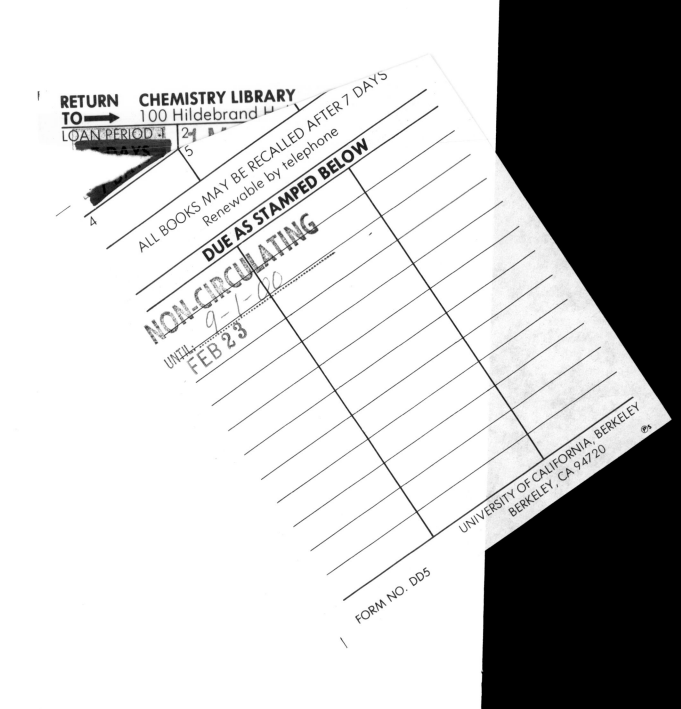

RETURN TO ➡ **CHEMISTRY LIBRARY**
100 Hildebrand H

LOAN PERIOD 1 | 2 | 3
DAYS
4 | 5 | 6

ALL BOOKS MAY BE RECALLED AFTER 7 DAYS
Renewable by telephone

DUE AS STAMPED BELOW

NON-CIRCULATING

UNTIL 9-1-00

FEB 23

FORM NO. DD5

UNIVERSITY OF CALIFORNIA, BERKELEY
BERKELEY, CA 94720